The Transformed School Counselor

Carolyn Bishop Stone
University of North Florida

Carol A. Dahir
New York Institute of Technology

Lahaska Press
Houghton Mifflin Company
Boston   New York

This book is dedicated to Elsie and Silas Bishop, Laura and Mitchell Dahir, and John Douglas Stone, because of the people they are.

Publisher, Lahaska Press: Barry Fetterolf
Senior Editor, Lahaska Press: Mary Falcon
Editorial Assistant: Lindsey Gentel
Senior Project Editor: Margaret Park Bridges
Senior Manufacturing Coordinator: Renee Ostrowski
Executive Marketing Manager: Brenda L. Bravener-Greville
Marketing Manager: Barbara LeBuhn

Cover image: © Hamish MacEwan / Superstock

Various quotes and excerpts throughout the book are from Stone, Carolyn B., and Dahir, Carol A., *School Counselor Accountability: A Measure of Student Success*, 1st Edition, © 2004. Reprinted by permission of Pearson Education, Inc., Upper Saddle River, NJ.

Lahaska Press was established as an imprint of Houghton Mifflin Company in 1999. It is dedicated to publishing textbooks and instructional media for counseling and the helping professions. The editorial offices of the imprint are located in the small town of Lahaska, Pennsylvania. "Lahaska" is a Native American Lenape word meaning "source of much writing."

Printed in the U.S.A.

Library of Congress Control Number: 2005923830

ISBN: 0-618-59061-7

123456789-MP-09 08 07 06 05

Contents

Chapter 3

Counseling Practice in Schools   62

Chapter 4

School Counselors as Leaders   90

Chapter 5

School Counselors as Advocates   **119**

Chapter 6

School Counselors as Consultants   **145**

Chapter 7

School Counselors as Coordinators, Collaborators, and Managers of Resources   **177**

Chapter 13

Promoting a Safe and Respectful Learning Environment   362

Chapter 14

Transitioning Into the Field of School Counseling   396

Preface

School counseling continues to evolve. Since the Transforming School Counseling Initiative (Education Trust, 1997) was launched, the school counseling profession has become a focal point of this nation's educational agenda. Transformed school counselors use leadership, advocacy, collaboration, and data-driven decision making to improve student achievement and success in school. With a solid foundation in counseling theory and techniques and consultation skills, the transformed school counselor delivers comprehensive school counseling programs, contributes to keeping our schools safe and respectful, and offers challenging educational opportunities to every student. The American School Counselor Association's National Model (2003) endorses this new way of thinking and working.

Through the process of implementing the transforming school counselor initiative at our respective universities, we (the authors of this book) have helped the next generation of school counselors acquire the skills and knowledge necessary to become transformed practitioners who are invested in school improvement. Writing this text gave us the opportunity to blend contemporary and traditional theory and practice to help both practitioners and degree candidates understand and implement the work of this new paradigm.

We have incorporated into our book the real-world experiences of dozens of practicing counselors who are successfully delivering accountable, data-driven school counseling programs. Through the voices of these counseling practitioners we bring the transformed practice alive.

From Vision to Action

> Vision without action is meaningless
>
> — *Spinetta, 2002, p. 24*

The transformed school counselor acts, influences, and impacts. Throughout this textbook, you, the school-counselor-in-training, will be challenged to take your personal vision of student success and connect it to the day-to-day realities in the place we call school. As a member of the next generation of school counselors, you are charged with the responsibility to ensure that every child will leave your school building prepared for the next transitional phase of her or his school and career plan.

Your studies this semester will challenge you to view your sphere of influence from a systems perspective. School counselors traditionally have not seen themselves as players in systemic change. Many problems that individual students bring to the school counseling center are symptomatic of larger issues. Linking school counseling with the mission of schools connects the school counselor and the school counseling program to the achievement of *all* students.

Transformed school counselors examine their practice and look at ways of working beyond one student at a time, focusing their attention on raising student aspirations and facilitating effective working relationships among students, faculty, parents, and community members. Transformed school counselors use data to inform their practice, and use data-driven decision making to respond to the needs of today's students and schools. Helping you to understand this new way of working is a key goal of this book.

The Basis for Knowledge and Skills

The goal of this book is to guide you in your acquisition of knowledge and understanding in the core content areas of the Council for Accreditation of Counseling and Related Educational Programs (CACREP) and the requirements of the National Council for Accreditation of Teacher Education (NCATE).

This Textbook	CACREP Core Content	CACREP School Counseling Specialty	NCATE
Chapter 1	Social and cultural foundations. Professional orientation and ethics.	Contextual Dimensions of School Counseling	1. Candidate knowledge 4. Diversity
Chapter 2	Social and cultural foundations. Counseling theory. The helping relationship and therapeutic process.	A. Foundations of School Counseling C. Knowledge and Skills Requirements for School Counselors 2. Counseling and Guidance	1. Candidate knowledge 4. Diversity
Chapter 3	Social and cultural foundations. Counseling theory. The helping relationship and therapeutic process. Professional orientation and ethics. Group dynamics and counseling. Technology.	A. Foundations of School Counseling B. Contextual Dimensions of School Counseling C. Knowledge and Skills Requirements for School Counselors 1. Program Development, Implementation, and Evaluation 2. Counseling and Guidance	1. Candidate knowledge 2. Candidate skills and dispositions 3. Field experience and clinical practice 4. Diversity

This Textbook	CACREP Core Content	CACREP School Counseling Specialty	NCATE
Chapter 4	Professional orientation and ethics. Group dynamics and counseling. Research and evaluation. Technology.	B. Contextual Dimensions of School Counseling C. Knowledge and Skills Requirements for School Counselors 1. Program Development, Implementation, and Evaluation 2. Counseling and Guidance 3. Consultation	1. Candidate knowledge 2. Candidate skills and dispositions 4. Diversity
Chapter 5	Social and cultural foundations. Professional orientation and ethics. Group dynamics and counseling.	B. Contextual Dimensions of School Counseling C. Knowledge and Skills Requirements for School Counselors 1. Program Development, Implementation, and Evaluation 2. Counseling and Guidance 3. Consultation	1. Candidate knowledge 2. Candidate skills and dispositions 4. Diversity
Chapter 6	Professional orientation and ethics. The helping relationship and therapeutic process. Group dynamics and counseling.	B. Contextual Dimensions of School Counseling C. Knowledge and Skills Requirements for School Counselors 2. Counseling and Guidance 3. Consultation	1. Candidate knowledge 2. Candidate skills and dispositions 3. Field experience and clinical practice 4. Diversity
Chapter 7	Social and cultural foundations. Professional orientation and ethics. Group dynamics and counseling. Technology.	B. Contextual Dimensions of School Counseling C. Knowledge and Skills Requirements for School Counselors 1. Program Development, Implementation, and Evaluation 2. Counseling and Guidance 3. Consultation	1. Candidate knowledge 2. Candidate skills and dispositions 4. Diversity

(*continued*)

This Textbook	CACREP Core Content	CACREP School Counseling Specialty	NCATE
Chapter 8	Social and cultural foundations. Professional orientation and ethics. Career development and decision making. Research and evaluation. Technology.	A. Foundations of School Counseling B. Contextual Dimensions of School Counseling C. Knowledge and Skills Requirements for School Counselors 1. Program Development, Implementation, and Evaluation 2. Counseling and Guidance	1. Candidate knowledge 2. Candidate skills and dispositions 3. Field experience and clinical practice 4. Diversity
Chapter 9	Professional orientation and ethics. Group dynamics and counseling. Research and evaluation. Appraisal and assessment. Technology.	B. Contextual Dimensions of School Counseling C. Knowledge and Skills Requirements for School Counselors 1. Program Development, Implementation, and Evaluation 2. Counseling and Guidance 3. Consultation	1. Candidate knowledge 2. Candidate skills and dispositions 3. Field experience and clinical practice 4. Diversity
Chapter 10	Social and cultural foundations. Professional orientation and ethics. Research and evaluation. Appraisal and assessment. Technology.	A. Foundations of School Counseling B. Contextual Dimensions of School Counseling C. Knowledge and Skills Requirements for School Counselors 3. Consultation	1. Candidate knowledge 2. Candidate skills and dispositions 4. Diversity
Chapter 11	Professional orientation and ethics. Research and evaluation. Technology.	B. Contextual Dimensions of School Counseling C. Knowledge and Skills Requirements for School Counselors 2. Counseling and Guidance 3. Consultation	1. Candidate knowledge 2. Candidate skills and dispositions 4. Diversity
Chapter 12	Social and cultural foundations. Counseling theory.	A. Foundations of School Counseling B. Contextual Dimensions of School Counseling	1. Candidate knowledge. 2. Candidate skills and dispositions.

This Textbook	CACREP Core Content	CACREP School Counseling Specialty	NCATE
	Career development and decision making. Appraisal and assessment. Technology.	C. Knowledge and Skills Requirements for School Counselors 2. Counseling and Guidance	4. Diversity
Chapter 13	Social and cultural foundations. Professional orientation and ethics. Group dynamics and counseling. Research and evaluation. Technology.	B. Contextual Dimensions of School Counseling C. Knowledge and Skills Requirements for School Counselors 1. Program Development, Implementation, and Evaluation 2. Counseling and Guidance 3. Consultation	1. Candidate knowledge 2. Candidate skills and dispositions 4. Diversity
Chapter 14	Social and cultural foundations. Professional orientation and ethics. Technology.	B. Contextual Dimensions of School Counseling 1. Program Development, Implementation, and Evaluation 2. Counseling and Guidance	3. Field experience and clinical practice 4. Diversity

Overview of This Textbook

Whether you are a first-semester graduate student acquiring an initial understanding of the scope and practice of the profession, or a professional school counselor motivated to acquire new knowledge and enhance your skills, *The Transformed School Counselor* will help you to

- embrace a leadership mindset, acting on your beliefs and advocating for the success of every student;
- use counseling, consultation, and the coordination of services to impact the climate and culture of your school;
- advocate for a social justice agenda and promote equitable access to quality education for all students;
- implement comprehensive, standards-based accountable school counseling programs;

- examine data to effectively identify patterns and behaviors that impede student success;
- use technology to efficiently and effectively expand the delivery of services and communication among all stakeholders, including parents.

Our focus on connecting school counseling to student achievement is not intended to be at the expense of attending to the mental health needs of students. Transformed school counseling offers us new ways of working with individuals and groups that ensure balance in providing academic, career, and personal-social development.

Content Overview

Chapter 1 Working in 21st-Century Schools

This chapter presents the challenges of the educational reform agenda of the past 20 years and explains how schools and school counselors proactively responded to the call for providing every child with a quality education. A context is established to address what school counselors need to know and be able to do to impact the teaching and learning process.

Chapter 2 Counseling Theory in Schools

Eight major counseling theories, including gestalt, person-centered, individual psychology, behavioral, reality therapy, rational emotive behavior therapy, cognitive behavior, and existential approaches are summarized. Each theory is followed by applications for the school setting. Counseling techniques and skills are presented as they apply to the child and adolescent in a school setting.

Chapter 3 Counseling Practice in Schools

This chapter addresses the use of individual and group counseling as well as classroom guidance with students for the purpose of developmental growth, prevention, and intervention. Teaming and collaboration among student support professionals, the use of the developmental assets, and building resiliency skills are presented as an important component of counseling in schools.

Chapter 4 School Counselors as Leaders

Leadership is becoming an increasingly valued and shared phenomenon at the school level. This chapter explores the unique opportunities school counselors have to assert leadership to support success in academic achievement for all students.

Chapter 5 School Counselors as Advocates

Involvement in social action and social intervention and a commitment to institutional improvement of schools are critical functions of the school counselor. This chapter examines social justice and advocacy roles for school counselors and addresses the skills that counselors need to examine and challenge the status quo.

Chapter 6 School Counselors as Consultants

Various models of consultation appropriate for the school setting are presented to help you develop the skills needed to be an effective consultant. An emphasis is placed on the benefits of the consultation role, relationship building, strategies for consultation with teachers and other school personnel, working effectively with parents, and gathering critical student information.

Chapter 7 School Counselors as Coordinators, Collaborators, and Managers of Resources

School counselors must balance providing direct services and managing resources to offer an expanded array of opportunities for students. Particular emphasis is placed on working with student support professionals, teachers, and mental health providers in the schools and in community-based organizations.

Chapter 8 Implementing the National Standards and the ASCA Model

The National Standards for School Counseling Program (ASCA, 1997) are the statements of the attitudes, knowledge, and skills that students should acquire as a result of participating in a school counseling program. Included in this discussion is an overview of the comprehensive program process as presented in the ASCA Model (2003), which provides a template for the development, implementation, and evaluation of a school counseling program.

Chapter 9 Accountability and Data-Driven Decision Making

School counselors must understand and manage data to make informed decisions about student needs and to set priorities in the school counseling program and in the school improvement plan. MEASURE (Stone & Dahir, 2004), a six-step process for school counselor accountability, is introduced to show how to collect and analyze data to inform, improve, and evaluate the effectiveness of school counseling on school improvement.

Chapter 10 Addressing Diversity in Schools

Conversations about diversity in today's schools must consider the influences of culture, class, race, ethnicity, gender, socioeconomic status, sexual orientation, learning ability, and language. Consideration is also given to cognitive differences that impact student learning, such as learning styles, and to special education, including the accommodations and assessment tools that help school counselors better understand student learning differences.

Chapter 11 Legal and Ethical Issues for School Counselors

School counselors function in an environment regulated by state and federal laws, court decisions, certification boards, and school boards. This chapter is a survey of the ethical, legal, and professional issues facing the school counselor. A case approach helps the student apply the American Counseling Association Code of Ethics and Standards of Practice (2005) and the American School Counselor Association's Ethical Standards (2004) in situations impacted by federal law, court case law, state statutes, community standards, and school board rules.

Chapter 12 Career Planning and Student Transitions

Preparing students to select a career goal and guiding them to enroll in the appropriate course work that will lead them to achieve their future aspirations is an important component of the work of school counselors. This chapter emphasizes the importance of developing a career guidance program as an integral component of your comprehensive school counseling program.

Chapter 13 Promoting a Safe and Respectful Learning Environment

The school counselor's collaboration with the principal, teachers, and parents to help individual students and classroom groups communicate caring and respect for one another is essential in today's rapidly changing world. This chapter helps school counselors understand the importance of climate and culture in creating positive learning communities.

Chapter 14 Transitioning Into the Field of School Counseling

In addition to practical suggestions to prepare counselors-in-training for induction into the school counseling profession, this chapter offers insight into the influences and trends that are driving the evolving professional orientation and the impact of the transforming school counseling initiative on school improvement.

Chapter Format

To enhance the usability of this book, each chapter follows a consistent format.

At the beginning of each chapter:

- *Chapter Outline*—A list of headings serves as an advance organizer for reading the chapter.
- *Chapter Objectives*—Learning objectives help you focus on key chapter content.
- *School Counselor Casebook: Getting Started*—A scenario concerning a contemporary school-based issue—such as the achievement gap or bullying—is followed by questions that prompt you to grapple with the issue as you read through the chapter.

Throughout each chapter:

- *Tables and Graphs*—Enhance your understanding of the text narrative.
- *Case Studies and Examples*—Bring real counselor and student scenarios alive.
- *Counselors Making a Difference*—Featured success stories demonstrate how real-life school counselors applied transformed practice to face challenges and solve problems. For example, in Chapter 5, *School Counselors as Advocates*, we see how high-school counselor Bernadette Willette, acting as a systemic change agent, was able to get Advanced Placement courses for her students.

At the end of each chapter:

- *TechTools*—An annotated list of technology resources related to chapter content.
- *School Counselor Casebook: Voices From the Field*—Practicing school counselors respond to the scenario presented at the beginning of the chapter.
- *Chapter Summary*—A review of key chapter content.
- *Key Terms*—A list of important terms and the page number where each is defined in the chapter.
- *Learning Extensions*—Exercises and activities designed to reinforce your comprehension and extend your understanding.

Wherein Lies the Future . . .

> As child advocates, let's take risks, disarm our personal and organizational egos, try new strategies, work with new networks, and leave our comfort zones of business as usual.
>
> — *Children's Defense Fund, 2002, p. xix*

The future of the school counseling profession resides in your hands, the next generation of school counselors. It is your words, behaviors, and actions that will transform school counseling as you contribute to school improvement and design and deliver student interventions that intervene, support, prevent, and motivate. The challenge is yours to become a school counselor who works systemically to achieve educational equity and excellence for all students. Today you begin your journey to join the ranks of the next generation. Are you up to the challenge?

Acknowledgments

We wish to extend our sincere appreciation to the thousands of counselor educators and school counselors across this country who inspired and encouraged us to create this textbook. They too believe that this next generation of school counselors will become the leaders, advocates, and systemic change agents who will continue to transform the profession of school counseling and make a significant difference in the lives of students.

A special note of appreciation to all of our "Voices From the Field," who generously gave their time to respond to school-based scenarios: Gloria Dansby-Giles, Linda Eby, Pamela Gabbard, Katie Gray, Deborah Hardy, Karen Kolkedy, Susan McCarthy, Shirin Mitsis, Joan Mudge, Patricia Nailor, Sejal Parikh, Philip Petrone, Michael Pines, Lin Roy, Mickie Stricker, Robert Tyra, Julie Van Nostrand, Barbara Webster, Dorothy Youngs, and Mary Zilko.

A special thank-you to the systemic change agents, leaders, and advocates whose work is highlighted throughout the text: Chris Bryan, Judy Cromartie, Mary Ann Dyal, Cindy Funkhouser, Melissa Hippensteel Howell, Kerryann Jannotte, Lee Kinard, Jim MacGregor, Kathy Morgan, Lou Nussbaum, Carol McLeod-Orso, LeAnn Pollard, Linda Quinn, Patricia Schneider, Michaele Sein-Ryan, Joni Shook, Penny Studstill, Robert Turba, Edith Vanderhoek, Bernadette Willette, and Nan Worowicz. We appreciate the school counselors of Jacksonville, Florida; Louisville, Kentucky; Memphis, Tennessee; Charleston, South Carolina; and Piscataway, New Jersey, who shared their struggles and commitment to ensure that every one of their students benefited from the work of school counselors.

Thank you to Amy Colvin, Lorene Gibson, Shirin Mitsis, Nancy Perry, Cheri Smith, Julie Van Nostrand, Michael Varady, and Dorothy Youngs, for your insightful comments and helpful suggestions throughout the development process. A special thank-you to Jan R. Bartlett, Oklahoma State University; Mary Ann Clark, University of Florida; and Lonnie Rowell, University of San Diego, for your thoughtful review and critique that furthered the development of the final manuscript.

A special acknowledgment and thank-you goes to Senior Editor Mary Falcon for working so closely with us to polish our diamond-in-the-rough manuscript into a sparkling jewel, and to Barry Fetterolf, publisher of Lahaska Press, for believing in our vision of preparing the next generation of school counselors. We thank Merrill Peterson and Kate Petrella for their meticulous attention to editing and production details.

We wish to acknowledge pioneers in the school counseling field: Norman Gysbers, Curly Johnson, Patricia Martin, and Robert Myrick, whose contributions provided solid pathways to a brighter future for all students. Finally, to our families and friends who patiently supported and encouraged us every step of the way, we cannot thank you enough!

Chapter 1

Working in 21st-Century Schools

Chapter Objectives

By the time you have completed this chapter, you should be able to:

- Explain the impact of educational reform and school improvement on students, teachers, and parents.
- Describe the role of counseling in today's schools.

- Describe how school counseling programs can support student achievement.
- Identify the many roles that the school counselor plays in a school environment that include advocate, leader, consultant, and as a collaborator and team member with students, faculty, parents, and community.

School Counselor Casebook: Getting Started

The Scenario

Many of the students in your school are English language learners (ELL) and students of color. Approximately 60% are eligible for the free or reduced lunch program. The state test scores are low and your school has been targeted by the state education department as a school under review (SUR) site. Under threat of a state takeover, the school must show improvement immediately. You know that school improvement is a shared responsibility. Your colleagues are busily planning and implementing new strategies.

Thinking About Solutions

As you read this chapter, think about how you as a school counselor in this situation might work with your colleagues to devise solutions and promote the necessary changes. When you come to the end of the chapter, you will have the opportunity to see how your ideas compare with a practicing school counselor's approach.

The Changing Direction of 21st-Century Schools

Education in America has changed. School buildings and classrooms may look the same as they did years ago, but a multitude of influences driving the contemporary educational reform agenda have had a significant impact on the teaching and learning process. In addition to promoting academic achievement, schools today are expected to promote good citizenship by addressing the affective and personal-social developmental needs of children and youth. Violent acts in our schools are increasingly receiving attention as incidents of trauma, tragedy, and terrorism have moved from the community into the schoolhouse.

The daily vernacular of educators today includes such phrases as **accountability,** standards-based education, **high stakes testing,** and closing the gap. In every state, school building, and community, educational reform initiatives have become the standard. The multitude of reform efforts since the mid-1990s continues to raise the expected level of achievement for students. Accountability is a driving force, and pressure weighs heavily on each school's staff to produce the desired results and improve in unprecedented ways. Teachers, principals, school support staff, and school counselors are actively engaged in developing and implementing annual **school improvement** plans to make their school a better place for children to strive and thrive.

Educational reform and school improvement are not new. Federal legislation historically has pressured school systems to examine practices and seek improvement. Twenty years ago, policymakers began drawing public attention to the mediocrity threatening American education (U.S. Department of Education, 1983). Monographs such as *A Nation at Risk: The Imperative for Educational Reform* (1983), *What Works: Research About Teaching and Learning* (1987), and *The Forgotten Half: Pathways to Success for America's Youth and Young Families* (1988) challenged student achievement. In 1989, the National Governor's Association (NGA) called for an unprecedented education summit to undertake a nationwide effort at educational renewal. The NGA generated broad-based objectives, which ultimately became the foundation for six national goals for education. These efforts resulted in *America 2000: An Education Strategy* (1990) which was considered at that time to be the most significant statement of a federal role and responsibility in the conduct of public education since the Elementary and Secondary Education Act of 1965 (Clinchy, 1991).

As high-school graduation requirements for students of all backgrounds and levels of performance became more rigorous (Sewall, 1991), public attention shifted to the back-to-basics components of education: curriculum, teaching, and administration. Also incorporated into America 2000 (1990) was the concept of developing world-class **standards** which intended to describe what students should know and be able to do across the curriculum areas.

> In the absence of well defined and demanding standards, education in the United States has gravitated toward de facto minimum expectations. Standards would provide the basic understandings that all students need to acquire, but not everything a student should learn.
> — *National Council on Education Standards and Testing, 1992, D-56*

The legislative iteration, Goals 2000: The Educate America Act (1994), promoted "raising the bar" to improve educational achievement for all students. Goals 2000 (1994) established expectations for student performance and school accountability that led to sweeping educational changes including the development of national voluntary academic standards across all disciplines. New curriculum standards and new measures of high stakes testing spun out of reform following Goals 2000, resulting in every state establishing standards, which for most have translated into increased graduation requirements. It is expected that the standards movement will continue to strengthen during this decade (Marzano, 2000).

With the change in the presidential administration in 2000, Congressional bipartisan support for continuous comprehensive school improvement resulted in the

No Child Left Behind Act (2001), which had as its expressed purpose, closing the achievement gap between minority students and their peers. No Child Left Behind (NCLB) embodies four basic principles:

1. Stronger accountability for results in each state determines what a child should know specifically in reading and math in grades 3–8. Student progress and achievement will be measured according to tests based upon those state standards and given to every child, every year.

2. Expanded flexibility and local control allows for local school districts to have more flexibility and a greater say in how federal funds are used in their schools to meet student needs.

3. Expanded options are available for parents of children from disadvantaged backgrounds whose children are trapped in failing schools. Funds are provided to students in failing schools to use for supplemental educational services, including tutoring, afterschool services, summer school programs, and charter schools.

4. The use of teaching methods that have been proven to work, strengthening teacher quality, and promoting English proficiency are essential to school improvement.

These principles underpin five primary goals to be realized by 2013–2014 (see Table 1.1). The first three goals focus on the improvement of curriculum, learning, and achievement. Goals 4 and 5 address affective development, school climate and culture, and the ability to ensure that every child will graduate from high school.

No Child Left Behind (2001) acknowledged the importance of equitable access to educational opportunities and sought to create settings in which all children are held to high expectations and are given the conditions necessary to achieve this

Table 1.1 No Child Left Behind (2001)
(Elementary and Secondary Education Act [ESEA])

ESEA Goal 1	By 2013–2014, all students will reach high standards, at a minimum attaining proficiency or better in reading/language arts and mathematics.
ESEA Goal 2	All limited English proficient students will become proficient in English and reach high academic standards, at a minimum attaining proficiency or better in reading/language arts and mathematics.
ESEA Goal 3	By 2005–2006, all students will be taught by highly qualified teachers.
ESEA Goal 4	All students will be educated in learning environments that are safe, drug free, and conducive to learning.
ESEA Goal 5	All students will graduate from high school.

Source: U.S. Department of Education, Office of Elementary and Secondary Education (2002).

goal. Student opportunities are frequently stratified by race, ethnicity, and socioeconomic status (Haycock, 2001). Student diversity, including ethnicity, language, and economic means, continues to challenge educators and community-based professionals (Sapon-Shevin, 2001), as depicted in Figure 1.1.

The quality of our public schools affects every citizen, and yet too many children in America are segregated by low expectations, low literacy, and self-doubt (NCLB, 2001). Today's educational agenda speaks to high expectations for all students regardless of race, ethnicity, and socioeconomic status (SES). Merely legislating requirements to promote change in expectations for students will not produce the desired outcomes. Although the number of high-school graduates is projected to increase by 11% between 2002 and 2013 (National Center for Education Statistics [NCES], 2004), far more needs to be accomplished to guarantee each student, regardless of ethnicity, race, or income, an equitable opportunity to a quality educational experience.

High stakes testing has put new and unprecedented pressure on teachers, students, and parents. Legislators, school board members, teachers, school site and district level administrators, parents, employers, and other school and community members feel the pressure of raising academic standards and improving student academic success. Quality Counts (Education Week, 2003) encouraged state education departments to balance policies to ensure that resources are available for students and schools to meet these higher expectations, especially when the futures of individual children are at stake. School administrators are required to constantly rethink the allocation of existing resources and maximize the potential of school staff to help all students achieve at these higher levels of academic success.

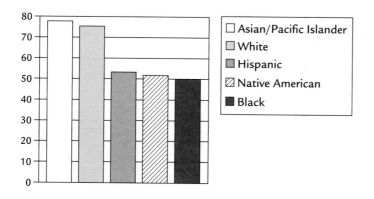

Figure 1.1 National Graduation Rates by Race
Source: Losing Our Future: How Minority Students Are Being Left Behind by the Graduation Rate Crisis, 2004.

As schools throughout the United States struggle with the demands of federal legislation, many will concur that raising student achievement is the primary focus of school improvement (Martin, 2004). Higher levels of expectations have resulted in many states revising and increasing the graduation requirements and eliminating the differentiation between college preparation and regular high school courses (Carnevale & Desrochers, 2003).

> It is recognized, even by the federal government, that we have a genuine national crisis. More and more, we are divided into two nations. One that reads, and one that doesn't. One that dreams, and one that doesn't.
>
> *— Bush, 2001, p.1*

The commitment to higher levels of student achievement and continuous improvement is a responsibility shared by all of the critical stakeholders, including school counselors. School counselors have an important role to play. As potential key players in furthering the primary goals of 21st-century schools, school counselors can become partners in systemic change and identify those students who need more support and assistance to achieve at expected levels. Many students are caught in the dichotomy of weak educational foundations and the expectations of rigorous academic standards; often, except for the school counselor's intervention, they may remain anonymous in their struggle to survive and succeed.

The 21st-century approach to standards-based reform and working in schools has dramatically changed the way every educator works to improve student performance. When school counselors operate under the premise that they are key players in the academic success story for students, then school counseling programs are viewed as integral to student achievement (Stone & Dahir, 2004). Impacting the instructional program, motivating and raising student aspirations to achieve at high levels, and collaborating to create safe school environments are some of the ways in which school counselors can fully participate in all aspects of the implementation of the No Child Left Behind Act (NCLB) and document efforts to help all children succeed.

School Counseling: Changing With the Times

Throughout this most recent wave of **educational reform** and legislative changes, relatively few areas of public education escaped the scrutiny of national attention. Yet school counseling programs and school counselors were absent from many of the early conversations that spoke to changes in curriculum, instruction, and pedagogy. Thankfully this is no longer the situation. Since the mid-1990s, the school counseling profession has undergone a transformation that parallels the call for change in schools (Education Trust, 1997). A brief retrospective examination of the history of school counseling offers insight into past perspectives and current initiatives that ultimately will influence the future.

The counseling profession first took a seat in the American schoolhouse in the late 19th century (Schmidt, 1999). Jesse Davis introduced a guidance program into a Detroit high-school curriculum in 1898 to help students develop character, avoid problems, and relate vocational interests to course work (Brewer, 1932). These efforts established the beginnings of what was to evolve from vocational guidance to school counseling. Frank Parsons, often cited as the "father of guidance," is credited as the person who began this movement. Parsons's attention to vocational guidance was coupled with his concern about society's failure to provide resources for human growth and development, especially for young people (Schmidt, 1999). In working with youth, Parsons and his followers emphasized that

- the individual must have a clear understanding of her or his abilities, interests, ambitions, and limitations. Thus, the counselor assisted individuals in learning about their personal characteristics.
- the individual must have knowledge of the world, the opportunities and options available, and an understanding of the requirements for the chosen field. The counselor assumed an information dissemination role.
- the individual must bring together knowledge of self and the awareness of the world of work. The counselor served as a guide to help the individual develop a clear and logical path to reach his or her goal.

Parsons's influence was long reaching and became the impetus and direction for expanding the concept of vocational guidance. World War I and its aftermath, which led to the Great Depression, resulted in a greater need for assisting students with vocational selection and placement. The term *vocational counselor*, rarely heard before the Depression, entered the educational vocabulary (Wittmer, 2000). Attempts to organize and expand guidance in the school setting in the 1930s led to the addition of educational and personal-social services (Gysbers & Henderson, 2000). The traditional way of describing guidance as a vocational service was no longer in vogue; these newer views broadened the goals of the program and added to it the elements of counseling.

Between the Great Depression and the outbreak of World War II, new assessment instruments such as intelligence tests and vocational aptitude tests appeared on the market for employment purposes and then for use in the military. High schools began to administer intelligence measurements for children and welcomed group testing for purposes of pupil evaluation. The use of these new instruments led to the development of counseling approaches that related student traits to interest and ability. The progressive education movement, although short lived, encouraged the school to play a greater role in the personal and social development of students (Nugent, 1994). In the 1940s, major events such as the impact of World War II, the influence of Carl Rogers's client-centered theory, and the government's renewed involvement in education strongly impacted the future direction of guidance and counseling (Gladding, 2004). The influence of mental measurement instruments and vocational guidance further shaped the delivery and orientation of guidance services. The George-Barden Act of 1946 provided funds to support guidance and counseling in the schools and other settings.

By the middle of the 20th century, psychological assessment, mental health approaches, counseling theorists, and the beginnings of educational reform began to influence school guidance and counseling. In the 1950s, the public became fascinated with the term *IQ* (intelligence quotient), and parents thought this data would better help them understand their children's school performance. Rogerian theory focused attention almost exclusively on individual counseling with an emphasis on the counselor-client relationship. Societal pressures resulting from the stresses of the Korean War also added to the need for mental health and vocational support for adults and students alike.

Professional associations emerged as strong influences, and the American School Counselor Association (ASCA) became a division of the American Personnel and Guidance Association in the 1950s. Guidance work in schools continued to grow and the numbers of counselors increased significantly due to a major stimulus, the National Defense Education Act of 1958 (Herr, 1979). The primary purpose of the National Defense Education Act (NDEA) was to increase funding to education to help the United States regain a competitive edge in mathematics and the sciences. Part of this funding was earmarked to augment the number of secondary school counselors. This generation of counselors was expected to have skill in therapeutic interventions that would support the student in resolving personal problems that might be a barrier to academic success; they also were required to have expertise in providing college admissions information (Perry & Schwallie-Giddis, 1993). The ultimate goal was to increase the numbers of students going on to college and pursuing careers related to math and science. This emphasis on postsecondary opportunities and individual personal support brought attention to the fact that guidance and counseling was available only to the college bound or for those with personal problems. Also during the mid-1950s, access to guidance and counseling in the junior and senior high schools became very limited (Perry & Schwallie-Giddis, 1993; Rosenbaum, 1976). Increased funding for the guidance provision in NDEA in the early 1960s added elementary guidance and counseling programs as the missing link in the continuum of services from kindergarten through high school (Gysbers, 2000). The expansion of services to elementary schools ultimately led to a broader professional focus on programs and services (Schmidt, 1999).

Gilbert Wrenn's (1962) book, *The Counselor in a Changing World*, may have influenced school guidance and counseling more than any other publication (Wittmer, 2000). Wrenn asserted that the primary emphasis in counseling students should be on individual developmental needs and not only on the remedial and crisis situations in their lives. Wrenn also suggested that counselors needed to expand their knowledge of human behavior to better serve the complex needs of students. As guidance services expanded across the country, Mathewson (1962) promoted school guidance as a process that moves with the individual student and in a developmental sequence through the age of maturity (Wittmer, 2000). Although the strong influences of Rogerian theory on school counselor training continued (Wittmer, 2000), no longer was mental health practice considered the primary responsibility of the counselor in a school setting. Social pressures and the emphasis on educational student support refocused the emphasis of school counseling from individual student response and crisis intervention to a proactive series of strategies that engage every student. This resulted in the development of new models for program design and delivery systems.

The 1970s saw the advent of guidance as a comprehensive program (Dinkmeyer & Caldwell, 1970; Gysbers & Henderson, 2000; Myrick, 2000). The comprehensive program approach de-emphasized clerical and administrative tasks and promoted guidance as a structured program with specific student outcomes (Gysbers & Henderson, 1994, 2000; Sink & McDonald, 1998). Consequently, the vast majority of state departments of education have adopted or endorsed a comprehensive approach to school counseling. Coupled with the expansion of the comprehensive model was the American School Counselor Association's proactive response to Goals 2000, the development of the National Standards for School Counseling Programs (American School Counselor Association [ASCA], 1997), which positioned school counseling to play an increasingly important role in contemporary school improvement (Dahir, 2004). The widespread use of the National Standards (ASCA, 1997), the Education Trust's Transforming School Counseling Initiative (1997), and the ASCA National Model (2003) defined the vision and goals for the 21st-century school counseling programs and placed the programs in a critical position to effectively complement academic rigor with affective development.

Defining the Role of School Counseling in School Improvement

Despite the presence of more than 100,000 school counselors in school districts across the 50 states, the school counseling profession was omitted from the educational reform agendas of the past. Was this omission an oversight or was it intentional? Because school counselors have always focused their efforts on assisting students to improve their attitude and/or behavior in order to achieve greater school success and championing student personal-social needs, the omission was confusing and troublesome. Perhaps, because school counseling was a relatively young profession in comparison to its educational counterparts, a natural confusion existed as to its nature, function, purpose, and role. Mathewson (1962) once referred to guidance and counseling as a search for a system characterized by statements of objectives and goals. Ryan and Zeran (1972) suggested that guidance and counseling suffered from the lack of a systematic theory to guide the practical applications of services, which significantly differ from the curriculum delivery of the academic disciplines. This could be attributed to the relatively small size of the counseling community or the poor public and professional understanding of the roles performed by school counselors (Burtnett, 1993).

Boyer (1988), in his description of the school counselor, stated:

> Today, in most high schools, counselors are not only expected to advise students about college, they are also asked to police for drugs, keep records of dropouts, reduce teenage pregnancy, check traffic in the halls, smooth out the tempers of irate parents, and give aid and comfort to battered and neglected children. School counselors are expected to do what our communities, our homes, and our churches have not been able to accomplish, and if they cannot, we condemn them for failing to fulfill our high minded expectations.
>
> — Exploring the Future, *1988, p.3*

School district administrators, educational organizations, and foundations and state departments of education had clearly dictated the functions, activities, and programs that professional school counselors should deliver to students. The assignment of non-counseling activities suggested that the role of the school counselor and the school counseling program were poorly defined and not valued by the school administration (Hart & Jacobi, 1992). This resulted in many new duties added to a counselor's already existing responsibilities (Gysbers & Henderson, 1997), including tasks that were administrative or clerical in nature. "When schools fail to clearly define the counselor's role, school administrators, parents with special interests, teachers or others may feel their agenda ought to be the school counseling program's priority. The results often lead to confusion and criticisms when they are disappointed" (Cunanan & Maddy-Bernstein, 1994, p. 1). Counselors focusing their attention on the delivery of a constellation of responsive and reactive activities, and performing "random acts of guidance" (Bilzing, 1996) will only service a small percentage of the student population.

School counselors felt compelled to accept the responsibility to address societal issues that continued to impact school-aged children (Boyer, 1988). The school counselor and the school counseling program regularly reacted, responded, and expanded to meet these needs and challenges. Thus the scope of school counseling practice continued to encompass a wide variety of diverse services offered to students from kindergarten through high school (Gysbers & Henderson, 2000). Services and activities varied from school to school and from state to state and resulted in ambiguity in the organization of school counseling (guidance) services. School counseling often was viewed as an ancillary service to support the academic goals of schooling (Gerler, 1992). From the multitude of external and internal forces influencing the profession, it is natural that school counselors have grappled with issues regarding professional title, scope of practice, and role and responsibilities as the profession defines and refines itself in 21st-century schools.

In the era following publication of *A Nation at Risk* (1983), the American Counseling Association (ACA), concerned about the future of counseling in schools, put forth a series of recommendations in a report entitled *School Coun-*

seling: A Profession at Risk (ACA, 1987). Six years later, ACA convened a "think tank," which proposed a series of activities and functions that more clearly establish the role and relationship of the school counselor in reference to the educational system. Organizations produced and widely distributed monographs, such as the College Entrance Examination Board's *Keeping the Options Open: Recommendations* (1986), that spoke to the ability of guidance and counseling to support and encourage student success. The ASCA continued to define the role and function of school counselors through position statements and monographs. The association (ASCA, 1994) encouraged school counselors to become agents of change and assume a leadership role in educational reform. As student advocates and allies of teachers in identifying student needs, school counselors were encouraged to help create positive change.

However, there was no external call from the educational or legislative arenas to take action, and responses to these recommendations remained solely within the confines of the school counseling community.

With a minimal amount of empirical evidence that addressed and demonstrated the impact of school counseling on student achievement, confusion about the contributions of school counseling programs to student achievement persisted. Borders and Drury (1992) suggested that school counselors played an important role in shaping the design and implementation of counseling programs to best meet individual student needs, while Whiston and Sexton (1998) noted that more research had been conducted in the areas of remediation and intervention rather than in preventing problems. A number of studies (Brigman & Campbell, 2003; Dimmitt, 2003; Gerler, Kinney, & Anderson 1985; Lehmanowsky, 1991; Sheldon & Morgan, 1984; Sink & Stroh, 2003; Sprinthall, 1981; Stevens-Smith & Remley, 1994; Thornburg, 1986) have demonstrated the positive impact of school counseling on student success. Although researchers have sought to identify and promote the value of counseling in the schools, the movement for the acceptance of school counseling as a legitimate and recognized component of the educational system by policymakers remained an uphill struggle. More recent federal funding initiatives including Gaining Early Awareness and Readiness for Undergraduate Programs (GEAR UP, 1998) and the Elementary and Secondary School Counseling Demonstration Act (ESCDA, 1998, 2001) offered financial support and recognized the contributions of school counseling to student educational attainment and achievement. Several recent monographs and reports (Jackson & Davis, 2000; National Association of Secondary School Principals, 1996, 2004) address the importance of incorporating affective development in the schooling process, especially during the adolescent and teenage years. Most recently, department of education school improvement plans have addressed and recognized the role and the impact of school counseling programs on student success and student achievement in states including Alabama, Delaware, Florida, Massachusetts, New Jersey, Nevada, and West Virginia. Recent empirical evidence suggests that the school counseling profession is responding successfully to the changing educational philosophies, social movements, economic trends, pressures of accountability, and the significant issues that impact school improvement (Feller, 2003).

Issues Impacting Today's Schools

Pressures From the Global Economy

More than twenty years have passed since *A Nation at Risk* (1983), and as a nation we continue the concerted effort to raise the standards in K–12 education. This push is driven by the educational needs of a 21st-century economy, rather than by the educational failures or deficiencies of the past or present (Carnevale & Desrochers, 2003). Without efforts to better prepare today's students for postsecondary education and increase their access to college, America's economic position and global competitiveness could be in jeopardy. The restructuring of the American economy initiated in the early 1980s has made postsecondary education or technical training the threshold requirement for employment, resulting in academic readiness for postsecondary education becoming the standard for adequacy in K–12 education (Education Trust, 2001). Two decades of concerted state efforts to strengthen the high school curriculum have encouraged a stronger academic foundation in the K–8 arena, and an intent to broaden the scope of assessment to progressively higher levels including high-school graduation (Postsecondary Education Opportunity, 2000, p.1) and the demand for highly skilled and educated workers has risen faster than the supply. Since 1979 the economic premium paid to workers with at least some college has increased from 42% to 62% even as the supply of workers with at least some college has doubled as a share of all workers (Bureau of Labor Statistics, 2004).

The purpose of schooling goes well beyond the means to the end of preparing students for the work force. The implications are broad for all educators, including school counselors.

> Educators have cultural and political missions to ensure there is an educated citizenry to continue to defend and promote America's democratic ideals. Nevertheless, the inescapable reality is that ours is a society based on individual economic autonomy. Those who are not equipped with the knowledge and skills necessary to get, and keep, a good job are denied full social inclusion and tend to drop out of the mainstream culture, polity, and enconomy. Hence, if the standards-based reform movement cannot fulfill its economic mission to help youth and adults become successful workers, it also will fail in its cultural and political missions to create good neighbors and good citizens.
>
> — *Carnevale & Desrochers, 2003, vii*

High-school graduation is now the minimum ticket to exit the cycle of poverty and provides the opportunity to earn a salary to escape the circumstances that are associated with earning a minimal income (Carey, 2004). Despite the economic realities, students continue to drop out of school and endanger their economic future (Greene, 2002). The dropout rate could be as high as one student in three (Greene, 2002; Mortenson, 2001), although the figure more frequently cited is one in four (Education Trust, 2002).

Because high school education is the minimum requirement for accessing postsecondary education, training, or the labor force, the economic consequences of leaving high school without a diploma are severe (NCES, 2001, p.1). The cumulative effect of hundreds of thousands of youths and teens leaving school each year short of finishing a high-school program translates into several million young people who are out of school, yet lack a high school credential (p. 23). The increased importance of a high-school education for entry to both the labor market and postsecondary education will impact their future economic success.

Students from poor families are considerably more likely to leave high school than are students from middle income and affluent families (Education Trust, 2001).

The data in Figure 1.2 reveal that the impact of poverty on students' desire and ability to pursue postsecondary education is powerful, and certainly an important consideration when working with students and addressing issues of equity and access. The higher the student's family income, the more likely it is that he or she will enroll in postsecondary education. Students whose families fall into the higher quartiles also have a greater chance of accessing and completing college. Conversely, students whose families are in the 4th quartile of income earnings are accessing postsecondary education at significantly lower levels, thus also reducing opportunities to complete a bachelor's degree.

During the past decade, poverty continued to blanket the lives of one in four children (Children's Defense Fund, 2004) despite the greatest economic boom the nation had ever seen. The data in Table 1.2 suggest how other variables, including ethnicity and gender, also influence educational attainment.

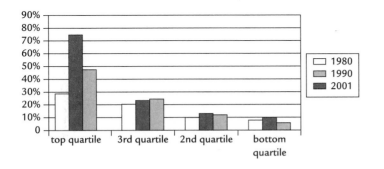

Figure 1.2 Estimated Baccalaureate Degree Attainment by Age 24 by Family Income Quartile 1980 to 2001

Source: Postsecondary Education Opportunity; November 2003.

Table 1.2 Too Few College Freshmen Ever Graduate

	Six-Year Graduation Rate
Total Population	63%
Caucasian	67%
African American	46%
Latino	47%
Asian	15.1%
Male	59%
Female	66%
Low income	54%
High income	77%

Source: U.S. Department of Education, National Center for Educational Statistics, 2002

The data presented send a clear message. Future earning power, education, family income, and race and ethnicity influence a student's choice of postsecondary options. Similar tables and charts can depict the story of students you will soon work with. Consider using information such as that presented here to raise the aspirations of your future students, their parents, and the community.

Twenty-first-century schools must ensure that all students acquire the attitudes, knowledge, and skills necessary to make successful transitions from grade level to grade level, to postsecondary education, and to the world after high school. Ninety percent of this year's kindergarten students will find themselves in jobs we know nothing about today (Hoye, 1998). By working closely with students and their families or caregivers, school counselors can help ensure that students will understand the options they have after high school and maximize their postsecondary opportunities.

The Power of Technology

Technology has changed not only the way students and adults access information, but more important, the way they communicate with each other. Multitasking is a way of life for teenagers who use the Internet, instant messaging, and their cell phones in simultaneous synchronous real time while doing their homework. The Internet has created a language all its own, which is embraced by the youth culture. This new form of peer-to-peer communication can be highly impersonal. Many youth see "net speak," chatrooms, blogs, and e-mail as safe havens or anonymous hangouts in which they can test their sexual identity, escape from loneliness, and find a peer group to identify with. Others throw their thoughts into cyberspace without considering the consequences. For today's youth it is a complex, exciting, and dangerous new age of exchanging information and engaging in "conversation."

However, not all youth have access to the technology needed for the socialization aspects described here. Many have only limited access to technology and the Internet in their schools. U.S. Secretary of State Colin Powell referred to the problem as digital apartheid, not the digital divide, and further suggested "there is a huge gap between those who have access to the wonders of digital technology and the Internet and those who do not . . . if we don't bridge the gap between the two, the 'have nots' will be poorer and more resentful and the 'haves' will find themselves lacking the skilled workers and potential customers they need" (Sanford, 2001, p. 32). Educational technology for many students from poor communities is a tool for liberation (Sistek-Chandler, 2001).

Television, MTV, computer and video games, movies, and DVDs also are major influences on the lives of students. The media impacting their world can often become a primary source for role models and developing career awareness. Students' dreams of their future goals revolve around snapshots of superheroes, sports figures, rock stars, and sit-com characters. This millennial generation has grown up with video games the way that baby boomers grew up with board games (Howe & Strauss, 2000). The media also have exposed youth to violent acts over and over in video games, on television, and in the movies (U.S. Department of Education, 2002).

Swings and Shifts in Societal Issues and Values

Children and youth have a wider exposure to lifestyles and career choices than ever before in our society, and the economic boom of the past ten years has created an affluence previously not experienced by middle- and upper-income families. Purchases by children age 4 to 12 tripled by the year 2000, and although not every child benefited from this age of affluence, the influence of media branding has resulted in tremendous peer pressure (Howe & Strauss, 2000).

American youth have been made aware of the fragile nature of human life by the tragic events of September 11, 2001. The attitudes of our youth toward terrorism and respect for human life have been influenced in ways that at this time cannot be predicted. Terrorism threats also are impacting our youth's connectivity to the community and eradicating some of the apathy that had previously stigmatized this generation. School violence, which once was reserved to large inner-city systems, has erupted in our rural and suburban schools (Sandhu, 2000). Concerns for safety in school have become a national priority and are addressed in one of the five goals of No Child Left Behind (2001).

With youth behavior and attitudes a primary source of concern, character education was promoted as a key component of the education platform of 2000. This agenda recently has translated into a new wave of character education program mandates in a majority of our 50 states (NCLB, 2001). Addressing sexual harassment and bully-proofing strategies has become part of the daily concern of school counselors in every elementary, middle/junior high, and high school across the nation. Schools now implement drug and alcohol education in elementary school. Many parents have left the responsibility of sex education to school personnel. Students questioning their sexual identity frequently find school an unsafe place. According to the National Center for Missing and Exploited Children, approximately one in five children received a sexual solicitation or were approached over the Internet during the past year (2001). Changing demographics and new waves of immigration no longer are the bane of urban centers. Schools have turned to teaching tolerance, respect, equity, and acceptance.

A complex and ever-changing economy, technological innovation, and the multidimensional influences of societal values all have significantly impacted the way educators will work with the millennial generation in 21st-century schools. The school counselor, a specialist in student growth and academic, career, and personal-social development, is essential to the goals of improving schools as well as the teaching and learning process.

The Important Role of 21st-Century School Counselors

Counseling in schools in the United States shifted its focus from a responsive services approach to one that is proactively and integrally tied to student achievement and student success. The new paradigm for school counseling is based on a comprehensive, national standards-based defined program that emphasizes student growth, learning, and results, and also recognizes that all children growing up in America face the normal challenges of coping with everyday problems. On a daily basis, school personnel encounter students who are abused, neglected, frustrated by the cycle of personal and academic failure, disabled, drug addicted, homeless, or suffering from feelings of worthlessness. Many students face emotional, physical, social, and economic barriers that inhibit successful learning.

Students who present these significant needs challenge educators. These challenges raise a series of questions, such as: How do we provide a quality and equitable education for students who face emotional and academic challenges? What is the responsibility of the school counselor for addressing the emotional and social barriers that inhibit student learning?

Supporting Student Success

The purpose of the counseling program in a school setting is to impart specific skills and facilitate learning opportunities in a proactive and preventive manner to help all students achieve school success through academic, career, and personal-social development experiences. The school counseling program promotes and enhances the learning process (Campbell & Dahir, 1997) as an integral part of the total school

The State of America's Children Yearbook 2004

Key Facts About American Children

1 in 3 is born to unmarried parents.

1 in 3 will be poor at some point in their childhood.

1 in 3 is behind a year or more in school.

1 in 4 lives with only one parent.

1 in 5 is born to a mother who did not graduate from high school.

1 in 6 children in the United States continues to live in poverty.

1 in 8 has no health insurance.

1 in 8 lives in a family receiving food stamps.

1 in 8 is born to a teenage mother.

1 in 10 teens ages 16 to 19 is a school dropout.

1 in 12 has a disability.

1 in 24 lives with neither parent.

1 in 60 sees their parents divorce in any year.

31% of fourth graders read at or above grade level.

7 out of 10 fourth graders cannot read or do math at grade level.

8 children and teens die from gunfire in the U.S. each day—one child every 3 hours.

3 million children are reported abused or neglected and referred for investigation or assessment each year; close to 900,000 of them are confirmed as victims of child maltreatment.

Source: Children's Defense Fund 2004, p. 13.

program (Clark & Stone, 2000). The comprehensive national standards-based school counseling program empowers school counselors to place themselves at the front and center of the restructuring process in their school systems and establish a rationale and motivation for providing students with an affective, child centered education. Competency-based learning in academic, career, and personal-social development sets high expectations of achievement for every student. By addressing barriers to learning and social-emotional health, school counseling programs can successfully bridge the gap between student needs and expectations for learning (AEL, Inc., 2000).

Helping All Children Achieve at a Higher Level

Concerns about equitable access to educational programs are major issues that warrant investigation as the current school improvement agenda unfolds. New mechanisms have been established to help all students reach the new standards. What are the effective teaching practices that will help all children achieve at a higher level? Not all students come to the school environment prepared, properly nourished, and ready to learn. Table 1.3 is a point of contention for discussion for those who are concerned that equal opportunity exists for all students.

Over a decade ago, *The School Counselor's Role in Educational Reform* (ASCA, 1994) encouraged school counselors to become catalysts for educational change and to assume and to accept a leadership role in educational reform. School counselors, as partners in student achievement, also face the test of preparing students to meet the expectations of higher academic standards and to become productive and contributing members of society. Recognizing the importance of this message, the following revised definition of school counseling was adopted by the ASCA Governing Board:

> Counseling is a process of helping people by assisting them in making decisions and changing behavior. School counselors work with all students, school staff, families, and members of the community as an integral part of the education program. School counseling programs promote school success through a focus on academic achievement, prevention and intervention activities, advocacy and social-emotional and career development.
>
> *— ASCA, 1997*

Table 1.3 Who Takes Advanced Placement Tests?

	Public K–12 Enrollment	Calculus AP	English Language and Composition	Biology
African American	17%	5%	6%	6%
Asian	4%	16%	11%	19%
Latino	17%	8%	12%	8%
Native American	1%	0%	1%	0%
White	60%	72%	69%	67%
Total	100%	100%	100%	100%

Source: Education Trust EdWatch Online 2004 State Summary Reports.

Leaders and Advocates for School Improvement

Through a leadership and social advocacy role, school counselors ensure that all students have equal access to quality academic programs and the needed support to meet the demands of these challenges. School counselors call attention to situations in schools that are defeating or frustrating students, thereby hindering the students' success. These situations, supported by data, present an opportunity for school counselors to lead a schoolwide effort to promote equity and provide opportunity. Measurable success resulting from this effort can be documented by an increased number of students completing school with the academic preparation, the career awareness, and the personal-social growth essential to choosing from a wide range of substantial postsecondary options, including college (Education Trust, 1997).

Partners in Educational Excellence

In collaboration with principals, teachers, other school professionals, parents, and caregivers, school counselors share the challenge of preparing students to meet the expectations of higher academic standards and become productive and contributing members of society. School counselors working toward the common goal of successful schools can provide an equitable, excellent, and challenging education for every child. As key partners in educational excellence, school counselors share the responsibility of educating all children. The school counselor is in a unique position to interact with students, faculty, administration, parents, and the community in order to help students build resiliency and overcome barriers to academic achievement.

Ensuring Every Stakeholder Benefits

When school counselors implement comprehensive school counseling programs, they demonstrate a commitment to collaboration and to student success and school improvement.

This way of work also demonstrates a strong commitment on the part of school counselors to ensure that every student will fully participate in the school counseling program. As a result of these efforts everyone, school counselors too, benefit from a shift in focus from delivering services to an organized program. Each group of stakeholders will benefit in a different manner.

Benefits of comprehensive school counseling for school counselors:

- Clarifies responsibilities within the context of a school counseling program;
- Eliminates non-school-counseling program activities;

- Ensures that every student has access to developmental and comprehensive school counseling programs;
- Offers the opportunity to design, deliver, and manage an accountable school counseling program;
- Demonstrates the school counselor's role as a leader, advocate, team player, and collaborator in the school setting;
- Shows the school counseling program's contribution to the mission of the school;
- Connects the work of the school counselor to school improvement and school climate; and,
- Documents students' achievement and growth in academic, career, and personal-social development.

Benefits of comprehensive school counseling for students:

- Provides a focused effort to improve student success and achievement as well as school climate;
- Involves students in targeted interventions aimed at closing the achievement gap;
- Addresses policies and practices that stratify student opportunities;
- Encourages high aspirations for every student;
- Helps students focus on the future;
- Focuses on rigor and results;
- Emphasizes the attitudes, knowledge, and skills that students acquire as a result of participating in a school counseling program;
- Ensures students' involvement in academic, career, and personal-social development;
- Promotes a rigorous academic curriculum for every student;
- Addresses equitable access to educational opportunities for all students.

Benefits of comprehensive school counseling for parents and caregivers:

- Provides them with knowledge about their children's academic, career, and personal-social development;
- Encourages parents and caregivers to partner with school counselors regarding their children's learning and career goals;
- Provides parents and caregivers with the necessary support to help their children successfully transition from grade level to grade level;
- Offers information and assistance with the postsecondary planning process;
- Encourages and assists with access to school and community resources;
- Offers training and informational workshops;
- Demonstrates the connection for continuous information about student progress.

Benefits of comprehensive school counseling for teachers:

- Encourages an interdisciplinary team approach to address student needs and educational goals;
- Ensures collaboration among school counselors and teachers;
- Encourages consultation for student needs and interventions;
- Lends support for student behavior management in the classroom and hallways;
- Offers a collaborative model for sharing classroom guidance lessons;
- Encourages collaboration to improve student achievement;
- Provides assistance with data analysis to improve school climate and school improvement.

Benefits of comprehensive school counseling for student services personnel:

- Defines the school counseling program as a model of collaboration;
- Uses school data to develop prevention and intervention strategies;
- Encourages collaboration for utilizing and coordinating school and community resources;
- Identifies ways to share strategies and coordinate services;
- Encourages teaming in designing and implementing prevention and intervention services.

Benefits of comprehensive school counseling for administrators:

- Demonstrates the alignment of the school counseling program with the school's academic mission;
- Documents the link between the school counseling program and student success;
- Aligns school counseling with school climate and culture;
- Promotes collaboration and support for the use of data in school improvement;
- Provides for an accountability process to measure success for the school counseling program;
- Demonstrates students' growth and achievement in academic, career, and personal-social development;
- Shows the alignment of the program with the National Standards for School Counseling Programs;
- Demonstrates school counselor support and involvement in the goals of No Child Left Behind.

Benefits of comprehensive school counseling for the boards and departments of education:

- Shows the connection of school counseling to school improvement;
- Demonstrates the involvement of school counselors in data-driven decision making;

- Promotes the equitable access to a quality school counseling program for every student;
- Supports the rationale for appropriate levels of funding and resources for school counseling;
- Offers awareness about the appropriate credential and staffing ratios;
- Provides the community with an awareness of comprehensive and developmental school counseling;
- Connects school counseling to standards-based reform;
- Documents measurable results and accountability for shared responsibility for student success.

Benefits of comprehensive school counseling for postsecondary educational institutions:

- Provides for articulation and transition of students to postsecondary institutions;
- Builds collaboration with all educators to prepare every student for postsecondary opportunities;
- Encourages every student to seek a wide range of substantial postsecondary options, including college;
- Endorses and supports high aspirations and rigorous academic preparation;
- Promotes equitable access to postsecondary education for every student.

Benefits of comprehensive school counseling for community members (community organizations, business, and industry):

- Offers opportunities for all community stakeholders to actively participate in the development and implementation of the school counseling program;
- Promotes collaboration and teaming to encourage citizenship, high achievement, and community pride;
- Encourages students to take pride in their community;
- Demonstrates the role that the community plays in a student's education;
- Shows community support, commitment to, and involvement in school improvement.

From the moment I stepped onto a school campus, I identified not with other therapists but with other educators, and like them, felt I was at the heart and soul of the educational process; not a visitor whose job it was to be a clinician, but an educator who brought unique counseling skills and specialized knowledge. As an educator, I need my counseling skills but I impact my students through a repertoire of other powerful roles: leader, advocate, collaborator, team builder, consultant, data analyzer/consumer, systemic change agent, steward of equity and access, manager of resources, career and academic adviser, and didactic counselor. We are in a setting called schools and as a school counselor I owe a duty to my clients, students, to help them become successful learners through the application of a wide range of exciting skills.

— Stone, C., ACA, 2003, p. 15

School counselors working in today's schools share the commitment, the responsibility, and the accountability for student educational success. As key players in the school improvement arena, 21st-century school counselors can contribute in powerful ways to creating schools that nurture respect, have high aspirations, and are committed to ensuring that every child, regardless of socioeconomic status, race, ethnicity, or gender has access to an equitable education. Helping to close the achievement gap is a primary purpose for the work of counselors in schools and an important focus of their programs.

TechTools

Effective school counselors use the power of technology to maximize their efficiency. Here are six "tech tools" you can use to maximize your own effectiveness:

- Use the World Wide Web to keep abreast of educational reform initiatives and find out more about the requirements of No Child Left Behind.
- Contact the office of your school district that manages student information and discuss how you can get data in a form that will be useful to you, such as attendance data disaggregated by grade level, day of the week, and so on.
- Examine your local school district's website. How can you use the website to improve communication to parents and other stakeholders?
- Access your district's school report card, which describes critical student data in your school system. Use this to develop a presentation on "Student Progress in My School District."
- Explore the Education Trust's website (www.Edtrust.org) and review the data slide section called Achievement in America which reveals student academic progress.
- Explore Postsecondary.org (www.postsecondary.org) and other websites that provide you with data that inform you about patterns in higher education enrollment. Use this information to compare these trends and patterns to those in your local high school and to inspire others to help your school improve.

School Counselor Casebook: *Voices From the Field*

The Scenario Reviewed

Many of the students in your school are English language learners (ELL) and students of color. Approximately 60% are eligible for the free or reduced lunch program. The state test scores are low and your school has been targeted by the state education department as a school under review (SUR) site. Under threat of a state takeover, the school must show improvement immediately. You know that school improvement is a shared responsibility. Your colleagues are busily planning and implementing new strategies.

A Practitioner's Approach

Here's how a practicing school counselor approached this challenge.

As a professional school counselor, I know how important it is that a climate of understanding and pride in cultivating community diversity be established as quickly as possible. Because the English language learners (ELL) work in both their primary language and in English to make academic progress, our other students and faculty focused on ways to make school a welcoming environment in order to facilitate learning for the ELL students. A majority of the ELL parents may be struggling to learn English themselves, and may be workers who receive minimal wages or are without a job. Because the family and community resources (including time and money) have been stretched to the maximum, the other school counselors and I decided to find new ways to use existing resources.

We knew that time was of the essence when submitting our action plan to the state. Our next step was to review the National Standards for School Counseling Programs before selecting competencies for the students, and to use school and community resources, including school data, to meet the goals of the action plan. We agreed that every counselor would make sure to keep abreast of new expectations, programs, and trends that might impact students, faculty, parents, and school counselors.

We made an inquiry to see if all of the counselors could attend the next School Improvement Team meeting to present additional strategies to be implemented simultaneously on several levels. With a large group sitting at the table, we brainstormed several strategies: The teachers suggested involving the PTA, community/business leaders, and legislators to network for sharing new programs and ideas. The high school principal volunteered the Honor Society students to tutor the younger ones. One idea included inviting parents to an evening event to talk about how to help their teens with homework. We planned for dinner and child care to be provided in order to facilitate participation for parents and caregivers. Our principal suggested a grant investigation to provide resources for teachers who were will-ing to set up a study/homework club before or after school.

The school improvement team planned to host a meeting of the total faculty and staff to secure their commitment and involvement in developing strategies that were needed to raise student aspirations and motivation. Parents, bus drivers, cafeteria workers, and custodians were included in the plan.

We agreed to investigate additional resources in our school and in our community. The school counselors, school psychologist, and school social worker volunteered to talk with school and community members about the specific roles they can play in helping our students achieve and to ensure that our school met the expected level of student performance. We involved district curriculum coordinators, community and faith group leaders, legislators, other district administrators, school coun-selors, school psychologists, school social workers, community mental health work-ers, drug and alcohol counselors, and health care workers in these conversations.

For our next school improvement team meeting, we have plans to pull the strate-gies together in order to show the State Department of Education our plan of ac-tion, which addresses necessary improvements and sequential benchmarks to accomplish our plan's goals. We understand the need to share the responsibility to improve student achievement and to make sure our students leave our school with a solid foundation for the future. The professional school counselor can be an effective catalyst and serve as an advocate, leader, and team player when school improvement is the goal and everyone accepts their fair share of responsi-bilities.

Barbara Webster, former elementary and middle school counselor and past Central Region vice president of the American School Counselor Association, has been a professional school counselor for more than 20 years in several settings, including the elementary through university levels. Her current studies at the University of Colorado at Denver include the Education Specialty program in Culturally and Linguistically Diverse (CLD) populations. Reprinted with permission by Barbara Webster.

Chapter Summary

The Changing Direction of 21st-Century Schools

The most recent educational reform agenda, which took a strong hold in the mid-1990s, focused its attention on developing national standards across all curriculum areas. This emphasis on what students should know and be able to do has also resulted in high stakes testing in every state across the nation. Coupled with this is a growing concern over the achievement gap, which appears to be rooted in socioeconomic, racial, and ethnic differences. The shared purpose of creating schools in which all children are held to high expectations must be addressed if we are going to prepare all students to meet the challenges of the 21st century.

School Counseling: Changing With the Times

Throughout the earlier years of educational reform and debate, school counseling was largely ignored as part of the solution to improve student achievement and success in school. Recently, counseling in schools has been acknowledged for the greater role it plays in contributing to student aspirations and educational achievement.

Issues Impacting Today's Schools: Pressures From the Global Economy; The Power of Technology; Swings and Shifts in Societal Issues and Values

All stakeholders have expectations of higher levels of academic achievement as standards-based education is the norm. The pressure is on from an ever-changing global economy. Business and industry continue to expect more from education.

There is a demonstrated need for academic and affective competence in all aspects of K–12 education, and there is a direct link between a person's knowledge and skills and income level. Changing technology impacts all aspects of our lives. The millennial generation spends its entertainment and leisure time in ways that adults cannot always identify with. Shifting societal issues and values impact the way we work with youth.

The Important Roles of 21st-Century School Counselors: Supporting Student Success; Helping All Children Achieve at a Higher Level; Leaders and Advocates for School Improvement; Partners in Educational Excellence; Ensuring Every Stakeholder Benefits

The purpose of the counseling program in schools is to impart specific skills and facilitate learning opportunities in a proactive and preventive manner to help all students achieve school success through academic, career, and personal-social development experiences. As school counselors establish a foundation for effective education, they also commit to contributing to a climate of high expectations of achievement for every student. In the 21st century, school counselors support student success; help all children achieve at a higher level; change attitudes and beliefs about students' ability to achieve; and are partners in educational excellence. Everyone benefits from school counseling programs, and implementing a comprehensive standards-based school counseling program empowers school counselors to place themselves front and center in the restructuring process of their school systems.

Key Terms

Accountability p. 2

Educational reform p. 6

High stakes testing p. 2

National Standards for School
  Counseling Programs p. 9

No Child Left Behind p. 4

School improvement p. 3

Standards p. 3

Standards-based education p. 2

Learning Extensions

1. Education professionals are talking (and writing) about the No Child Left Behind Act (2001). This latest reauthorization of the Elementary and Secondary Education Act is driving the educational agenda in our states, districts, and schools. Use a search engine like Google or Yahoo to find out what principals, school board members, superintendents, and parents are thinking about No Child Left Behind.

2. Read *A Nation at Risk*, which can be found online at http://www.ed.gov/pubs/NatAtRsk. How does this paper, written two decades ago, apply to the state of education in America today?

3. Locate your state department of education's website to review the *Educational Requirements for Students*. Create a table to summarize what is required at each level in elementary, middle/junior high, and high school. Carefully examine the new curriculum, assessment, promotion, and graduation requirements.

4. Think back to your high-school days. Were you placed in a particular academic track? Which type of academic program did you follow? Which academic program did your friends follow? Did you notice differences in the various plans of study among students in your school? How did tracking impact your expectations of yourself and of your friends?

5. Talk to someone you know who works for a large organization and also to someone who works in a small business or company. Show them the Secretary's Commission on Achieving Necessary Skills (SCANS) competencies. Ask them how the SCANS competencies could be used in their organization.

6. To explore the current state of student achievement, go to the website http://www.edtrust.org. Explore the slide show "Achievement in America." Why is this information important to your preparation as a school counselor?

7. The National Center for Education Statistics (NCES) maintains comprehensive data on the state of education across our nation. Find three positive improvements in your state's data and identify three areas that require additional improvement.

8. Examine your local school district/system's report card. What does this tell you about levels of students' performance in your community? What else might you want to know?

Chapter 2

Counseling Theory in Schools

Chapter Objectives

By the time you have completed this chapter, you should be able to:

- Understand the purpose of counseling in schools.
- Demonstrate an understanding of the major theoretical approaches to counseling that are relevant in a school setting.
- Apply counseling theory to case studies.
- Identify counseling techniques that are appropriate to your style and a school setting.
- Explain how to utilize counseling theories and techniques to help each student achieve academic, career, and personal-social success.
- Understand how to address the diverse counseling needs of students including race, ethnicity, culture, religion, sexual orientation, learning differences, and/or physical or emotional disabilities.
- Explain the importance of utilizing community-based mental health resources.
- Demonstrate the knowledge to identify counseling interventions appropriate to the specific needs of the student and the issue, problem, or challenge that he or she faces.

School Counselor Casebook: Getting Started

The Scenario

Faithfully each morning a group of seventh graders meets with you to touch base and get focused for the day. This 10-minute daily check-in seems to work well for you and these 12 academically at-risk students. This is the third day that Raymond has missed, though he is coming to school. When you ask the group if anyone has seen Raymond, you are told that Raymond won't come to your office any more because his friends are making fun of him. You go in search of Raymond and find him hanging around outside the front door with a small group of boys who are frequently seen in the in-school suspension room for cutting and fighting.

Thinking About Solutions

As you read this chapter, think about how you as a school counselor would handle this situation. What plan of action might you follow? How might you use your knowledge of counseling theory and techniques to help Raymond? When you come to the end of the chapter, you will have the opportunity to see how your ideas compare with a practicing school counselor's approach.

Counseling in the Complex World of Schools

On a daily basis, students face a fast-paced world replete with multiple personal and emotional concerns. Coping with day-to-day pressures such as trauma, grief, loss, economic stressors, temptations of substance abuse, peer influence, and aggression in school hallways are part of the challenges of growing up in the 21st century.

Schools are microcosms of our communities. Some children, streetwise and sophisticated in their knowledge about sex, drugs, and alcohol, learn to adjust. They develop coping mechanisms and acquire resiliency skills to find balance in their school, family, and community lives. Nevertheless, academic success often is depressed by the stressors of the world in which children live. Students move through the developmental stages of physical and emotional growth faced with multiple dilemmas and complex choices. Abuse, dysfunctional home environments, blended families, hunger, poverty, violence, harassment, bullying, peer pressure, and homelessness are just some of the pressures they encounter and struggle with on a daily basis (Children's Defense Fund, 2004). For some students, the school building is a safe haven.

Schools are complex institutions, and daily routines are at times confusing and frustrating for many children. Students may walk through the front door each day ready and willing to learn, but when met by external and internal pressures, their motivation, drive, and concentration are tempered or crushed. Although many children have developed the coping and resiliency skills needed to survive and even thrive, a growing number develop emotional, social, and behavioral problems that necessitate intervention. Children struggle with behavioral reconciliation whether challenged by peers, parents, teachers, or other figures of authority. Escapism has become an alternative via the world of alcohol and drugs or immersion in a world of video games and media (Howe & Strauss, 2000).

Counseling is a complex helping process in which the counselor establishes a trusting and confidential working relationship with a student or groups of students (ASCA, 1997) to help students set goals and make changes in behavior. Students bring acting-out behaviors, lack of motivation, poor achievement, learning problems, sadness, depression, social isolation, and pressure and stress to the **counseling process**. Counseling goals address, analyze, and explore behaviors and attitudes that impact a student's ability to perform successfully in the learning community. The focus of counseling in the educational setting is on problem solving, decision making, social-emotional development, and the personal issues and concerns that impact learning and development.

The foundation and basis for the school counseling program reside in **counseling theory** and those processes and techniques relevant to the school setting. Not to be confused with advising or guidance or therapy, counseling is the most significant component of the school counseling program, and the one by which the counselor's professional identity often is established.

When trying to address the needs of an overwhelming number of students, the teachers and administrators sometimes send students to the school counselor to be "cured." Where counseling is considered a quick fix, disappointment and confusion follow when students continue to pose problems for themselves and others (Cunanan & Maddy-Bernstein, 1994). It is difficult to eliminate or even remediate students' presenting problems when you work with the students in isolation. School counselors are needed not to provide a panacea but rather to provide counseling for students toward change as well as support to teachers, administrators, and parents in the form of facilitative, collaborative interventions. Oftentimes, the person who is the most highly trained to prevent, intervene, and remediate student behavior is the school counselor.

Counseling Students: Purpose and Limitations

> Counseling is a confidential relationship which the counselor conducts with students individually and in small groups to help them resolve their problems and developmental concerns.
>
> *— ASCA, 1999b, p.1*

Counseling is a professional skill. Unlike conversations between friends, or working with students in a guidance or advisory role, counseling is a complex process and is far more involved than simply establishing a relationship with a student and setting goals for behavioral changes. Schmidt (1999) reminded us that counseling requires the use of the helping relationship to focus on concerns that can be developmental or problem-based, help a student make decisions to correct a situation, or learn or acquire new behavioral skills to improve one's image of self.

Clear goals are needed when counseling students (Schmidt, 1999). George and Cristiani (1990) identified five major goals that are at the heart of most counseling theories and models:

1. facilitate a change in behavior

2. improve social and personal relationships

3. increase one's ability to cope

4. learn and apply the decision-making process

5. enrich personal growth and self-development

These same goals can serve as a good guide for you when you become a school counselor because they are applicable to helping students—our "clients"—learn to help themselves, make good decisions, and bring about positive changes in behavior.

Counseling in schools differs from therapeutic treatment in purpose and process. Counseling in schools usually involves short-term goals, while psychotherapeutic intervention relies on a positive therapeutic alliance influenced by the commitment of the client and the skill and talents of the clinician (Seligman, 2001). The focus of counseling with students is to address prevention, intervention, and developmental concerns, assist with mild disorders in educational or developmental settings, and engage students in dealing with personal, social, emotional, career, and educational decisions and behaviors (Thompson & Rudolph, 2000). When the goals of counseling are complex and require therapeutic intervention, school counselors will refer students to a mental health professional in an agency, clinic, or private practice setting.

Theoretical Underpinnings of Counseling

In order to professionally and skillfully move a student through the counseling process, the school counselor needs a broad-based awareness, knowledge, and understanding of theory. Counseling is first and foremost guided by theory (Gladding, 2004). Counseling theories provide a point of reference from which the counselor develops a personal perspective of human growth, development, and behavior. The counselor selects different theories and approaches according to the models used and the assistance that a student needs. Counseling requires the acquisition of requisite skills and knowledge so that counselors can facilitate, process, and construct appropriate intervention plans. Counselors use techniques and strategies that best match their theoretical approach, philosophical orientation, the needs of their clientele, and the setting in which they work.

There are more than 250 documented counseling and psychotherapy systems (Corsini & Wedding, 1995) to study, analyze, and incorporate into practice. In this chapter you will be introduced to eight theories that were carefully chosen as those having the greatest potential for counseling work with minors in a school setting. These eight theories are presented in a brief and concise manner that is not intended to replace comprehensive reading, study, and analysis. As you read each theory, consider referencing a counseling textbook that is specifically devoted to the study of theory. This will provide you with a much deeper intellectual awareness and understanding of theories, interventions, treatment systems, and the skills associated with each. In-depth study and supervised practice in applying student growth and developmental theories will increase your confidence and effectiveness.

The Gestalt Approach

The Gestalt approach was developed by Fritz Perls and promotes the importance of wholeness and completeness in day-to-day living. Perls (1969) purported that people strive to accomplish all that they can in their lifetime. **Gestalt theory** emphasizes the present and supports the equation *now = experience = awareness = reality*. Only the *now* exists, because the past is no more and the future has not yet revealed itself.

The phrase "the whole is greater than the sum of its parts" emphasizes the importance of wholeness or completeness. Through Gestalt therapy, the client learns to identify and analyze the smaller issues in relationship to the larger problem or situation. The client works with the present to resolve past issues and seeks her or his self-actualization, which emerges through personal interaction with the environment. Problems can arise in five different ways: (a) loss of contact with the environment; (b) loss of touch with self by becoming too involved with the environment; (c) failure to put aside unfinished business; (d) finding oneself moving in several different directions; and (e) being caught in conflict between doing what one thinks one should do versus what one wants to do.

Techniques

The Gestalt approach uses a repertoire of exercises and experiments. When exercises are used, the counselor guides the student through experiences that include enactment of fantasies, role-play, and psychodrama. Exercises such as the "empty chair," "I take responsibility," and "may I feed you a sentence" are intended to help the student acquire and apply newly honed skills. Other examples of different Gestalt approaches include:

Dream Work—the student fantasizes what it would be like in different parts of the dream in order to better understand the multiple ways of interacting with the environment.

Empty Chair—the student talks to an empty chair to better understand rational and irrational ways of communicating.

Confrontation—the student is challenged by the counselor for his or her actions or words. For example, the student is constantly smiling and masking anger or frustration.

Making the Rounds—often used in group counseling, this technique involves expressing an emotion or feeling to each person in the group. The student becomes more aware of internal emotions and feelings through verbal expression

I Take Responsibility—the student makes a statement about an issue or perception and completes the sentence with ". . . and I take responsibility for it."

May I Feed You a Sentence—the counselor supplies the student with a sentence to help him or her clarify thoughts and responses.

Although Gestalt techniques include free association, the school counselor does not interpret or analyze. Rather, the purpose is to help students get in touch with their emotions through self-exploration.

Theory Into Practice

Gestalt therapy is complex and sophisticated and requires a high level of cognitive and behavioral development in students. Because life does not unfold in a controlled environment, young students may not be able to apply what they have learned in a counseling situation to a real-life challenge. Techniques such as "I take responsibility" can help students sort through blaming and enabling by making them aware that the solution lies within them and does not lie with their parents, peers, or teachers.

The Gestalt approach helps to address situations that are current in a student's life. There is an emphasis on immediacy to make choices in the present that will impact the future, and there is no room for procrastination or putting off until tomorrow or indefinitely. However, Gestalt theory is a difficult concept for most young people and many adults to grasp.

Practical Application

During a parent–student conference, you are well aware that your seventh-grade student is sending out mixed messages. Jennifer verbally states her desire to succeed but is not doing anything concrete to get assignments in on time either during class or for homework. Her mom talks about her procrastination, laziness, and even indifference to her schoolwork. When the three of you reviewed Jennifer's school records, there was nothing apparent that indicated a learning problem. Up until this year, Jennifer was a solid B to B+ student.

Using a Gestalt approach, what techniques might work in this situation?

The Person-Centered Approach

This theory, which evolved from the work of Carl Rogers (1961), focuses on the "core conditions" of genuineness, empathy, positive regard, and concreteness, all of which are essential to all helping relationships and the counseling process. Humans are characteristically positive, forward moving, constructive, realistic, and trustworthy. Rogers also believed that each person is aware, inner directed, and moving toward self-actualization from the time they are born. Rogerians believe that self-actualization is the most prevalent and motivating drive of existence and that it encompasses actions that influence the total person.

Person-centered theory stresses that each person is capable of finding personal meaning and purpose in life, and that the self is an outgrowth of what a person experiences. Self-awareness helps a person differentiate herself or himself from others;

however, a person needs positive regard in his or her life for a healthy self to emerge. Positive regard is love, warmth, care, respect, and acceptance.

Through the counseling process, the client learns how to deal with and cope with situations. As the client begins to free herself or himself of defense mechanisms and past experiences, she or he approaches counseling with openness to self-exploration and self-awareness. Person-centered counseling assists the client to develop into a more mature, confident, and well-adapted decision maker. The client embraces a more realistic sense of self, can adapt and recover quickly from situations, and is less stressed by everyday events.

Techniques

There are three different stages of application of the theory. The nondirective stage emphasizes the development of the relationship with the student by creating a permissive and noninterventive atmosphere that creates a climate of acceptance and clarification. The second stage is known as the reflective period. During this time the student, with the counselor's help, tries to create nonthreatening relationships in his or her life. The counselor concentrates on responding to the student's feelings and reflects the underlying affect back to the student. During the third application, called the experimental stage, positive regard (acceptance) and congruence (genuineness) are emphasized. Other overall techniques that are used are active and passive listening, accurate reflection of thoughts and feelings, clarification, summarization, confrontation, and general and open-ended leads.

Theory Into Practice

The person-centered approach works well when treating students who exhibit mild to moderate anxiety, adjustment, and interpersonal disorders. This therapy requires students to have a complete understanding of themselves and their experiences. Therefore, it may not work well with young children or students with learning or emotional disabilities.

Students with minor behavioral adjustments or mild anxiety, and older students who are just generally confused about their future direction may benefit from this approach, which can be effective in a relatively short time. However, behavioral change also may be short term. The person-centered approach may address only surface issues and not challenge the student to explore deeper. When the ultimate goal is to develop a long-lasting impact on the student, person-centered counseling may be too optimistic and the solution too short-lived for today's complex societal issues.

Practical Application

Michael's parents are going through a separation. Although Michael cannot remember a time in his 10 years when his parents were not arguing and fighting, he feels he is to blame and that somehow he has contributed to the problem. At least three times this week, Michael started to cry in class when corrected for small errors on homework or class work. His teacher also noticed that Michael does not seem to be hanging out with his friends as much in the lunchroom and on the playground. Michael's teacher asked you to talk with Michael.

How could you use person-centered techniques to help Michael?

The Individual Psychology Approach

Individual psychology was developed by Alfred Adler. However, one cannot discuss Adler's work without reference to the influence of Sigmund Freud. Adler, initially one of Freud's disciples, eventually became one of his strongest dissidents. Freud invited Adler to participate in discussion circles until such time that Adler rejected Freud's emphasis on sex, the unconscious, and the influence of the past. Although Freud's theory of psychoanalysis suggested new ways of understanding love, hate, emotions, family relations, fantasy, and sexuality, Adler purported that personality difficulties are rooted in feelings of inferiority and are derived from an individual's need for self-assertion. Adler termed his theory "individual psychology" to distinguish his work from that of Freud. Central to Adler's theory is the concept that social interest drives behavior. Terms such as *inferiority complex, social interest, empathy,* and *lifestyle* were coined by Adler and quickly adopted by other theorists and scholars (Gladding, 2004).

Human beings desire success; thus, all behavior is purposeful and goal-oriented. The Adlerian approach encourages the client to be well aware of his or her surroundings and environment, and the theory supports healthy emotional development to overcome any feelings of inferiority. This theoretical orientation stresses the influence of subjective feelings as a primary motivator. The client learns to grapple with conscious levels of thought and assumes responsibility for taking charge of changing behaviors.

Behavior and misbehavior are the externals and are symptomatic of the feelings that the client has internalized. Especially when dealing with misbehavior, school counselors can pay particular attention to the reasons for the behavior, such as looking for attention, seeking power, revenge, or compensating for feelings of inadequacy (Dreikurs & Soltz, 1990). Schools present vast opportunity for students to experiment with different types of behaviors and gain a sense of belonging and connectedness (Sciarra, 2004).

Techniques

Counselors who consider themselves "Adlerian" demonstrate empathy, support, and genuine warmth toward students. However, the counselor uses a variety of techniques to assist and encourage change in behavior, such as confrontation. Confrontation challenges students to examine their logic and behavior and to look at the situation they are in. Asking questions and attending are used to explore possibilities. For

example, when a student is asked "What would be different if you _____?"
the student can respond with an answer based on what he or she wants ideally. The
counselor listens and encourages the student to embrace good, positive, and realistic behaviors. Encouragement motivates the student to believe that change is possible. "Catching oneself" is a technique that teaches the student to become aware of
self-destructive behaviors and thoughts.

Other specialized strategies such as "pushing buttons" help students to develop
an awareness of what prompts their reactions and to recognize when they are acting in an inappropriate manner. Students also are encouraged to set tasks and establish short-term goals to ultimately establish and attain a long-term but realistic
change in behavior.

Theory Into Practice

Adlerians approach behavior as goal directed; the focus for children is on immediate behavior targets rather than long-term objectives. Play therapy helps young children learn how to better express themselves, socialize, and interact with others, and
it provides a vehicle for differentiating between good and bad behaviors. Drawings
also are helpful to discern a child's pattern of behavior.

The Adlerian method helps students to identify more successful ways of resolving problems than what they currently are doing in school, play, and social interactions. The counselor works with the assumption that the students can assume
responsibility and acquire better ways to meet personal goals. The counselor uses
questioning to frame the structured interview and explore the perspective that the
students have of their own lives. Students explore their orientation in their families,
confront negative behavior, establish goals, and examine social interactions. Encouragement is a critical part of the counseling process, and the Adlerian method
subscribes to the belief that students misbehave when they are frustrated and discouraged and have no other means to succeed. School counselors use these techniques to facilitate, change, and encourage appropriate behaviors while disregarding
unwanted and unhealthy ways of responding.

Practical Application

*Katie feels that she is unable to do anything well. She is only comfortable in class when the
teacher expects nothing from her. You ask Katie, "What do you want your teacher and classmates to know about you? Are there some things in class that you are really good at and would
like everyone to know? How can we make that happen?"*

How would you approach this counseling situation if your professional orientation is Adlerian?

The Behavioral Approach

The behavioral approach to counseling is strongly influenced by the work of B. F. Skinner and is based on the processes closely associated with overt behavior. **Behavioral therapy** promotes the premise that all behavior is learned and that learning is effective in changing maladaptive behavior. The three main approaches in contemporary behavior therapy are the stimulus-response model, applied behavior analysis, and social-cognitive theory.

The stimulus-response (S-R) model approaches behavioral change through the conditioning of involuntary responses. It sometimes is also called respondent learning. The classic example that immediately comes to mind is Pavlov's dog. Salivation occurs when the bell is rung because the bell is associated with food. Behavior also can be "unlearned" through counter-conditioning, in which new associations take the place of old ones.

When behavioral analysis is applied, a person is rewarded or punished for her or his actions. This is an extension of operant conditioning. A person learns to repeat what was rewarded (reinforced) and not repeat the actions that were punished.

Social-cognitive theory purports that people acquire new knowledge and behavior by observing others. It emphasizes observational learning, imitation, social modeling, and vicarious learning. Social-cognitive theory is efficient in that it saves time, energy, and effort in acquiring new skills, and it is most effective if the observer can relate to the model. The counselor plays multiple roles as consultant, teacher, advisor, reinforcer, and facilitator, and responds in a concrete, objective, and collaborative manner. Additionally, the client is involved in every phase of counseling.

Behavioral counseling goals help clients make good adjustments to life circumstances and achieve personal and professional objectives by replacing unproductive actions (maladaptive behavior) with productive actions. The counselor and client mutually agree upon goals in these four basic steps:

1. Define the problem

2. Explore how past circumstances were handled through a developmental history

3. Establish specific goals in small achievable units and design learning experiences to acquire needed skills

4. Determine the best methods for change

Techniques

School counselors who subscribe to a behavioral approach will apply different techniques for various situations. Many of these techniques are adapted for classroom and group experiences. For example, teachers often use positive reinforcers to yield a desired result or action. This can be translated into intrinsic or extrinsic rewards. It is important to differentiate between negative reinforcers and punishment. Is there a difference between a teacher "yelling" at the class versus withholding a privilege? Would either technique result in the desired change in student behavior?

School counselors also work with students on "shaping" behavior, which is learning new ways of responding through successive approximation. In "generalization" the counselor helps students understand how they have applied the behavior outside of where it was initially learned. "Maintenance" means the student continues the behavior without anyone else's support. "Extinction" occurs when the student eliminates a behavior(s) due to the withdrawal of its reinforcement.

Additional techniques are used when a student has a greater need to further explore particular situations:

- Behavioral rehearsal is practicing a desired behavior until it is performed the way the student wishes.
- Environmental planning is establishing an environment to promote or limit certain behaviors and help the student avoid places that associate with painful memories.
- Systematic desensitization helps the student overcome anxiety in particular situations.
- Assertiveness training helps the student to express thoughts and feelings appropriately without feeling undue anxiety.
- Contingency contracts spell out the behavior to be performed, changed, or discontinued, and the rewards and/or stipulations involved in the agreement.

Theory Into Practice

School counselors using behavioral techniques are actively engaged in the teaching and learning process to help the student learn, unlearn, or modify behaviors. The teaching aspect of counseling is very much a part of behavioral theory. It can be very empowering to students, even young ones, when they see and feel tangible results for modifying or changing behavior. As a student learns to eliminate negative or distracting behavior, she or he simultaneously is encouraged to display positive behavior. With this approach, students are seen as capable of learning new ways of addressing situations, and they are empowered by the knowledge that they are capable of taking charge and learning control. Behavioral theory relies on a good working relationship between the students and the counselor. Although the students extend the effort to make the desired changes, they are encouraged, supported, and empowered to stay focused by the counselor.

Practical Application

Ms. Bishop has her hands full with 25 high-energy second graders. Although she feels she has created a stimulating and challenging learning environment, there are at least four students who have significant difficulty completing their assignments on time. Ms. Bishop thinks the students' problems stem from difficulties with organization and attending rather than a learning disability. You offer to help the teacher set up a positive reinforcement system that will benefit the entire class but will most specifically be targeted to help these four students.

How will you use behavioral techniques to bring about the desired results?

The Reality Therapy Approach

Reality therapy helps clients understand the need to be psychologically strong and make healthy, productive choices in their interpersonal and intrapersonal relationships. Attaining psychological strength and using productive decision making lead to autonomy and taking responsibility for the behaviors that affect oneself and others. Reality therapy encourages the client to learn how to make more effective choices and develop the skills to cope with daily stresses and problems. Individuals take ownership of realistic goals, thus accepting responsibility for their present and future. Most important, the counselor helps clients to realize that they cannot blame others for inappropriate decisions; reality therapy attempts to eliminate such excuses.

William Glasser, the father of reality therapy, believes that human beings operate on a conscious level and are not driven by unconscious forces or instinct (1965, 1989, 1998, 2000). Human learning is a lifelong process based on choice. Glasser suggests that there are six criteria for healthy behavior that a person must seek. Behavior is easily completed, individually driven, has value, improves lifestyle, is not self-critical, and is not competitive. Choice theory is the foundation of reality therapy. Individuals self-determine the way in which they meet their needs for survival, power, fun, freedom, and belonging, and they choose their thoughts, actions, and emotions accordingly (Corey, 2001). This approach concentrates so much on the present that it tends to ignore the past and the unconscious, unlike psychoanalytic theory, which is heavily immersed in both. The application of reality therapy is difficult to apply to individuals who have problems expressing themselves or their feelings.

Techniques

The school counselor uses active techniques such as humor, role-play, confrontation, feedback, goal setting, attending and teaching, designing plans, and composing contracts to help the students explore their options. The primary technique of reality therapy is teaching students how to become responsible for their actions. The counselor's role is to reinforce positive planning and action steps. Students then begin to see how their behavior is unrealistic and sometimes negative. Guided by the school counselor, the students begin to understand that they are in control of the desired change(s).

Confrontation and role-play help the students to accept responsibility for their behavior and bring past events into the here and now. Reviewing past behaviors helps students take charge in the present and plan for the future, while establishing realistic goals to change their behaviors. Humor can be an effective technique, but it must be used respectfully. Students have fragile egos and must not think the counselor is making fun of them. Used carefully, humor may help students to look at a situation differently and see how unrealistic it was.

Reality therapy uses the WDEP system (Wubbolding, 2000) to help the counselor and the student focus on the desired change and assess progress. The counselor identifies what the student *wants* early on in the session. The counselor shares what he or she *Wants* for the student. The student takes *Direction* over his or her life. Evaluation is the basis for reality therapy. Students learn to *Evaluate* their behaviors and begin to recognize which behaviors are unproductive. Students take action to create a *Plan* for changing behaviors. Reality therapy places the responsibility on the student to accomplish the goals set forth in the plan of action. The counselor never gives up on the student, and the student assumes responsibility to break the cycle of failure.

Theory Into Practice

Reality therapy requires students to accept the responsibility of determining the course of action they will follow. Reality therapy does not dwell on the past but rather projects the students forward toward a change in action and behavior. Students may view reality therapy as empowering, believing that they have choices and that there are alternatives to the way a situation or problem was approached in the past. Reality therapy keeps students focused on dealing with the "here and now," which helps them gain self-confidence and assurance. Using role-play helps bring the future or past into the present. Reality therapy seems to work best with older children who are capable of understanding choice and demonstrate the desire to change their behavior.

Practical Application

At the eighth-grade team meeting last week, Mrs. Riemer, social studies teacher, presented some concerns she has about Robbie. She discovered that in all of his classes, Robbie was seeking constant attention, mainly in the form of joking and clowning. Academically he is very inconsistent, performing well for some teachers and not for others. Robbie is in danger of failing four out of his eight classes. You agree to meet with Robbie and explore the reasons that he is successful in some classes and not in others.

How will you use reality therapy to help Robbie change his approach to his schoolwork and behavior?

The REBT (Rational Emotive Behavior Therapy) Approach

First introduced by Albert Ellis in 1962 as Rational Emotive Therapy (RET), the B for "behavior" was added later as Ellis found that the use of pleasurable behaviors helped to motivate the client to be vigilant in his or her new thinking patterns. **Rational emotive behavior therapy** (REBT) is intended to help people live balanced, productive, and more rational lives by limiting the demands that one makes on oneself. This theory concentrates on the relationship between thoughts and their impact and effect upon emotions and behaviors.

Ellis believes that if people gain insight into their thinking process, they can change, because thinking influences feelings and behavior. Ellis also suggests that people have within themselves the ability to control their thoughts, feelings, and actions. However, clients first must be aware of what they are telling themselves (self-talk) to gain control. It is the difference between saying "I act badly" rather than "I am bad." Demands and wishes, and words such as "should have," "must," "have to," and "need to," lead to irrational thoughts and unfulfilled emotions. As clients gain a more rational thought process and positive way of thinking, they gain the ability to focus on altering specific behaviors instead of making a total personality change. Clients begin to understand that they have the choice of what to say and do, and this becomes empowering.

Techniques

School counselors who subscribe to REBT believe that experiences directly affect one's feelings, whether they are positive, negative, neutral, or mixed. Techniques such as teaching and disputing help school counselors educate students about the anatomy of emotion. Feelings are viewed as a result of thoughts and students have the ability to change their way of thinking to positively impact their emotional well being. The counselor helps students dispute irrational thoughts and encourages students to facilitate change in their thought patterns. Often the irrational thought is not the thought presented by the student; the technique of inference chaining is then very valuable in revealing the true thought that needs to be confronted. School counselors guide students to come to an understanding of their behaviors through cognitive processing, guided imagery, and behavioral disputing. Each of these techniques invokes direct questions, logical reasoning, imagining real situations, and attempting behavior that is not within the students' norm. Students may experience role-play, homework assignments, journal writing, and bibliotherapy as part of the counseling process.

The counselor also uses the cognitive theory of disturbance to help students understand how irrational beliefs lead to negative consequences. The ABC equation is central to REBT practice. A is the fact, an activating event, or the behavior or attitude on the part of a student. B is the student's belief about A, which causes C, the emotional and/or behavioral consequence. However, students must come to understand that the reaction could be healthy or not; appropriate or not, A does not cause C. Students learn to acknowledge that they are largely responsible for creating their own problems and to accept that they have the ability to change the outcome. Ultimately, the student understands that the problem stems from an irrational belief, works hard to counteract the irrationality, and engages in rational, emotive behavior as a way of life.

Theory Into Practice

REBT helps to restore emotional balance. This approach helps students learn new ways of thinking, behaving, and feeling, and ultimately to take control of the direction in which their lives are going. REBT can be used with other behavioral techniques to effectively assist students who have anxiety and adjustment disorders. The intent of REBT is to complete the process in a short-term period; therefore it is considered a viable theory in a school setting in which time is limited. REBT is best applied with older children and adolescents who are mature enough and intellectually able to discern reality from fictional thought processing. REBT is considered ineffective with mentally or severely emotionally disabled students or with very young children.

Changing thought patterns may not be the simplest or most compelling way to reframe emotions or behaviors. Accountability for behavior requires that students must become responsible for their own actions. Although an event can create a thought, which can lead to a consequence of action, students must assume responsibility for their own actions. REBT encourages students to be more tolerant of themselves and to strive to achieve their personal goals.

Practical Application

It is senior year and the college selection process is under way. Amanda is feeling very pressured as to what schools she should apply to. In her community, there is a lot of pressure on getting into the "right" college. It seems to be more of an issue with the parents than with the students. Although she ranks number 3 in her class and has an exceptional high-school resumé, Amanda has asked for your help in explaining to her parents that she is not interested in applying to an "Ivy League school." She very much wants to study in an environment that will not put as much pressure on her and will allow her to participate in co-op experiences and internships as part of her studies. With early-decision deadline dates looming ahead, Amanda is very stressed out over the conversation she needs to have with her parents before she can submit her applications.

How can using the REBT approach help Amanda communicate her personal goals to her parents?

Meet Eric Katz

Using REBT Techniques in a School Setting

Eric Katz is a high-school counselor who uses REBT techniques in a school setting at the Newburgh Free Academy. Eric studied part-time at The Albert Ellis Institute for Rational Emotive Behavioral Therapy in New York City.

REBT theory provided me with a strategy that helped me to address some of the prevalent challenges, such as developing a locus of control (i.e., the teacher failed me vs. what did I do that contributed to my failing) and the all-or-nothing thinking, which is so much a part of the adolescent mindset.

Last year two of my juniors in particular seemed to be very responsive to an REBT approach. The first student, Paul, suffered from chronic generalized anxiety. He would get physically ill obsessing about taking his tests. He would start with a dozen "what if I fail" type questions days before and continuing up to the day of the exam. In attacking the irrational thoughts, which here were "I am going to fail this test and it will be *terrible, catastrophic*, and I will be a *total* nothing," I got Paul to start to challenge his thoughts (much like weighing the evidence in a court trial) and ask himself two questions: Where is the proof that I will fail this test? If I do, why will this specific exam be the one that will make me a "nothing"? We looked at the facts that would dispute his thoughts: first, Paul was getting the top grades in this class, and second, he had taken many tests in the past and always tested well. We went over his assets, other than exam scores, that made him an attractive candidate for college admissions and likely to be a success in later life.

Kelly's situation was a much more common scenario. Kelly had been an honor student up through junior high and then began to slip academically and her attendance deteriorated. When I spoke with Kelly, she revealed to me that her father had told her "college is not for you." Like many teens, she bought into this belief and told me that no college would want her. Here we went right to attacking her belief. In 20 minutes, I helped her find a list of 15 colleges that would admit her when she graduated. I continued meeting with her and providing a counter voice to that of her father. This year, for the first time in 3 years, Kelly passed all her classes and is back on track to graduate on time with her class.

In using REBT, I often utilize a lot of humor to defuse the catastrophic feeling of the student's beliefs. At times the humor is used to eliminate the thoughts, which can help the student start to see that the belief is not fact. I must advise anyone who wishes to use these techniques that great care is needed. The humor taken outside of context can border on sarcasm. I want to make clear that I am only able to work this way when the quality of the relationship between the student and me is firmly established as safe and mutually respectful.

Today, in the midst of my frustration trying to accommodate dozens of schedule changes and corrections, Paul stops by my office, looks at me, and says, "Remember to breathe, Mr. Katz, in through the nose and then let it out slowly through the mouth." Apparently, our relaxation breathing training sessions have borne fruit, and the student is now the teacher.

Reprinted with permission by Eric D. Katz.

The Cognitive Behavior Approach

Albert Bandura influenced behavioral therapy by applying the concept of conditioning to social development (1986). Social-cognitive theory builds on social-learning theory (Mitchell & Krumboltz, 1996) and self-efficacy; it assists clients to deal with life's events and accomplish personal and professional goals. Bandura purported that faulty thinking leads to emotional and behavioral disturbances. Cognitions are a major determinant of how we feel and act. This therapeutic approach is directed toward creating cognitive and behavioral change. While the cognitive aspect focuses on thinking and understanding why a person behaves a certain way, the behavioral component focuses on doing and how to change. The client confronts faulty beliefs with the evidence that she or he gathers and evaluates.

Cognitive behavior theory is direct in style, structured, goal oriented, time limited, and focused on problem solving. It is a process in which clients are taught to identify, evaluate, and change self-defeating or irrational thoughts that negatively impact behavior. It is a psycho-educational model that emphasizes the learning process to acquire and practice new skills, learn new ways of thinking, and acquire new ways of coping with problems.

The psycho-educational model includes four steps. The first step is defining the problem in order to resolve the issue. This step involves first identifying or observing what the behavior or the presenting problem is. The second step requires taking a developmental history in which both the client and the counselor are aware of past events and how behaviors and issues were addressed or resolved. The third step is to establish specific goals, beginning with smaller incremental steps that lead to achievement of the primary goal. The fourth step is to analyze the best method for change. Thus, the counselor and client can explore various behavior modifications and identify which strategies will best support an individual dealing with change.

Techniques

Counselors who practice the cognitive behavior approach must maintain objectivity and become well versed in a variety of strategies. Cognitive restructuring teaches students how to identify, evaluate, and change self-defeating, irrational thoughts that can negatively influence behavior. Reinforcers, both positive and negative, facilitate behavior change. Behavior modification is coupled with positive reinforcement, primarily based on behavioral conditioning. A good deed or correct response is rewarded. Shaping is another technique that counselors use to help achieve behavior adjustments. Once a new behavior is learned, the counselor can gradually help the student manage the new skill and build on it to improve or change behavior. Generalization helps the student transfer the learned behavior to the presenting situation at home or in school. Maintenance helps the student focus on self-control and self-managing the new or modified behaviors. Extinction occurs when the undesired behavior has been eliminated from the individual's daily routine and is no longer part of the repertoire of response. The counselor may use confrontation, time out, confirmation, and attending to facilitate the client's progress. Homework assignments and recording activities and responses aid in the purpose of understanding and changing behavior.

The cognitive aspect of this theory is more focused on "thinking"; the behavioral component supports the "doing" necessary to change behavior. However, both aspects are essential to work effectively. The presenting problem is framed in the present, and it is assumed that the student's belief system about his or her behavior is the primary cause of the disorder. The premise is simply to modify unwanted behavior. The cognitive behavior approach is perceived as a therapeutic timesaver because it does not need to delve into the past to deal with the present; it is a learning theory that is constantly evolving. Today's society is dynamic, and people and their surroundings are always in a state of flux. Students must always be conscious of falling back into bad patterns.

Theory Into Practice

Token reinforcement and behavior modification programs are familiar classroom interventions. Cognitive behavior theory adds the dimension of understanding, applying logic and using reasoning to modify and change behavioral response, going well beyond conditioning and rewards. Cognitive behavior theory focuses on problem-solving abilities; it helps students identify, evaluate, and change self-defeating or irrational thoughts that negatively influence their behavior by using cognitive restructuring. Students who are feeling defeated in learning, who have fallen prey to the cycle of failure or inappropriate behavior, or who easily succumb to peer pressure can learn and apply a new set of skills to modify or change how they respond or cope in the situation. By selecting a "choice goal" (Bandura, 1986) the student becomes determined to carry out a specific task or achieve a particular accomplishment.

Stress inoculation helps students acquire coping skills to help them handle stressful events. For example, a student with a chronic illness or disability is constantly dealing with stress events. This is partially because the student simply does not comprehend the nature of the illness or why the emotional, physical, or learning disability exists in the first place. Teaching a student about his or her illness or disability and the treatment involved is empowering. When a young person acquires skills to gain some control over a difficult situation, it is easier to cope with any negativity and challenges. Whether addressing maladaptive behaviors, stress, pressure, or disabling conditions, cognitive behavioral theory can help students change how they respond to situations by learning and then applying new and appropriate behaviors. Consideration must always be given to the developmental and maturity level of the students to ensure that the conceptual framework is within the realm of their cognitive thinking and understanding.

Practical Application

Jason is convinced that the high-school exit exam is the most important test that he will ever take. His parents, teachers, and you, his counselor, have reminded him that he still has several opportunities to pass—just in case. Jason is an average student and usually gets Cs and Bs in most of his subjects. He failed the test the first time he took it. He said he got overly anxious and could not think straight. Jason told you that if he cannot pass the test the next time he takes it, he will just have to quit high school. He does not know what he wants to do after high school; sometimes he thinks he wants to go to college, and other times he thinks that he wants a technical career. Now he thinks he should just go to work and not deal with any of this.

How can cognitive behavioral techniques help Jason reduce his test anxiety and pass the exit exam?

The Existential Approach

People live by the choices they make. Self-determination is freedom of choice. The founders of **existential theory** (Frankl, 1963; May, 1950; May & Yalom, 1995; Yalom, 1980) developed this theory to bring an awareness of being, responsibility, freedom, and potential to individuals. One goal of this theory is to encourage clients to take a more active role in shaping their personal reality and putting themselves first. Clients are taught to shift the process of thinking from an outward to an inward approach. This results in a better understanding of the relationship between decisions and present and future actions.

Existentialists emphasize the importance of anxiety, values, freedom, and responsibility as one searches to find meaning. Because people author their lives by the choices they make, no longer can life's choices depend on the judgment of others. The client uncovers life's meaning by doing a deed, experiencing a value, or by suffering.

Techniques

There are no specific techniques for the existential approach other than an assurance of the student's readiness to work in an open and inquiring manner. The counselor encourages the student to accept the truth and learn how to work through ambiguity. The counselor must remain open and self-revealing to help the student become more in touch with personal feelings and experiences. The emphasis in the relationship is on spontaneity, authenticity, and honesty. The use of confrontation, goal setting, and imagery helps the student see that each person is responsible for her or his own life and that the student should not allow outside influences to impact choice or behavior. Issues are presented not as problems, but rather as learning experiences that can motivate one to strive to succeed.

Existentialism respects diversity and places importance on an individual's ethnic and social background. Existentialism may be used in conjunction with other theories, such as behavior modification and cognitive theory, to assist in cases such as alcoholism and severe depression. This style of counseling is so individualized that each counselor practices in a different way and tends to be more philosophical than theoretical. Existentialism ascribes to the belief system that connects individuals to the universal problems faced by humankind, such as searching for peace and confronting life's challenges through honest expression. Feelings are not classified as negative or positive; they simply are accepted. Because no two individuals are alike, this theory focuses on uniqueness.

Existentialist philosophies also can be combined with other theoretical models, such as person-centered and Adlerian, that are sensitive to individual uniqueness and focus on the student's personal well-being and effective adjustment in society. The ultimate goal is for students to work and live productively and peacefully in their current environment.

Theory Into Practice

The debate continues as to whether existentialism is a philosophy or a counseling approach; this is not an easy discussion to resolve. However, let's consider that the existential approach helps students realize the importance of meaning, responsibility, awareness, freedom, and potential. The student cannot be merely an observer of life but a participant in meaningful personal activity. What matters most in the existential approach is the student's perception, not that of someone else.

In a school setting, the counselor must be both open and inquiring; however, the student must offer the same. In this approach, students assume responsibility for their own lives. Students participate in guided imagery and awareness exercises and goal-setting activities similar to those of other models.

Practical Application

You have been invited by the team of eighth-grade teachers to collaborate on developing a program that will help the students make a smooth transition from middle school to high school.

Which existential approaches would you propose for classroom activities and for group counseling?

Choosing a Theoretical Approach

School counselors must be fully cognizant of the theoretical applications or dominant approaches that are incorporated in the counseling process. School counselors who are confident in their knowledge, understanding, and application of theory will operate from a perspective that is compatible with their assumptions about student development progression, emotional well-being, and school appropriateness. The differential effectiveness of various approaches, a familiarity with a broad range of treatment systems (Seligman, 2001), and the melding of one's own knowledge and experiences in utilizing various theories has resulted in some clinicians choosing an eclectic or integrated approach. Taking an eclectic approach is a challenging choice; approaching treatment in an eclectic manner requires a solid foundation in knowledge and experience. School counselors do not always have the luxury of indefinite periods of time in which to work from a particular theoretical approach, and may choose to use more than one approach with the hope of seeking a quicker resolution to achieve the desired goal.

Acquiring Counseling Skills and Techniques

Counseling is a continuous process, a series of stages that begins with exploration and investigation and terminates at an appropriate time when the client's (student's) goals are achieved. The stages are not necessarily sequential or discrete, and overlap is common, but they offer a structure to help school counselors evaluate and monitor their level of skill and application of technique in the counseling process (Brammer, 1993; Carkhuff, 1985; Egan, 1994; Gladding, 2004; Ivey, Ivey, & Simek-Downing 1993).

1. Stage 1: Establishing a Relationship
2. Stage 2: Setting the Tone in a Counseling Setting
3. Stage 3: Exploring the Issues
4. Stage 4: Setting Goals
5. Stage 5: Transitioning to Independence

Establishing a Relationship

A strong relationship with a student is paramount in order to gain the student's commitment and willingness to establish and achieve the agreed-upon goals defined by the counseling relationship. Relationship building starts with the initial contact between counselor and student. The relationship builds during the exploration of the issues that directly affect and impact the student's state of mind, well-being, and motivation. The counselor's level of skill, selection of techniques, and theoretical orientation influence the counseling relationship and ultimately, the student's satisfaction and success.

Attending, an important counseling technique in the first stage, establishes the working relationship between client and counselor. The effective school counselor knows how to build rapport with students and considers all of the variables that affect a student's arrival at the counselor's door. Attending requires the school counselor to unilaterally focus on the student and avoid distractions and interruptions. Many students have learned to read adults, and they are highly intuitive, easily recognizing insincerity or lack of interest. Depending on their history and experiences, students may come to counseling with resistance.

The counseling relationship can be impacted by whether or not the student is referred by others or is a self-referral. Teachers and administrators may send a student to the counseling center and inadvertently or pointedly give the student the impression that he or she is going to see the school counselor for a disciplinary reproach, which creates a defensiveness toward counseling. A teacher also may send a student to seek remediation for a problem or apathetic behavior. Because appropriate referral approaches increase the likelihood of relationship building and success, counselors may suggest that learning about such approaches would be a useful staff development topic.

As a relationship begins to develop, consider the following:

- What is the student's motivation to engage in a counseling process?
- How does the student view the situation?
- Is the student open to learning new behaviors, motivated to seek alternative solutions, willing to make a change?
- Does the student see how counseling can help?

Students may enter the counseling situation reluctantly or with no desire to change. Engaging students in the process of exploring options to change behavior is a constant challenge. School counselors frequently encounter students' resistance to change and lack of commitment to becoming engaged in their education.

School counselors need to display unconditional acceptance and understanding to gain the confidence and trust of their young clients (Gladding, 2004). Accurately reflecting the students' feelings and capturing the content of what is shared facilitates the establishment of this trusting relationship. School counselors respond to students in a manner that helps them integrate feelings, behaviors, and thought processes to influence the desired outcome or change.

When counseling is effective, the school counselor directly impacts the student's ability to maximize the educational experience. The counselor intentionally can generate multiple alternatives and approach a problem from many vantage points using a multitude of skills and personal qualities while adapting styles to individualistic needs and cultures (Ivey, 2003).

Setting the Tone in a Counseling Setting

School counselor behavior, skills, and techniques are carefully chosen to set a tone in the counseling session that will provide optimum opportunity for growth. Unconditional positive regard, active listening, attending, empathy, and congruence are considered by many in the profession to be powerful tools in setting a tone conducive to client growth.

Unconditional positive regard   is primarily rooted in respect and requires that the counselor accept the student in an open and respectful manner. This sets the tone for the student to be able to reveal his or her thoughts in a manner that will not result in a judgmental response.

Active listening   is the counselor's way of showing the student that she or he is paying close attention to everything that the child is sharing in the counseling session. Active listening clarifies the counselor's ability to confirm the nature of the problem or presenting issue (Carkhuff, 1985).

Attending   is a way of behaving that attests to communication and understanding (Egan, 1994). The school counselor demonstrates by physical behavior that psychological contact is established. Body position, eye contact, nonverbal encouragement, and a relaxed and open posture all contribute to the student's perception of the counselor's involvement.

Empathy   is the counselor's ability to respond in such a way that the student realizes that the counselor understands his or her frame of reference and point of view (Egan, 1994). A skilled counselor perceives the worldview as the student sees it and has the ability to communicate that understanding. Empathy involves the skills of perception and communication (Rogers, 1961).

Congruence   displays genuineness and implies that the counselor is behaving in an open and honest manner (Rogers, 1980). There is no sense of artificiality about the manner in which the counselor is behaving. Congruence helps the student gain a sense of trust about the counseling relationship.

Exploring the Issues

Frequently, the school counselor needs to help a student identify and clarify what has brought him or her to the counseling office in the first place. Depending upon the developmental, cognitive, and social maturity level of the child, the process of exploring, identifying, and clarifying can be very complex. School counselors need to be cognizant of moving too quickly or too slowly and of making assumptions until the student reveals the problem. If the student defines the problem it increases ownership, which is a necessary step if progress is to be made (Perls, 1969). School counselors can utilize a variety of techniques to help students illuminate the issues for themselves.

Questioning   is both an art and a technique, and must be appropriate for the developmental level of the child (Garbarino & Stott, 1989). Questioning is not an interrogation with a string of "why" questions. Interrogations lead to defensiveness and withdrawal. Rather, questioning is selectively used to enhance the counselor's understanding of what the student is communicating and to cause the student to self-disclose. As opposed to closed questions, for which there is a "yes" or "no" response, open-ended questions support the conversation and engage the student.

Focusing,   bringing the conversation back to the salient issues, is sometimes necessary when students stray away from the issues for too long. For some students the school counselor is the only adult in their life who provides undivided attention. For others, rambling in the conversation is a diversionary tactic to avoid the issue or potential conflict.

Paraphrasing   is used to restate what the student has said using almost the same wording but capturing the intent of both the content and the meaning. This technique offers the student an opportunity to review or reexamine both the content and the intent of the statement.

Reflecting   helps the school counselor clarify the content of the student's statement. Reflecting means that the counselor synthesizes what was communicated, and accurately and correctly shares this with the student, thereby strengthening understanding, rapport, and communication.

Exploring alternatives   assists the student in identifying courses of action prior to making a commitment to any one solution. This exploration can be done by the student or counselor when gathering information, or it can be the result of the student's participation in a formal decision-making process. Exploring alternatives helps students understand the necessity of gathering information and exploring options to make needed changes.

Summarizing   offers the student a review of the thinking and processing that took place during the counseling session. Oftentimes the summary can "string together" or connect the multiplicity of issues, concerns, and explorations in a format that the student can understand and put into action.

Throughout the counseling process we constantly assess the student's ability to take control of the situation and make positive and constructive change. Students have minimal legal rights, little influence over the dysfunction in their families, and usually no control over the level of income in their households. However, with help, support and confidence, they can learn to successfully overcome many of the obstacles they face at home and encounter in a school setting. As school counselors explore the issues that impact school success, so too they help their students identify barriers and challenges, and address these in a plan of action.

Setting Goals

Counseling helps students define for themselves what personal achievement and personal best mean for them, and then set goals toward those ends. Counseling provides structure and a way of measuring the results of students' efforts toward goal attainment. A course of action is mutually agreed upon by the student and counselor and may involve negotiating and mediating. For most students, goals need to be clearly stated, positive in nature, and approached in small increments. School counselors celebrate all successes with students, whether minuscule or huge.

Transitioning to Independence

In the world of community-based organizations and mental health agencies, "terminating" the counseling relationship is a term that is often heard. Terminating the relationship is not as easily accomplished in a school setting. What will it take to maintain the appropriate level of support to ensure that the student can sustain the progress made to date, continue to grow in self-confidence, and achieve self-efficacy? Although the student may no longer need to engage in frequent or scheduled counseling sessions, monitoring and evaluating progress is still needed. The continuity of a school setting facilitates the transition process for counselor and student, as an abrupt termination of services would only be needed if the student leaves the school, parents refuse the counselor's involvement, or the relationship is otherwise interrupted.

How will you know that a student is ready to move on? A mutually developed transition plan will help the student assume independence and control. Students need to know that their counselor remains available even after the initial need has been reduced or eliminated (Corey, Corey, & Callanan, 1998). Because counseling is about change, it is necessary to make sure that the transition plan engages students in a process that can result in positive change, despite the situations and circumstances that envelop their day-to-day lives. The counseling process was intended to make the students personally stronger, teach them to make good choices, and assist them in clarifying what they want out of life, now and in the future. The transition plan will build on the students' coping and resiliency skills to allow them to continue their progress despite environmental and societal influences.

The Challenge of Counseling Individuals and Groups in Schools

Although the sphere of school counselor responsibility and influence has greatly expanded over the years, individual and group counseling in schools is not fully appreciated as an acceptable option to help students maximize the school experience. School counselors face limitations in the scope of counseling practice due to district policies and procedures, parental concerns, community values, time constraints, and sheer numbers of students. Faith groups may require an assurance that there is no encroachment on or interference with the moral or ethical dilemmas that school-aged children experience.

Successful school counseling programs are designed and organized by counseling professionals who have a deep understanding of the factors that impinge on their ability to deliver individual and group counseling services to students. Through collaboration and teaming, school psychologists, school social workers, agency-based counselors, and school counselors can address the culture and norms and seek solutions as partners in prevention and intervention.

In addition to an in-depth knowledge and application of counseling theory, techniques, and process, school counselors must consider all aspects of diversity in their work with students, including gender, race, culture, religion, learning ability and disability, and sexual orientation. Appreciating diversity helps counselors to effectively develop a trusting relationship with students who present a variety of different learning styles, cultural issues, attitudes, family pressures, and social mores and customs (Holcomb, 2004; Lee, 2002).

As societal issues continue to grow in complexity and as peer pressure dominates the decision-making ability of most children, adolescents, and teenagers, educators and families alike turn to the school counselor for insight and assistance. Each student requires a different set of goals, presents a different set of challenges, and demands a different set of counseling skills and techniques (Sciarra, 2004). It is the school counselor who can make the difference in the lives of these students by supporting them as they cope with developmental and emotional challenges, and by nurturing them as they achieve their goals and seek balance in their lives. Making a difference is the reason we choose the profession of school counseling.

TechTools

When you become a school counselor, use the power of technology to maximize the grounding of your practice in counseling theory.

- Surf the American Counseling Association (ACA) website to find out more about the various divisions and specialties within the counseling field. http://www.counseling.org/

- Design a database to help you maintain and categorize your student contacts and interventions.
- Establish an electronic forum with your colleagues to discuss strategies and techniques to help you more effectively do your job.
- Maintain an electronic journal of your applications of theory into practice.
- Use a database to categorize your practicum observations. Which theoretical approaches were most frequently used by school counselors?
- Construct "virtual" simulation activities for future role play with students. Presentation software tools like PowerPoint have easy to use graphics, sound and animation that can help you capture your students' attention more easily. Game-like simulations help break down barriers and give students a comfortable and familiar medium to explore.
- Use the Internet to learn more about the major counseling theorists. Easy-to-find summaries can be located by using search engines such as Google and Yahoo.
- Search websites of organizations including the Association of Supervision and Curriculum Development or the National Association of Secondary School principals to learn more about how the work of William Glasser, Abraham Maslow, and others is used in a school settings.

Internet Resources

Teen issues: www.saviodsilva.net/dir/teenadvice.htm

Connect for Kids: www.connectforkids.org

Helping Children Deal with Scary News:
 http://pbskids.org/rogers/parents/sept11a.htm
 www.aap.org/advocacy/releases/disastercomm.htm

 www.apahelpcenter.org/featuredtopics/

Tragic Times, Healing Words: www.sesameworkshop.org

Talking with Children, Tips for Parents: www.nasponline.org

Trauma and the Attacks on the United States: www.aboutourkids.org

Children and Grief: www.aacap.org/publications/factsfam/grief.htm

All Kids Grieve: www.allkidsgrieve.org

Talking to Public School Students About Disaster:
 www.k12.dc.us/dcps/emergency/emergprephome.html

Crisis Communications Guide and Toolkit: www.nea.org/crisis

Cinematherapy: www.cinematherapy.com

School Counselor Casebook: *Voices From the Field*

The Scenario Reviewed

Faithfully each morning a group of seventh graders meets with you to touch base and get focused for the day. This ten-minute daily check-in seems to work well for you and these 12 academically at-risk students. This is the third day that Raymond has missed, though he is coming to school. When you ask the group if anyone has seen Raymond, you are told that Raymond won't come to your office any more because his friends are making fun of him. You go in search of Raymond and find him hanging around outside the front door with a small group of boys who are frequently seen in the in-school suspension room for cutting and fighting.

A Practitioner's Approach

Here's how a practicing school counselor responded to the school counselor casebook challenge:

As a proactive counselor with a history of a positive relationship with Raymond, I would approach him and ask to speak with him. I would then tell him I miss him at the daily Breakfast Club. I would invite him to attend the special breakfast that I am serving tomorrow during first period to honor the Breakfast Club members. I would suggest that he invite his friends as guests but let him know that I need a commitment so I can order the right amount of food. I would also share with him my plans to have the Breakfast Club members appear in a new orientation video, "Piscataway—the School of Choice," as well as have them travel with me to the middle schools to answer the eighth graders' questions about high school. I also would tell Raymond that I am forming a new weekly academic support group (self-referrals) that I will describe at tomorrow's breakfast. Believing in the power of the group process, I would suggest that some of his friends may be interested in being in a weekly group—with the hope of recruiting Raymond and a few of his friends for the support group. After interviewing perspective members individually, I would have a kickoff breakfast and invite the participants' families as a way to involve them in the strategy as well as strengthen the family-school connection. As a cognitive behavioral counselor, I am interested in helping my counselee make changes in his behaviors and thoughts by providing activities to reinforce positive behavior and challenge his beliefs as well as offer choices.

My plan of action is based on:

- The importance of mutual respect between counselor and counselee and the fact that I have been Raymond's counselor since ninth grade.

- Using a cognitive behavioral counseling theory approach, which will help Raymond learn new ways of thinking and acquire new ways of coping with challenging situations and problems.
- The power of the group process and working collaboratively with his peers on problem solving.
- A strong, active, and proactive approach by the school counselor.
- Family outreach and engagement, which is so important in every adolescent's life.
- Making sure that adolescents have choices.

Dr. Dorothy Youngs has been a district supervisor of counseling, K–12, for 11 years. Prior to that she served as a middle school counselor. She has presented on the local, state, and national levels on school counseling standards-based programs, bullying, and multicultural counseling skills. She has received awards from the American School Counselor Association, the New Jersey School Counselor Association, Seton Hall University, and the Middlesex County Commission on the Status of Women. Reprinted with permission by Dorothy Youngs, Ph.D.

Chapter Summary

Counseling in the Complex World of Schools

Abuse, dysfunctional home environments, blended families, hunger, poverty, violence, harassment, bullying, peer pressure, and homelessness are just some of the issues and pressures that students encounter and struggle with on a daily basis. Although many children have developed the coping and resiliency skills needed to survive and even thrive, a growing number develop emotional, social, and behavioral problems that necessitate intervention.

Counseling Students: Purpose and Limitations

Counseling in schools is a complex helping process in which the counselor establishes a trusting and confidential working relationship. The focus of counseling in schools is on making positive change, goal setting, problem solving, decision making, and discovering personal meaning related to learning and development (ASCA, 1998). School counselors can assess the need for counseling services and establish clear goals with students to create benefits for all involved, including parents.

Theoretical Underpinnings of Counseling

Counseling theories provide a point of reference from which the counselor develops a personal perspective of human growth, development and behavior. Counselors must recognize and choose the appropriate behaviors and strategies that best match their theoretical approach and philosophical orientation and select different theories and approaches according to the models used and the assistance that a student needs.

Gestalt theory   emphasizes the present and supports the equation *now = experience = awareness = reality.*

Person-centered theory   focuses on the "core conditions" of genuineness, empathy, positive regard, and concreteness, all of which are considered universally essential to all helping relationships and the counseling process.

Individual psychology   encourages clients to be well aware of their surroundings and environment, and supports healthy emotional development to overcome any feelings of inferiority.

Behavioral counseling   works under the premise that all behavior is learned and that learning is effective in changing maladaptive behavior.

Reality therapy   encourages clients to set realistic goals and take ownership of goals, thus accepting responsibility for their choices in life and to obtain what they want in the present and future.

Rational emotive behavior therapy   focuses on helping people live balanced, productive, and more rational lives by limiting the demands that one makes on oneself.

Cognitive behavior therapy   assists clients in being able to deal with life and accomplish personal and professional goals.

Existential theory   emphasizes the importance of examining anxiety, values, freedom, and responsibility to find meaning. The client uncovers life's meaning by doing a deed, experiencing a value, or by suffering.

Acquiring Counseling Skills and Techniques

Counseling, like the other key elements of a school counseling program, is a process, a series of sequential stages that begins with exploration and investigation and ends when the goals are achieved. Many factors will influence the counseling process and the success of the client, including the skill, techniques, and theoretical orientation of the counselor

The Challenge of Counseling in Schools

Counseling is one component of a school counseling program. It is paramount to counselor training, to interactions with students and other stakeholders, and to acquiring a professional identity. Specialized training in counseling is what differentiates the work of counselors from those who advise or guide.

Key Terms

Behavioral therapy p. 39
Cognitive behavioral therapy p. 46
Counseling p. 31
Counseling process p. 31
Counseling theory p. 31
Existential theory p. 48

Gestalt theory p. 33
Individual psychology p. 37
Person-centered theory p. 35
Rational emotive behavior therapy
  p. 43
Reality therapy p. 41

Learning Extensions

1. Reflect on the personal qualities that a school counselor should possess to successfully engage students in the counseling process. Which qualities do you need to further develop? How will you do this?

2. How would you conduct a first counseling session with an elementary, middle, or high-school student? What preparation needs to be done in advance? Outline the steps that you would follow.

3. Reflect on your personal experience(s) with counseling involving you or someone close to you, in a school setting or in a private/agency setting. Consider the insecurities, anxieties, and uncertainties faced when the process began. As a counselor in school, what can you do to engage the student early on in the session and to alleviate some of her or his anxiety?

4. Create a theory summary chart for your personal use. The chart should have five columns: Theory, Summary, Goals of Therapy, Techniques, and Applications in the School Setting.

5. Name the theory from which each of the following techniques is derived. Give an example of a situation in which it could be used:

   a. Saying to the student: "You feel _____ because you _____ and you want _____."

   b. Expressing genuine confidence in the student and using encouragement.

   c. Asking the student to complete this sentence: I take responsibility for _____.

   d. Discussing the difference between friendly competition and "one-upmanship."

   e. Saying to the student: "How can you remove those self-defeating thoughts, which are holding you back from doing better?"

Chapter 3

Counseling Practice in Schools

Applying Counseling Theory in the Comprehensive School Counseling Program
> Brief Solution-Focused Counseling

Applications of Counseling in Schools
> Counseling and the Comprehensive Model
> Individual Counseling
> Group Counseling
> Classroom Guidance

Applications of Testing and Assessment

Counseling: Contributing to Student Development
> Resiliency
> Developmental Assets

Chapter Objectives

By the time you have completed this chapter, you should be able to:

- Articulate the role of counseling in a comprehensive school counseling program;
- Define the multidimensions of counseling in schools, including individual counseling, group counseling, and the school counseling curriculum;
- Explain the use of brief solution-focused counseling in a school setting;

- Discuss the school counselor's role in gathering, interpreting, and presenting testing and assessment data;
- Describe how to help students build resiliency and acquire coping skills.

School Counselor Casebook: Getting Started

The Scenario

You have just left the school improvement team meeting at your intermediate school, and your head is spinning. The primary topic of conversation was the increased number of reported incidents of sexual harassment. Your principal suggested that individual counseling for all of the students involved would be the perfect remedy. You responded that individual counseling is only a small part of the solution. You volunteered to pull a group of staff together to look seriously at creating a prevention and intervention plan. You reminded your principal that alleviating sexual harassment required a commitment from the entire faculty and staff to realize any impact or improvement. With your caseload of 925 fourth through sixth graders you are feeling pretty overwhelmed.

Thinking About Solutions

As you read this chapter, reflect on these questions: As the counselor in this scenario, how might you get at the underlying causes of sexual harassment? How might this initiative fit into your comprehensive school counseling model? What resources might be available (people and materials)? Which counseling theories and approaches would you apply in this situation?

When you come to the end of the chapter, you will have the opportunity to see how your ideas compare with a practicing school counselor's approach.

Applying Counseling Theory in the Comprehensive School Counseling Program

The Starfish

There was a young man walking down a deserted beach before dawn. In the distance he saw a frail old man. As he approached the old man, he saw him picking up stranded starfish and tossing them back into the sea. The young man gazed in disbelief and watched as the old man carefully picked up the starfish, one by one, and gently tossed them back into the water. He asked, "Why do you spend *so much energy doing what seems* to be a waste of time?" The old man replied that the stranded starfish would die if left in the morning sun. "But there must be thousands of beaches and millions of starfish," exclaimed the young man. "How can you make a difference?" The old man looked down at the small starfish in his hand, and as he threw it to the safety of the sea, he said, "I just made a difference to this one."

— *Source unknown*

There was a time when it was expected that a school counselor would spend the preponderant amount of her or his time working with students, one at a time. Students who were in crisis or in trouble often were sent to the school counselor. As the old man did with the starfish, the school counselor picked up the students one by one, used the very best counseling skills possible, and then set them back on their feet. The focus of attention was on individual intervention; with large caseloads, the sphere of influence remained small. Counselors expended energy predominantly on those who sought assistance or with those students who were brought to the school counselor's office for immediate attention and needed an intervention. Counselors recognized that effectiveness was limited by time constraints; the ability to intervene and impact more students remained elusive.

School counselors know that much more needs to be accomplished than saving one starfish at a time by picking it up, supporting it, and placing it gently back into the sea. Is there an assurance that the starfish won't end up back on the beach after being returned to the sea? How can we prevent the starfish from washing up on shore in the first place?

The comprehensive process encourages school counselors to look at the cause-and-effect relationship that lies at the root of the problem. Why are so many starfish (or children) finding their way to our shores (our offices)? What is the fundamental cause of this dilemma? Oftentimes, the answers lie not with the individual student, but in the systemic issues that cloud our schools and community. Why are so many students adrift, or worse, left to survive on their own? We must value the importance of working with some students one on one, but when we look deeply within the system, we will discover that we can reduce and eliminate academic, career, and personal-social barriers by implementing strategies and techniques that will impact the greatest number of students and utilizing effective prevention and intervention methods.

Counseling, the term that defines our profession, is preeminent in the work of school counselors. Counseling skills and techniques underpin the skills of leadership, advocacy, using data, and teaming and collaboration. Counseling theory and technique hold a paramount position in training, in interactions with students and other stakeholders, and most important, is the key indicator of one's professional identity. Specialized training in counseling differentiates the work of school counselors from those who advise or guide. Counseling and the counseling relationship is the foundation upon which candidates are prepared to be school counselors in the majority of our university programs.

The increased need for students to have counseling in schools and agencies has become more apparent as documented occurrences of children's emotional difficulties have been evidenced in violent, disruptive, and aggressive behavior (Luongo, 2000). Schools are a significant source of referrals of young people to mental health agencies for increasingly complex problems (Atkins, Mc Kay, Arvanitis, et al., 1998). Adolescent suicide rates continue to be a major concern for counselors working with adolescents, and suicide follows accidents and homicide as the third leading cause of death for youth (Children's Defense Fund, 2004). Homelessness, poverty, domestic and community violence, and alcohol and drug abuse all impact the mental health and well-being of our children (Lockhart & Keys, 1998). The lines have blurred between school and community, with problems flowing back and forth.

> Research suggests that high-quality counseling services can have long-term effects on a child's well-being and can prevent a student from turning to violence and drug or alcohol abuse. High-quality school counseling services can improve a student's academic achievement. Studies on the effects of school counseling have shown positive effects on student's grades, reducing classroom disruptions, and enhancing teachers' abilities to manage classroom behavior effectively. High-quality school counseling services also can help address students' mental health needs.
> — *U.S. Dept. of Education, 2002, p. 117*

A comprehensive and developmental approach ensures that the impact and influence of prevention and intervention reaches every student, and extends well beyond interventions with a few students through individual counseling, group work, or classroom guidance (Borders & Drury, 1992; Dahir & Stone, 2003; Dimmitt, 2003; Lapan, 2001; Whiston, 2002; Whiston & Sexton, 1998).

In Chapter 2, Counseling in the Complex World of Schools, key theoretical models were presented that can be applied to counseling in a school setting. Skilled school counselors select theoretical approaches that consider the age and mental and emotional maturity of students who are in need of individual or group counseling. The application of specific theoretical orientations will influence the design and delivery of the entire comprehensive school counseling program, from prevention and intervention (responsive) services to system support. Whether school counselors apply reality therapy, rational emotive behavior therapy, or cognitive-behavioral theory, the growth and learning benefit to the student cannot be minimized.

For example, person-centered theory (Rogers, 1961) promotes the use of unconditional positive regard, which implies a deep and genuine concern for the individual. When utilizing unconditional positive regard, the counselor would create an environment that is safe and nonjudgmental in an individual, group counseling, or student planning session. School counselors can apply the same principle to the creation of a safe and respectful school climate and can use system support to foster collaboration and teaming. In a classroom guidance situation, the school counselor ensures that every student's opinion is valid and that all contributions are welcome. This is just one example of applying theory to the delivery components of the comprehensive school counseling program.

As you recall from Chapter 2, counseling knowledge and theoretical orientation influences the selection of techniques, strategies, and approaches and informs practice across all the components of a comprehensive program. Insight and instinct are best supported by knowledge, skills, and experience that are relevant to the needs of the student as well as to the presenting situation. School counselors who are secure in their knowledge and understanding of theory have the ability to transform theory and techniques into applications that provide for growth and development. The application and integration of theory is not owned exclusively by "responsive services" or perceived as magic-wand waving. Theory into practice is thus more fully aligned with the mission of each school and supports each student's academic, career, and personal-social development.

Brief Solution-Focused Counseling

Brief solution-focused counseling is a theoretical orientation and process that has become popular among school counselors primarily because of its focused approach and short duration (Littrell, 1998; Murphy, 1997; Sklare, 1997). For purposes of this textbook, the authors considered brief solution-focused counseling as a model with specific strategic purposes and techniques. In our opinion, it draws upon a rich source of various theoretical constructs, including reality therapy, REBT, cognitive, and cognitive behavioral theory. Research continues to uncover new information about the therapeutic aspects of this model and about its ability to remediate mental health concerns (Seligman, 2001). Brief counseling is not a "quick fix" or an efficient approach to problem solving. The emphasis on the developmental and comprehensive approach to school counseling requires school counselors to serve all students (Galassi & Akos, 2004). The use of brief solution-focused interventions tailored to a school setting is a valuable approach when time constraints are always an issue (Murphy, 1997; Sklare, 1997).

Brief counseling is not new. Freud himself conducted brief, time-limited therapeutic sessions in the early 1900s. However, as psychoanalysis and therapy became more complex, attempts to apply a brief paradigm became more challenging and complicated. More recently, especially within the last 20 years, short-term solution-focused counseling became more predominant. Solution-focused counseling was originally conceived by de Shazer (1985) and was grounded in the work of Erickson (1963) and family systems theory. Solution-focused counseling demonstrates the counselor's confidence in the student's ability to make positive changes by accessing inner resources. This counseling process does not dissect and rehash the problem; rather, it constructs solutions that capitalize on the exceptions to the problem. Metcalf (1995) reminds us that "knowing why we are the way we are doesn't offer solutions. As students discover why they are sad, angry or shy, they often use the information as a symptom and reason for not succeeding" (p. 19).

Brief counseling is by intent; it is not brief by accident (Bruce, 1995). Hoyt (1995) further explained that brief counseling could refer to fewer sessions, sessions of a lesser duration, or a less frequent scheduling of sessions, but cautioned us to address the time-sensitive connotation of "brief" as it applies to the school setting. School counselors with limited access and limited time to work with students need to address the importance of making the most out of each minute. The student and counselor agree on realistic and achievable goals and strategies. See Table 3.1 for a

Table 3.1 Benefits of Brief Counseling

Researcher	Benefits
Koss & Butcher (1986)	• Limited time
	• Limited goals
	• High level of counselor activity
	• Interventions are introduced early
	• Assessments are applied early
	• Counselor flexibility
Steenbarger (1992)	• Maximize use of time and limited students access
	• Sensitive to the constraints in a school setting
	• Goals established for positive changes
Bloom (1992, 1997)	• Interventions are introduced early
	• Specific but limited goals are introduced
	• A clear focus for counseling is established and maintained
	• Time limits are set
Koss & Shiang (1994)	• Counseling focus is clear and maintained
	• Counselor flexibility
	• High level of counselor activity
	• Interventions are introduced promptly
	• Termination is discussed early on
Bruce (1995)	• Counselor and students build working relationship
	• Counselor works with students on strengths and resources
	• High level of counselor and student activity
	• Counselor and student establish clear and concrete goals
Sklare (1997)	• Solution talk rather than problem talk
	• Problems have identifiable exceptions that can be parlayed into solutions
	• Small changes have ripple effect and lead to larger changes
	• Students have what it takes to solve their difficulties

summary of the benefits of brief counseling in the school setting, as enumerated by six researchers.

Characteristics of Brief Counseling

According to Davis & Osborne (2000), there are eight principles that guide brief solution-focused approaches:

1. Students have strengths and resources needed for change, and it is more important to focus on strengths rather than weaknesses.

2. Accepting the student's point of view reduces resistance and helps to establish a cooperative working relationship.

3. Students need help to see that repeating a pattern of behavior will not result in any change to eliminate the problem. School counselors need to challenge the student to try to do something different.

4. Solutions are based on developing "non problem" behavior.

5. Students often know what the solution is although they may not be able to verbalize it. Oftentimes a student may not know that the solution lies within or may not have the confidence to solve the problem.

6. There are many paths to achieve the same goal. School counselors and students need to explore all of the options.

7. You do not have to know everything about a problem to be able to seek solutions.

8. Small changes are reasons to celebrate and can make a positive impact on other parts of a student's life.

The ultimate purpose of brief counseling is for students to gain control and experience success. Students can assess the problem in concrete and developmentally appropriate terms, explore attempts previously used to correct the problem, establish short-term goals, and implement the intervention (Bruce, 1995).

Sklare's (1997) model emphasizes four concepts that are key to implementation:

1. Avoid problem analysis and focus on what does work.

2. Be efficient with designing interventions and develop solutions that can work, and work immediately.

3. Focus on the present and the future and eliminate the tendency to analyze the past.

4. Focus on actions, rather than insights, which may be more helpful in working with children who may have limited developmental ability to delve deeply.

Although brief solution-focused counseling may not be appropriate for every student in every situation, many of the principles are applicable to individual counseling and also can be used in small group counseling situations. In the real world of school counseling, with telephones and school bells ringing, with meetings to make and deadlines to meet, brief solution-focused strategies offer an approach that seeks to promote changes in a short period of time. The respect and utilization of what the student can bring to the session lies at the heart of the solution-focused approach (Murphy, 1997). Additionally, some of these very same strategies can be applied to working with colleagues in problem-solving situations.

Acquiring expertise in brief solution-focused counseling requires years of study and experience. School counselors can take professional development workshops and graduate courses to refine and improve their skills in individual and group counseling, whether in utilizing a traditional approach or a solution-focused approach. Most important, school counselors can utilize counseling theory to proactively promote positive growth in students.

Applications of Counseling in Schools

ASCA (1999b) defines counseling as "a confidential relationship in which the counselor meets with students individually and in small groups to help them resolve or cope constructively with their problems and developmental concerns" (www.schoolcounselor.org/content.asp?contentid=133). Counseling, often equated with emotional well-being, is flexible in its approach and is applied to a wide variety of academic, career, and personal-social issues. School counselors typically serve large numbers of students, parents, and teachers; it is critical to assess who will benefit from the individual and group counseling relationships in a school setting (ASCA, 2003). The scope and extensiveness of counseling services are affected by many factors, including to what degree counseling is considered appropriate in a school setting (Geroski & Knauss, 2000). Local policies influence how often and for what purpose a counselor can engage a student in counseling. Parents and community school boards have in some instances claimed that it is beyond the school's authority to provide mental health services in the schools (Kaplan, 1996). School counselors need to be aware of the climate of the community with regard to the parameters of providing individual and group counseling in school and follow the appropriate protocols and procedures to deliver the services, including the parent's right to have their child "opt out."

Counselors become aware of student issues, concerns, needs, and problems through a variety of sources including student self-referral as well as referrals from faculty, family members, or other acquaintances of the student. School counselors always consider the reason for referral, the development stage and cognitive processing skills of the child, and the cultural background and influences when selecting a theoretical approach or techniques. Counselors must also ensure that students understand the purpose of counseling, because confusion or distress can result if a child is unsure of why she or he has been called to the counseling center. Resentment of the reason for the referral can lead to student resistance to counseling. Counseling in schools often is equated with "having a problem" or "being in trouble," and the resulting stigma must be taken into consideration and eliminated.

Traditional counseling practice has been perceived as reactive and remedial rather than proactive and positive. Newer schools of thought view counseling in schools as an opportunity for students to move from the negative emotions generated by involvement in certain situations to acquiring the positive emotions that could be generated by the same situation (Fredrickson, 2001). As counselors work with students on identifying the issues necessary to be more successful, decision making is often at the core of behavioral change. Choices can be overwhelming, and peer influences play heavily in a child's ability to choose wisely and act in his or her best interests. Counseling also is used with individuals and groups to address issues such as grief, substance abuse, socialization issues, learning frustrations, interpersonal skills, stress, and behavior modification.

Transformed school counselors can shift from the traditional individual remediation model to a proactive counseling process that places greater emphasis on skill building rather than deficit reduction (Galassi & Akos, 2004). Counseling in schools is then viewed as learning, as a problem-solving process, and as a developmental growth process (ASCA, 2003; Campbell & Dahir, 1997; Gysbers & Henderson, 2002; Myrick, 2000).

Counseling and the Comprehensive Model

Gysbers and Henderson (2000) and the ASCA model (2003) classify individual and group counseling as responsive services, a key component of the delivery process, one of the four quadrants in the comprehensive school counseling program. Responsive services support students experiencing personal, social, career, or academic problems. Interventions are categorized as preventive, remedial, or crisis oriented (Gysbers & Henderson, 2000) and these prevention and intervention (responsive) services are designed to meet the immediate needs and concerns of students. Responsive services can include but are not limited to individual and group counseling. The school counseling curriculum also can be considered a proactive service and response to a demonstrated need.

Individual Counseling

Individual counseling is both a proactive and a reactive response to student needs. The counselor explores a problem or topic of interest through a personal and private interaction with a student. This face-to-face meeting with a school counselor provides the student maximum privacy to freely explore ideas, feelings, and behaviors. School counselors convey trust and confidence by their actions and words, always considering the rights, integrity, and welfare of students.

Individual counseling also can be considered part of the individual planning process in which a student establishes personal, career, or academic goals. The goals of individual counseling vary from that of the student who seeks assistance with relationships, emotional balance, or behavior management to the student needing help with motivation and decision making. Individual counseling remains an important component of the role for school counselors, especially academic counseling, which results in improving student success (House & Hayes, 2002).

Group Counseling

In **group counseling** a counselor works with two or more students simultaneously, which is an efficient way of addressing common concerns or problem behavior. The discussions may be relatively unstructured or quite formal in focus, with specified goals for each session. Group topics can range from common school success topics such as motivation to more dire topics such as anger management or dealing with separation and loss. Group counseling requires a high degree of complex counseling skills and techniques to manage and organize group sessions and facilitate appropriate topic and age-group interaction.

Group members have an opportunity to learn from each other. They can share ideas, give and receive feedback, increase their awareness, gain new knowledge, practice skills, and think about their goals and actions. Students also gain insight from exploring their feelings, attitudes, and behaviors. Group counseling can reduce social isolation and build skills in peer relations to create a sense of belonging (Arman, 2000). Group counseling specifically engages the students in behavioral analysis, change, and adjustment.

Group counseling can be proactive or reactive in addressing problems, or it can be growth-centered, which relates general topics to personal and academic development. Group counseling also can help students to acquire the skills, attitudes, and knowledge that are associated with healthy youth development (Galassi & Akos, 2004).

School counselors can also use their group process in working with parents or teachers. Evening parenting groups on skill-building topics, and specialized task- or knowledge-building groups for teachers are examples of using counseling skills to provide system support services as part of the comprehensive program.

Classroom Guidance

Classroom guidance, which is also known as the school counseling curriculum, is a component in the delivery quadrant of the ASCA model (2003). The school counseling (guidance) curriculum is a sequence of learning activities and strategies that address the academic, career, and personal-social development of every K–12 student (Gysbers & Henderson, 2000). The school counseling curriculum is most frequently delivered in collaboration with the classroom teacher. These learning units are linked to the national standards and identified student competencies, are outcome based, and are articulated with the school's core academic curriculum (ASCA, 2003).

Implementing a school counseling curriculum is not counseling in the pure sense. Through classroom guidance, school counselors impact students' thinking and influence their choices. However, it does not have as a primary goal the development of the counselor-client relationship, which is the trademark of counseling. The school counseling curriculum is constructed by the school counselor in collaboration with teachers and other specialists and connected to the school improvement goals. The curriculum has a specific purpose and goal in mind and is intended to be instructive and cognitive in nature.

School counseling curriculum is a tool to educate students on a particular topic and can also help identify those in need of group and/or individual counseling. For example, a school counselor in a middle school may use classroom guidance lessons to "teach" students how to protect themselves from sexual harassment. The counselor also would visit the same class to address a sexual harassment incident that involved many of the students. As a result of the lessons and the observations of the counselor and the classroom teacher, some students may present themselves needing further support and intervention. These students would be supported through group and individual counseling. Classroom guidance programs are most successful when they are developed as a result of demonstrated need and connected to specific classroom or school improvement goals.

Counselors also need skill development to deliver classroom guidance including lesson design, assessment strategies, and classroom management techniques. New counselors without previous classroom teaching experience can benefit from collaborating and teaming with more experienced professionals. Classroom guidance is an effective and efficient way of abiding by the law of parsimony and allows for a large number of students to benefit from prevention and intervention strategies. Some students will need additional "reinforcement" or group counseling, while a few students may require one-on-one support through individual counseling. In classroom instruction teachers often deliver a lesson as whole-group instruction. Some students may need a small group follow-up lesson; a few may need one-on-one tutoring. A similar analogy can be used for the counseling process:

	FROM CLASSROOM TEACHER	FROM SCHOOL COUNSELOR
All Students Receive ———>	Subject Classroom Lesson	School Counseling Curriculum
Some Students Receive———>	Small Group Remediation	Group Counseling
A Few Students Receive———>	Individual Extra Help	Individual Counseling

Box 3.1

Connecting the National Standards
to the Comprehensive Model

Academic Development Standard A: Students will acquire the attitudes, knowledge, and skills that contribute to effective learning in school and across the life span.

Student Competency: Students will apply knowledge of learning styles to positively influence school performance.
   The counseling skills necessary to deliver this student competency are applicable to all areas of the comprehensive model.

Individual Student Planning   offers an opportunity for the same students to apply this knowledge of learning styles to course selection and to establishing career goals.

Prevention and Intervention (Responsive) Services   will benefit students who are experiencing frustration by providing group counseling to help them apply what they know about their learning styles to the classroom situation. Students might benefit from individual counseling and begin to work on changing attitudes and behaviors toward a teacher whose teaching style is at odds with the student's learning style.

School Counseling Curriculum   will support all students to gain an understanding of how they learn, how to approach note taking and studying, and how to get the most from the classroom experience.

System Support   presents school counselors with the opportunity to provide staff development on the differences between teacher styles and student learning styles. Teachers can brainstorm as to how to help their students adapt and adjust as needed to the classroom instruction. Distributing a brief article about learning styles in the school and/or in the PTA newsletter could be both informative and anxiety reducing for students and parents.

Applications of Testing and Assessment

Testing and assessment significantly impact every member of the student population and are important components of the work of school counselors (Whiston, 2000). Absent a school psychologist, the school counselor may be the only professional with a background in testing and assessment (Neukrig, 1999). It is not uncommon for school counselors to find themselves involved in situations that require different levels of assessment; they also must be prepared to administer tests and interpret the results. With the proliferation of students undergoing assessment as well as testing for special education and/or 504 accommodations, school counselors must understand the nature and purpose of the different tests. As advocates for students and their families, they also need the competence to interpret the data that is used for placements, classification, or assignment of services (Guindon, 2003).

Assessment can involve gathering data and information, researching and interviewing, analyzing the entire variable, looking for patterns, and organizing the results in a way that has meaning for decision making and/or problem solving. School counselors can teach students how to conduct a self-assessment that includes their interests, achievement, aptitude, and motivation to help them further plan for their futures. Testing, on the other hand, is a subset of assessment for the purposes of measuring cognitive ability, personality, career preferences, and achievement (Anastasi, 1992). Testing in schools is most frequently aligned with achievement. With the current demand for results, decisions regarding student and school performance are often based on test data (Guindon, 2003).

Testing and assessment has evolved over the years from an initial focus on vocational guidance to the more complex processes of psychological appraisal and evaluation. The impact of testing on schools was more dramatic in the mid-1950s, when the National Defense Education Act (NDEA) provided funding incentives to identify students with the aptitude to successfully pursue mathematics and science careers. The current mandates of No Child Left Behind (2001) have placed significant pressure on schools for accountability of results, as demonstrated especially by the proliferation of high stakes testing from grade 3 onward to high-school graduation. NCLB requires state-developed annual assessments in grades 3 through 8, and additional high-school testing is required for achieving a diploma. The results of high stakes testing impact annual promotion from grade level to grade level as well as the adequate yearly progress made which determines each school's level of success in educating its students. With this greater emphasis on testing, school counselors more than ever before are assigned the coordination, administration, and interpretation of test results (Schmidt, 1999).

A test can only depict a moment in time; it is a snapshot of a performance. As advocates, school counselors can remind teachers, parents, and students that a single test score does not provide enough information to make significant and important decisions. ASCA and ACA position statements recognize the use of standardized testing as one of a range of measures used to assess student performance and learning (ACA, 2005; ASCA, 2002).

There are many different kinds of standardized tests, and descriptions can be found in the Mental Measurement Yearbook, first published in 1938 by Oscar Buros. The latest edition (Conoley & Impara, 1998) contains reviews for more than 400 newly published or revised tests and is a comprehensive resource to identify and evaluate various type of instruments.

Standardized tests are commonly used in a school setting and are categorized in the following ways: achievement, intelligence, aptitude, career, personality, and diagnostic.

Achievement tests   measure a student's knowledge of a subject or task. These tests often are normed, which means one can compare progress of an individual or group of students as compared to other individuals or groups. Achievement tests may be teacher designed or standardized. Standardized tests are most often used to assess knowledge and growth, measure academic progress, and demonstrate progress in a particular subject or across the content areas.

Intelligence tests   are used to define a student's intelligence potential. Commonly used intelligence tests are the Stanford-Binet Intelligence Test and the Otis-Lennon Intelligence Test. Intelligence tests measure learning, which is one aspect of aptitude.

Aptitude or ability tests   are defined as a capability for a particular skill (Aiken, 2000). Single skills such as manual dexterity, spatial perception, gross motor coordination, and eye-hand coordination are tested either individually or in a battery that comprises several subtests (Guindon, 2003). The Armed Services Vocational Aptitude Battery (ASVAB) is a test to assess readiness for various military and civilian occupations. The Differential Aptitude Test (Psychological Corporation, 1991) is widely used in middle, junior high, and high schools to assess career readiness.

Career and interest inventories   help to determine a student's preference for specific activities or areas of interest. There are numerous interest inventories available for elementary, middle, and high-school students to help students gain career awareness and explore career opportunities. Some career interest inventories, such as those developed by John Holland, include assessments of personality characteristics and temperaments in addition to a like or dislike scale.

Personality tests   measure emotions, feelings, inclinations, individual characteristics, attitudes, and opinions (Anastasi & Urbina, 1997); however, the uniqueness of the nature of individual personalities makes assessment difficult. The most widely used and researched instrument is the Minnesota Multiphasic Personality Inventory-2 (Butcher, Dahlstrom, Graham, Tellegen, & Kraemmer, 1989). An adolescent version for youth ages 14–18 was developed three years later (Butcher et al. 1989). The MMPI-2 manual stresses that the purpose of the instrument is to differentiate among the various patterns of personality and emotional disorders (Butcher et al., 1989, p. 2).

Another widely used instrument, the Myers-Briggs Type Indicator, is based on the work of Jung. His theories suggest that differences in behaviors are related to the ways in which individuals prefer to perceive and the ways that they judge their perceptions. The Myers-Briggs is intended to help people understand their preferences and is used by counselors and school district administrators to better understand the dynamics of human interaction.

Other personality assessments are structured and projective in nature. School counselors generally do not administer tests such as the Rorschach Thematic

Apperception Test (TAT) or House-Tree-Person Test (H-T-P) due to the additional specialized training required for administration and interpretation. A student in need of a complex personality assessment may be referred by the school counselor to the school psychologist or a mental health professional specially trained to interpret the complex scoring and analysis procedure.

Diagnostic assessments   are used to assess student ability and disability for learning problems, emotional disorder, and mental illness. Assessments are used to assess suicide risk, eating-disorder behaviors, substance abuse, and violent tendencies. Psychologists, psychiatrists, and specially trained professional counselors use a variety of tools for diagnostic purposes. The Diagnostic and Statistical Manual: Mental Disorder (DSM-IV-TR) published by the American Psychiatric Association (2000), includes 13 major categories of mental disorders and addresses the role of culture in diagnosis and assessment. Understanding the scope of the DSM-IV-TR is invaluable knowledge for school counselors, and helps to inform communication and consultation with other mental health care professionals.

Considerations for school counselors   The use of testing, which often creates anxiety and stress in students, is extensive (Cheek, Bradley, Reynolds, & Coy, 2002). One of the common uses of testing and assessment is for classroom and grade-level placement. Test results frequently are used to label students and group them in instructional "tracks." High stakes tests such as the SAT or the ACT are used for college admissions or serve as an exit exam for high-school graduation. Educators continue to debate the value of homogeneous groups (grouping of students of similar learning characteristics) versus heterogeneous groups (grouping of students with dissimilar learning characteristics), and use testing as a vehicle for placement.

The accountability component of No Child Left Behind (2001) has placed an all-consuming emphasis on testing and assessment. With this increased emphasis also comes the need to more closely examine the bigger view of assessment with respect for all aspects of diversity, taking gender, ethnicity, culture, and language into account as well (Baker, 2000).

Reasonable accommodations, modifications, and/or alternative assessments must be considered also for students who have limited English capability as well as for students with disabilities (American Counseling Association, 2004). Test bias is almost impossible to totally eradicate; thus it is important to use multiple measures of assessment (Gladding, 2004). School counselors have an ethical responsibility to look beyond the use of a single test score for decision making as well as to educate their colleagues to use multiple assessments in order to gain a broader view of a student's potential and prognosis for success. No decision about a student's educational status (graduation, promotion/retention, tracking, advanced placement, special education, postsecondary admission, and so on) should ever be unilaterally made on the basis of a single test score (ACA Task Force on High Stakes Testing, 2005).

Assessment goes far beyond paper-and-pencil tests. Observation must not be overlooked as a contributing element to any comprehensive assessment. Formal and informal observations conducted by school counselors and other education professionals offer the human dynamic and interactive component that cannot be gleaned from a paper-and-pencil diagnostic instrument. Observations in the classroom, on the playground, and in a multitude of situations offer insight into academic as well as social-emotional performance. The counselor, observing both behavior and verbal interaction, can look for patterns. Observations are often used in assessing students for disabilities, both learning and emotional.

Individual interviews of students also contribute to understanding behavior, thinking, and ways of responding. Careful attention must be given to crafting questions that provide thoughtful and insightful responses. Interviews remind us of the importance of adding the human dimensions to the reams of paper that often compose a comprehensive assessment. This use of qualitative data helps gather a broader view of the individual, not limited to any one paper-and-pencil tool.

School counselors are not clinicians with expertise in diagnosis, but rather developmental experts who gather information from a multitude of assessments, and work with colleagues to determine the best educational setting for each child. School counselors gather, interpret, and present data comprehensively, ethically, and fairly at all times. Assessment and testing are invaluable tools and resources when they are chosen wisely, administered carefully, and the results used in ways that open the door for students to new and appropriate opportunities.

Counseling: Contributing to Student Development

Counseling programs in schools can be considered the fifth discipline, with its strong emphasis on the affective needs of a large number of students rather than a remedial model of mental health interventions for a small number of students (Education Trust, 1999). With a national emphasis on character development and academic achievement, school counselors seek to optimize successful functioning and well-being through individual and group prevention and intervention strategies. Healthy student development is the result of the acquisition of knowledge and skills in the areas of academic, career, and personal-social development.

Resiliency

Fostering **resiliency** requires instilling in students the attitude that suggests strengths are more powerful than are problems (Henderson & Milstein, 1996). Students have reported that they find school to daily be a consistently open and safe place (Banach, 2004). When the school climate and culture create the perception of a safe haven, it is the ideal environment to assist children, youth, and teens to identify how they develop their inner strength. Grotberg (1998) identified fifteen key elements that are in a resilient youth's active voice (Table 3.2):

Table 3.2 Key Elements of Resiliency

I have	I am	I can
People around me	A person people can like and love	Talk to others about things that bother or frighten me
People who set limits for me	Glad to do nice things for others and show my concern	Find ways to solve problems that I face
People who show me how to do things right by the way they do things	Respectful of myself and others	Control myself when I feel like doing something not right or dangerous
People who help me even when I am sick, in danger, or need to learn	Willing to accept responsibility for what I do	Find someone to help me when I need it

Additionally, researchers have noted that youth who have bounced back from adversity also develop a level of competence in affective and personal-social development (Werner & Smith, 1992). Building resiliency is far more than the slogan we often hear: "Just Say No!". This simplistic approach is a strong undercurrent in many prevention programs, particularly those that address alcohol and substance abuse. Programs that demonstrate successful results have not stopped short with slogans and education but rather have included a cadre of adults who build strong and significant relationships with youth. Dryfoos (1994) identified the following common elements of successful programs:

1. positive adult-youth relationships;

2. youth involvement in community and service opportunities;

3. an established vision of high expectations for students;

4. affective and academic skills building;

5. school and community collaboration to provide information and support services; and,

6. positive connecting strategies that involve adults, peers, activities, recreation, and learning.

With these critical elements in place, school counselors can help each student assess his or her ability to cope, show determination, overcome, and succeed. Henderson and Milstein (1996) have identified protective factors that will help each individual build a strong, resilient foundation. These include a student's ability to:

- Use life skills
- Demonstrate perceptiveness
- Be self-motivated
- Persevere
- Show competence
- Have inner direction
- Have a sense of humor
- Build relationships
- Be flexible
- Have positive view of the future
- Develop a love of learning

These protective factors bear a strong resemblance to the personal-social development competencies in the ASCA model (2003) and, whether viewed through the eyes of a school counselor or mental health provider, have similar objectives for youth growth and development.

Developmental Assets

Building resiliency and acquiring protective factors is also about asset building. With the knowledge that healthy student development is at the core of school-community collaboration, the Search Institute in Minneapolis has conducted extensive research, identifying specific **developmental assets** as the foundation of healthy development for young people. *The 40 Developmental Assets* (1997) are indicators of healthy, caring, and responsible students. Assets are internally and externally based and are reflective of the willingness of school and community to mentor, guide, and nurture children. Parental involvement is essential to asset acquisition and youth development. The four major categories of external assets (Table 3.3) focus on positive experiences that young people receive from the people and institutions in their lives.

A community's responsibility for its youth does not end with the provision of external assets. There needs to be a similar commitment to nurturing the internal qualities that guide choices and create a sense of centeredness, purpose, and focus. Indeed, shaping internal dispositions that encourage wise, responsible, and compassionate judgments is particularly important in a society that prizes individualism. The four major categories of internal assets (Table 3.4) support a commitment to internal nurturing.

The developmental assets are the relationships, competencies, values, opportunities, and self-perceptions that are necessary for students to succeed in school, at home, and in the community. Research (Leffert & Scales, 1999) attributed performance and achievement to asset building. Students who reported acquiring 31 to 40 assets were more likely to achieve higher grades in school than were students who reported acquiring 11 to 20 assets. Significant relationships were found among

Table 3.3 External Assets

Category	Asset	Description
Support	Family support	Family life provides high levels of love and support.
	Positive family communication	Young person and her or his parent(s) communicate positively, and young person is willing to seek advice and counsel from parent(s).
	Other adult relationships	Young person receives support from three or more non-parent adults.
	Caring neighborhood	Young person experiences caring neighbors.
	Caring school climate	School provides a caring, encouraging environment.
	Parent involvement in schooling	Parent(s) are actively involved in helping young person succeed in school.
Empowerment	Community values youth	Young person perceives that adults in the community value youth.
	Youth as resources	Young people are given useful roles in the community.
	Service to others	Young person serves in the community one hour or more per week.
	Safety	Young person feels safe at home, at school, and in the neighborhood.
Boundaries and Expectations	Family boundaries	Family has clear rules and consequences, and monitors the young person's whereabouts.
	School boundaries	School provides clear rules and consequences.
	Neighborhood boundaries	Neighbors take responsibility for monitoring young people's behavior.
	Adult role models	Parent(s) and other adults model positive, responsible behavior.
	Positive peer influence	Young person's best friends model responsible behavior.
	High expectations	Both parent(s) and teachers encourage the young person to do well.

(continued)

Table 3.3 Continued

Category	Asset	Description
Constructive Use of Time	Creative activities	Young person spends three or more hours per week in lessons or practice in music, theater, or other arts.
	Youth programs	Young person spends three or more hours per week in sports, clubs, or organizations at school and/or in community organizations.
	Religious community	Young person spends one hour or more per week in activities in a religious institution.
	Time at home	Young person is out with friends "with nothing special to do" two or fewer nights per week.

variables such as academic goals, grades, graduation success, and beliefs about the value of education with asset building (Leffert & Scales, 1999). Asset acquisition has also been linked to lower reported instances of substance abuse and sexual intimacy.

The Search Institute identified more than 20 assets that schools can most directly influence. At the top of the list are student engagement in school, achievement motivation, positive peer influence, youth programs, and safety (Benson, Scales, Effort, & Roehikeepartain, 1999). A caring school climate with clearly established and enforced guidelines coupled with the strength of parental involvement appeared to be at the foundation of developing successful learners and future citizens. The premise of asset building is grounded in the potential of the "power of one" (Search Insitute, 2004), which is the ability of one individual to heal, to support, to challenge, and to change for the better the life of one young person.

Assets underscore the premise that students need to be prepared to face pressure and acquire skills to face the challenges of a world that with each day becomes more complex and complicated. Successful students acquire skills in coping, learn to adjust to new and different situations, and build resiliency skills to overcome barriers and obstacles that come their way, whether these are academic, personal-social, career, or environmentally related.

Resiliency is the capacity to spring back, rebound, successfully adapt in the face of adversity, and develop social competence despite exposure to stress (Leffert & Scales, 1999). Social competence, problem-solving ability, autonomy, and a sense of purpose and future are the individual traits and assets that resilient students carry as part of their middle school survival tool kit (Moe, 2001). Students who demonstrate characteristics of resiliency and acquire the majority of the internal and external assets are more likely to be successful throughout the middle and high-school years (Search Institute, 1997).

Table 3.4 Internal Assets

Category	Asset	The young person:
Commitment to Learning	Achievement motivation	is motivated to do well in school.
	School engagement	is actively engaged in learning.
	Homework	reports doing at least one hour of homework every school day.
	Bonding to school	cares about her or his school.
	Reading for pleasure	reads for pleasure three or more hours per week.
Positive Values	Caring	places high value on helping other people.
	Equality and social justice	places high value on promoting equality and reducing hunger and poverty.
	Integrity	acts on convictions and stands up for her or his beliefs.
	Honesty	"tells the truth even when it is not easy."
	Responsibility	accepts and takes personal responsibility.
	Restraint	believes it is important not to be sexually active or to use alcohol or other drugs.
Social Competencies	Planning and decision making	knows how to plan ahead and make choices.
	Interpersonal competence	has empathy, sensitivity, and friendship skills.
	Cultural competence	has knowledge of and comfort with people of different cultural/racial/ethnic backgrounds.
	Resistance skills	can resist negative peer pressure and dangerous situations.
	Peaceful conflict resolution	seeks to resolve conflict nonviolently.
Positive Identity	Personal power	feels he or she has control over "things that happen to me."
	Self-esteem	reports having a high self-esteem.
	Sense of purpose	reports that "my life has a purpose."
	Positive view of personal future	is optimistic about her or his personal future.

TechTools

When you become a school counselor, use the power of technology to maximize the efficiency and effectiveness of using counseling applications in a school context.

- Use technology to help you create a simple survey to identify issues that students have, or concerns that the faculty may have about students. Input the data into a spreadsheet, and use charts, graphs, and presentation software to share the results.
- Help your students get on the Road to Resilience. Explore http://www.apahelpcenter.org/featuredtopics/feature.php?id=6
- Go to www.search-institute.org to find out more about the work of the Search Institute and the 40 Developmental Assets.
- Review the ASCA website (www.schoolcounselor.org) to better understand how the national association serves members and makes resources available for a variety of counseling applications. Find the websites for your state school counselor association and your local professional associations.
- National School Counseling Week (NSCW) takes place the first week of February. Search the Web for ideas and resources and use presentation software to present five tips to your faculty that can help them in their work with students. Use your school's electronic or traditional bulletin board to highlight a different message for each day.

School Counselor Casebook: Voices From the Field

The Scenario Reviewed

You have just left the school improvement team meeting at your intermediate school, and your head is spinning. The primary topic of conversation was the increased number of reported incidents of sexual harassment. Your principal suggested that individual counseling for all of the students involved would be the perfect remedy. You responded that individual counseling is only a small part of the solution. You volunteered to pull a group of staff together to look seriously at creating a prevention and intervention plan. You reminded your principal that alleviating sexual harassment required a commitment from the entire faculty and staff to realize any impact or improvement. With your caseload of 925 fourth through sixth graders you are feeling pretty overwhelmed.

A Practitioner's Approach

Here's how two practicing school counselors responded to the school scenario:

1st Response

As a school counselor, I often encounter my principal making suggestions that might not necessarily be the most appropriate solution to the problem. At this point I have to be assertive and go to him with a plan that is practical and yet will, I hope, make a difference for the students and school climate.

How do I devise a plan? It involves thought, and sometimes research conducted by interviewing teachers, students, and parents. I also need to look at how it will fit in my comprehensive developmental program.

When there is a problem of sexual harassment in the school, I have found that a schoolwide plan seems to be the most effective solution. In other words, we totally integrate into the curriculum and involve all of the staff. A strong emphasis on the problem has positive results. For example, I deliver individual and group counseling and focus on students who have been identified as harassing others. I provide classroom guidance lessons with my teachers on topics such as "We Respect Each Other." I direct students to write skits about situations they encounter, and then they perform them on the morning news with help from the art and music teachers. I give open-response questions about sexual harassment to classroom teachers to be used for students' writing assignments. The art teachers encourage students to design posters with messages of respect for each other, and these are put in all the classrooms, cafeteria, gym, and hallways. Messages of "I Care Language" are strongly encouraged for all of the school family.

To accomplish any of these activities I must talk with teachers and help them make lesson plans, provide them with materials, send out memos, offer consultation and encouragement, and do role modeling. Finally, an assessment from the principal and staff must be conducted to see if the plan has helped harassment problems in our school. My hope is that the results will demonstrate to the principal and the site-based council that a whole-school effort yields better results than just focusing on individual counseling only.

Pam Gabbard, a past president of the American School Counselor Association, has been an elementary school counselor for 17 years and currently works in Ballard County Public Schools. She has presented programs all over the United States at various state counseling and career development oriented conferences. She has received several prestigious awards and has authored or contributed to many published works. Reprinted with permission by Pamela Kaye Gabbard.

2nd Response

I recognized from the discussion at the school improvement team meeting that sexual harassment was a growing problem in our building and in the district, and required a comprehensive response. We discussed the problem at our next counseling department meeting to gain a deeper understanding of the nature and severity of the problem, determine what was already being done, and identify the major barriers that had to be overcome. The counselors and I also decided to assess the current levels of parent and community involvement to address this problem, and will explore opportunities for increasing their involvement.

I spoke to our principal and asked if I could call a support team meeting (e.g., building administrator, school counselor, school psychologist, school nurse, classroom teacher, special education teacher, physical education teacher, parents, students) to make sure I had broad-based constituent representation to address this problem. Before we met, the counselors and I reviewed the relevant research regarding the problem and looked for solutions that are successfully being used in other districts.

At our meeting we decided to take the following actions:

1. Draft policy language on sexual harassment for approval by the superintendent and school board.

2. Develop and expand protocols for handling sexual harassment, and incorporate them into our Counseling Policies & Procedures Handbook.

3. Identify and review several programs on harassment prevention and then recommend to the school improvement team for inclusion in our school.

4. Set up professional development on sexual harassment.

5. Create an immediate plan to address specific instances of sexual harassment and a long-range plan to proactively address the problem as a schoolwide effort.

6. Communicate the results of our findings and efforts to central administration, and draft recommendations for adopting districtwide policies and procedures.

Our district is implementing a comprehensive developmental school counseling program based on the ASCA National Model. Part of our implementation strategy is to identify essential counseling activities that can help students succeed academically, in the world of work, and in their personal and social lives. Counseling activities related to sexual harassment are currently being documented as essential. These modules are an integral part of our professional development program for all counselors in the district.

We would utilize activities developed for inclusion in the district counseling framework to help students meet the personal-social standards regarding understanding and respecting themselves and others. We would draw upon techniques used in reality and cognitive behavior theories with students in large and small group sessions. With students accused of sexual harassment and their victims, we would work individually and perhaps in small groups to help them learn to take personal responsibility for their actions and develop action plans to practice new choices.

Patricia Nailor, EdD, has worked as a school counselor at the middle school and high-school levels. She also served as the elementary guidance coordinator prior to her current position as director of counseling and social services for Providence Public Schools. Pat did her doctoral research in effective school counseling programs and currently serves as an adjunct instructor in counselor education at Providence College in Rhode Island. Reprinted with permission by Patricia Nailor, Ed.D.

Chapter Summary

Respecting Tradition and Seeking Innovation

Documented occurrences of children's emotional difficulties have escalated in large numbers of violent, disruptive, and aggressive behaviors. Counseling skills and technique underpin the way school counselors approach and apply skills in leadership, advocacy, and teaming and collaboration. School counselors cannot overlook the paramount importance of counseling theory and techniques in our training, in our interactions with students and other stakeholders, and most important, to our professional identity as counselors in schools.

Counseling Theory and the Comprehensive Model

Comprehensive programs are grounded in developmental theories and are an assurance that student competencies and strategies are organized in a way that is stage- and age-appropriate to the learner. Developmental stages aid in the identification of the counseling theories and techniques that are the most effective considering the age and cognitive and emotional development of the student.

Brief Solution-Focused Counseling

Brief counseling is by intent; it is not brief by accident. The school counselor needs to address the importance of making the most out of each minute. By emphasizing intentionality and using the process that maximizes the availability of the client (the student), brief counseling takes into consideration the constraints of access in a school setting. The student and counselor agree on realistic and achievable goals and strategies.

The Many Applications of Counseling

Counseling is equated with emotional well-being, is flexible in its approach, and can be applied in a wide variety of student academic, career, and personal-social situations. Every student benefits from prevention and intervention knowledge, attitudes, and skills that are presented in the classroom guidance lesson. Some students will need specific group intervention to help them acquire and practice the skills. Others may need one-on-one counseling intervention.

Delivering Counseling in Schools

Individual and group counseling are responsive services, a key component of the comprehensive model delivery process. Responsive services include counseling to students experiencing personal, social, career, or academic problems. School counseling curriculum also can be considered a proactive service and response to a demonstrated need.

Applications of Testing and Assessment

Testing and assessment are important components of the work of school counselors. Oftentimes, absent a school psychologist, the school counselor is the only professional with a background in testing and assessment. School counselors, acting as advocates for their students, gather, interpret, and present data comprehensively, ethically, and fairly at all times.

Building Resiliency and Acquiring Assets

Fostering resiliency requires instilling in students the attitude that suggests strengths are more powerful than problems. School counselors can help each student assess her or his ability to cope, show determination, overcome, and succeed.

The developmental assets are the relationships, competencies, values, opportunities, and self-perceptions that are necessary for success in school, at home, and in the community. Assets are internally and externally based and are reflective of the willingness of school and community to mentor, guide, and nurture children

Counseling Applications in a School Context

Successful counseling relies not only on the skills of the counselor, but also is solidly grounded in the attitudes, knowledge, and skills that students bring to individual, group, and classroom guidance sessions. The application of counseling in a school setting is most impactful when faculty, administrators, and all student-support personnel recognize the unique role that counseling plays in a school setting. School counseling helps schools become learning communities in which students can thrive and grow academically and effectively.

Key Terms

Brief solution-focused counseling p. 66
Classroom guidance p. 71
Developmental assets p. 79

Group counseling p. 71
Individual counseling p. 70
Resiliency p. 77

Learning Extensions

1. Systemic involvement leads to systemic change. Reflect on the scenario at the beginning of the chapter. How did your strategies support individual student planning, prevention and intervention (responsive) services, system support, and classroom guidance?

2. Prevention is a critical component of every student's education. Proactive approaches to student issues can help to alleviate future pitfalls.

   You are concerned about the seniors in your caseload making a good transition to college life. You know that many students have difficulty adjusting the first year, and you have heard that the national dropout rate for freshmen is upwards of 30%. Students are beginning to receive their letters of acceptance and seem very excited about the independence that comes with leaving high school. There are still three months left before they graduate.

   How can counseling strategies address these issues?

   How will you use the dimensions of counseling—classroom guidance, group counseling, and individual counseling—in your school setting?

3. Intervention may be necessary to deal with crisis or at-risk behaviors. Remediation, which is a term often equated with teaching and learning, is about acquiring skills for learning new behaviors.

   Several students in Mr. Bryant's third-grade class have gotten into "trouble" repeatedly for fighting on the playground. The class has developed a reputation as being full of troublemakers. The majority of the students are concerned about how the other students and teachers in the school are talking about them. This situation has caused conflict in the classroom and Mr. Bryant has asked for your help.

   How will counseling help to alleviate the problem? Who needs to be involved? How will you use the dimensions of counseling to intervene and prevent future occurrences?

4. The primary topic at the faculty meeting last week focused on a child abuse case in a neighboring school district that received national attention. Your mid-

dle principal called you and your colleague into his office after the meeting and strongly suggested that the two of you organize a counseling program on child abuse prevention for all 1,000 of your sixth, seventh, and eighth graders. You left your principal's office with a sinking feeling. How will you add this important activity to your already busy schedule? Who else can you involve, and how?

5. Classroom guidance, used as a school counselor prevention and intervention strategy, is a vehicle for advocating for student success. Consider how classroom guidance will further help your commitment to creating a positive school climate. Future planning and career development are used to encourage a positive "mindset" for achievement and success for all students.

6. Often overlooked are the community-based organizations (CBOs) that specialize in prevention and intervention counseling and education about social issues and youth-related concerns. Go to your local yellow pages and identify 10 CBOs that can help support your local school counseling program.

7. How would you go about presenting the 40 Developmental Assets to your faculty as a school-community initiative?

Chapter 4

School Counselors as Leaders

Chapter Objectives

By the time you have completed this chapter, you should be able to:

- Define educational leadership and types of leadership and power.
- Describe the role of the school counselor as a leader in the school.
- Explain the school counselor's role on the principal's (or school's) leadership team.
- Describe how school counselors use leadership to holistically support academic, career, and personal-social development for every student.
- Identify the behaviors of a school counselor as a leader, advocate, and collaborator to: (a) change attitudes and beliefs; (b) contribute to successful instructional programs; (c) develop high aspirations; (d) influence course enrollment and tracking patterns; and (e) contribute to safe and respectful school climates.

School Counselor Casebook: Getting Started

The Scenario

In your school district, large numbers of students are considered for special education placement. The school where you've just begun your school counseling position seems to be especially entrenched in the practice of testing and placing students in special education as a natural intervention for students struggling academically. It has become an automatic practice to test for special student education when a student is in danger of failing.

Thinking About Solutions

As you read this chapter, think about how you as a school counselor would define your leadership role in this scenario. When you come to the end of the chapter, you will have the opportunity to see how your ideas compare with a practicing school counselor's approach.

Collaborative Leadership for the 21st-Century School

Collaborative leadership is building and sustaining relationships to accomplish the seemingly impossible task of helping all students match ever-rising expectations (Rubin, 2002). Collaborative leadership entails collaboration among multiple parties such as community, parents, teachers, school counselors, and others for the development, acceptance, and achievement of goals that lead to academic success for all students (Rubin, 2002). Leadership is increasingly recognized by businesses and educational institutions as too critical and too far reaching to be the lonely domain of a sole designee (Adelman, 2002; Hackman, 2002). In schools, collaborative leadership also has become an increasingly valued and shared phenomenon given the multiplicity of student needs. All community members with a stake in quality education are needed to bring their skills and talents to bear in support of students' academic, career, and personal-social success (American School Counselor Association, 2003; Bryan & Holcomb-McCoy, 2004).

Collaborative leadership places the principal at the hub; however, this type of leadership is extended to other players including teachers, counselors, and community members. Collaborative leadership fosters a school culture or climate that contributes to learning outcomes for students as defined by the educational reform agenda (or school improvement agenda). Collaboration for the sake of collaboration alone will not heighten achievement or reduce inequities. When educators bring their talents to bear around the right initiatives in a collaborative culture, the opportunity for success is significantly furthered. School counselors are exercising a central role in the collaborative culture toward educational reform (Bryan & Holcomb-McCoy, 2004; House, Martin, & Ward, 2002).

School principals shifted their leadership focus from middle management to instructional leadership in order to serve as collaborative problem-solvers around academic success issues. A similar shift also is occurring for school counselors since the American School Counselor Association (ASCA) developed a new school counseling model, which emphasizes a leadership role with the ultimate purpose of casting a wider net and impacting greater numbers of students. "Leadership is exactly what the American School Counselor Association's National Model is about. The model is a guide for all school counselors, in all settings, and with all populations. It is a model that is flexible and adaptable to meet the unique needs of schools and students" (Schwallie-Giddis, Maat, & Park, 2003, p. 170).

"Since school counselors are seen as having potential for leadership in educational reform and as advocates of student success, it is suggested that school counselors promote educational reform through leadership in partnerships between school, families, and communities" (Bryan & Holcomb-McCoy, 2004, p.162). As valued partners in leadership efforts, school counselors are placing themselves squarely in the center of educational reform (Adelman, 2002; Sears, 1999).

School Counselors as Collaborative Leaders

School counselors as leaders and critical change agents are key contributors to improving the conditions under which students learn (Coker & Schrader, 2004; House et al., 2002; Paisley, 1999; Perusse, Goodnough, & Noel, 2001; Stone & Clark,

2001). School counselors traditionally have been supported by the administration, faculty, and parents to assume the role of working with individual or small groups of students, educators, and parents. Educational-reform demands have allowed school counselors to be viewed through a wider lens, not only as the person who can make a difference in a child's life but also as a leader who supports the same school improvement agenda that teachers, administrators, and all other educators must sustain (Adelman, 2002; Coy, 1999; Sears, 1999; Sink, C. A. & McDonald G., 1998).

The school counselor as leader joins forces with other educators and the larger school community to positively impact the opportunities students will have to be successful learners, to achieve high standards, and to become productive citizens (Bemak, F., 2000; House & Hayes, 2002). Leadership for the school counselor is acting and fully participating as an integral part of the mission and function of schools, supporting each student and impacting the system to enable student success. Leadership for school counselors is not administration or management; as it is, many counselors already have the task of testing coordinator, which is an administrative task. School counselors try to avoid or reassign administrative tasks. Leadership for school counselors does not mean being involved in managing the day-to-day life of a school, such as overseeing the bus program, giving attention to the smooth running of the cafeteria program, evaluating teachers, or taking an active part in discipline. Rather, leadership for the school counselor is an exciting, powerful way to literally and figuratively wrap your arms around each student by influencing, and collaborating with, both the internal school community and the larger external community to break down institutional and environmental barriers in order to create the conditions that help students realize the potential of their lives (Clark & Stone, 2000).

Leadership is most easily carried out through collaboration with the significant people in the lives of students, including teachers, administrators, and family and community members (Bryan & Holcomb-McCoy, 2004). When the principal takes a stand on important educational issues, she or he is perceived as a strong leader and an advocate for continuous school improvement. More frequently, school counselors are exercising similar models and leadership behaviors (House et al., 2002). Counselors are change agents, a role made easier when they are seen as leaders in their schools. The more visible school counselors are in classrooms and in working side by side with teachers, parents, and administrators, the more credible they become (Ballard & Murgatroyd, 1999; Guerra, 1998).

Leadership as a Mindset

Leadership for school counselors does not necessarily equate with membership on a **leadership team** such as a school improvement team, committee, or task force. Rather, leadership for school counselors is a mindset, a way of thinking about how you can impact student success. Although school committees, teams, and task forces are excellent vehicles for school counselors to extend their leadership efforts, school counselors can use their leadership influence with or without membership on committees. The counselor who possesses a mindset for leadership is the school counselor who views his or her role as another person or additional set of eyes and ears looking for and identifying environmental and institutional barriers that stratify opportunities for student success. The **leadership mindset** means that the school counselor, along with colleagues who embrace leadership, views his or her position in the school as critical in supporting indicators of student success such as grades, attendance, discipline referrals, test scores, dropout rate, and student retention. This mindset also can impact conditions of learning such as school climate, the instructional program, and students' emotional well-being. Throughout this textbook, you will be introduced to practicing school counselors behaving as leaders, working with students individually, in small groups, in classroom guidance, and in their family, community, and educational systems to help impact students' success.

Leadership as a mindset calls for school counselors to behave and act in collaborative, proactive ways to support all students. Membership on the school improvement team and other critical committees gives counselors a mechanism for their voices to be heard. Membership on the school improvement team, albeit not a necessity in the leadership equation, is highly desirable to facilitate leadership efforts.

Personal-Social Consciousness Skills and Leadership

As a school counseling candidate, you have an opportunity to develop and grow those aspects of your personality that will enhance your ability to be a successful leader. School counselors are "people persons" and are drawn to the school counseling profession because of their strong personal-social consciousness skills. The school counselor as leader in the 21st-century school is someone who can "create a fundamental transformation in the learning cultures of schools" (Fullan, 2002, p. 15). Leadership in today's schools requires vision, the ability to develop others, collaboration skills, the willingness to be accountable, and the ability to see the big picture (Hay Management Consultants, 2000). "Successful leaders tend to engage others with their energy and are, in turn energized by the activities and accomplishments of the group" (Fullan, 2002, p.15). An effective school counselor as leader has a moral purpose and a mindset for action (Fullan, 2002). As Charles Handy (2002) observed: "A worthwhile life . . . requires that you have a purpose beyond yourself" (p.126).

Principals as Partners

School counselors working in partnership with the principal and other critical **stakeholders** toward common goals enhance each other's influence and thus increase the leadership potential of the school. Principals have one of the most difficult jobs in

America (Adelman, 2002; Hackman, 2002; Rubin, 2002). The changing face of American society and the fact that schools reflect all the social issues of the larger society often result in unrealistic expectations of principals. Just a few of the tasks principals are called on to perform on a daily basis are to

1. be the instructional leader;

2. take responsibility for the success and failure of all students;

3. keep the school climate safe and conducive to learning;

4. run a fiscally responsible school and balance the budget;

5. evaluate, motivate, and support faculty and staff;

6. effectively work with parents and be able to tell the truth even when it is going to be tough for parents to hear;

7. hold the line with parents and maintain control of the school;

8. understand teachers', parents', and students' rights;

9. understand the role and function of every school employee from the bus driver to the superintendent;

10. monitor student progress and know the patterns of students' failures and successes;

11. attend to students' physical health, emotional well-being, and social growth;

12. keep the school site clean and well maintained;

13. be a master at public relations and public image;

14. know how to negotiate legal landmines; and,

15. be willing to take the responsibility for all that can go wrong when hundreds of people gather under one roof each day.

The issues in our schools today and their complexity demand that many hands work together and many minds come to the table to solve problems (Dahir, 2000; Fink & Resnick, 2001). Principals are more frequently seeking collaboration with a leadership team because autonomous leadership makes the job daunting (Lawson & Barkdull, 2000). "No professional can succeed alone in addressing the multifaceted needs of students and their families" (Anderson-Butcher & Ashton, 2004b, p. 39).

The expectations of leadership in the schools has changed dramatically since its inception (Bass, 2000; Fink & Resnick, 2001; Silins & Mulford, 2002). With the change in the philosophy of school leadership some leaders were rendered incompetent, although these same leaders at one point had matched the socially determined expectations of an exemplary leader. The social ground of leadership in schools shifted under them, and these leaders did not shift with it (Fink & Resnick, 2001; Leithwood, Jantzi, & Steinbach, in press). The "social ground" has shifted for all educators, including school counselors, and the profession is turning its attention to the development of leadership skills for school counselors in order to equip these professionals with the tools needed in today's schools (Daggett, 2003).

The principal and school counselor are increasingly engaging in a leadership partnership, demonstrating by their collaborative efforts a commitment to delivering optimum educational opportunities (Clark & Stone, 2000; Ponec & Brock, 2000). This spirit of cooperation between school counselor and principal will garner support for the school's counseling program, considerably forward the school counselor's efforts to be viewed as a critical player in the school, and, more important, make a difference for students in school.

School Counselors and Power

School counselors have a number of natural entrées to promote leadership through power. **Power** is an opportunity for influence, and growth toward leadership can be facilitated by the exercise of power.

Authors have defined the power behind leadership roles in many ways (Leithwood, Begley, & Cousins, 1992). French and Raven's (1959) classical work can be applied to the school counseling role by looking at the congruence between the dominant themes and the school counselor role with respect to: (a) position power or jurisdictional power; (b) referent power or relationship power; (c) caring power; (d) transformational power or developmental power; (e) connection power; (f) reward power; and (g) technical, information, or expert power (French & Raven, 1959; Raven, 1965).

Position or jurisdictional power is power that comes from the authority invested in the job or position. In education, this power historically has been assigned to superintendents and principals (Leithwood et al., 1992). School counselors possess position power when they are placed in charge of committees such as the "child study team," composed of a school psychologist, social worker, and others who consider special education placements. Position power that comes with committee membership enables school counselors to exercise leadership on behalf of students. Other examples of position power for school counselors include leadership positions within their professional organizations, such as the American School Counselor Association and the teachers' union, or a counselor's movement into district-level positions, such as district supervisor for counseling.

Referent or relationship power is power that comes from positive relationships with others. The leader who relies on referent power hopes to influence through positive relationships with others. Referent power greatly depends upon the influence that leaders have on followers through supportive behavior such as encouragement and recognition. Other aspects of leadership involve community building, working with others, facilitating, exercising good listening skills, and persuasion, as the leader expresses concern about the vision and mission of the group. School counselors are in a unique position to focus on and develop relationships among members of the organization.

Because of their training in the facilitative skills, school counselors are likely to try to seek and explore the dynamics that exist among members of the organization, which in turn enhances referent power. This skill in understanding the dynamics of groups is an asset that school counselors can capitalize on to help move the school agenda forward. School counselors need referent power to capture and profit from furthering their work as consultants, change agents, and systemic reformers.

Caring power relies on the passion of the individual and one's ability to relate that deep-seated caring to further a mission and goals. Although closely related to referent power, caring power is different because of the influence that results even if the relationships are not optimal. The respect garnered for the school counselor who cares about the children in his or her charge can be used to optimize resources and opportunities for students. It is difficult to deny a passionate educator who is advocating for resources and opportunities to level the playing field of opportunity for all students. School counselors can capitalize on caring power more than any other type of leadership power, and can use it to maximum advantage in the leadership role. Caring power, often viewed as natural for a person who goes into the helping field of school counseling, serves the professional well, especially in the role of advocate. Caring power centers around motivating students, supporting teachers, and assisting the administration. An example of this is a middle school counselor in an urban setting who was able to persuade a local business to provide funds and people-power for an afterschool tutoring program that would impact the 32% failure rate of her eighth graders. Her caring power was apparent and caused people to respond generously with their time, talent, and money.

Transformational or developmental power is the ability to help others become empowered. This power is about enhancing the individual and collective problem-solving capacities of organizational members (Leithwood et al., 1992, p. 7). Transformational leadership occurs when the goals, vision, and motives of the followers are shaped and enhanced by the ability of the leader to empower others to be part of exercising a leadership role in furthering the collective mission of the school. School counselors have endless opportunities to exercise transformational leadership by establishing counseling programs whose purpose mirrors the mission of the school and assuming a leadership role to further that mission. The school improvement team (SIT) is where many school counselors are finding a voice for their transformational power. For example, if a determination is made by the SIT that the failure rate in the fifth grade is unacceptable, the school counselor, as part of the problem-solving or transformational leadership, may want to implement a mentoring program for students in danger of repeating the fifth grade.

Connection power is based on the school counselor's connections with others. Connections are defined as people of power or influence, or people holding the key to something that followers need or want. School counselors as a group may have no more or less connection power than do most other educators and thus rarely rely on this type of power. However, school counselors can look for opportunities to exercise connection power, especially with school board members, central administration staff, parent organizations, and others who are in a position to positively influence the future. Counseling organizations recognize the power of connection and in most states will seek connection power with legislators through "legislative days," during which counselors visit lawmakers and lobby for their causes. Much time, interest, and money is spent grooming a relationship in order to influence legislation. In particular, high-school counselors recognize the power of connections when they start advocating for their students with admissions representatives. When the counselor has been able to groom relationships with select admissions representatives, they have connection power and are in a better position to be effective advocates. The opportunities to help students are endless when school counselors pay attention to and utilize the power of connections.

Reward power means having the ability to lead through material or psychological rewards. Praise, support, recognition, promotions, and monetary rewards are a few of the forms of reward power. This power can influence and shape the behaviors of others. For school counselors, who do not possess the power to give raises or other types of monetary rewards, referent or relationship power can help to achieve reward power. When the school counselor has the respect of the person he or she is praising or acknowledging, this can serve to shape behavior in the desired direction. For example, an elementary school counselor who is respected in her school developed a recognition program to enhance effective teaching. Every two weeks this counselor's "spotlight on teaching" features a teacher who has been observed implementing an effective teaching technique. The counselor places the teacher's picture on a bulletin board, along with a write-up. In addition, the teacher is asked to briefly discuss his or her technique during the next faculty meeting. These spotlights (from someone the teachers respect) are very effective in disseminating a variety of effective techniques that enhance learning and reward the teachers' efforts.

Technical, information, or expert power is the power that derives from possession of specialized knowledge, information, or expertise. This power is bestowed on a leader by others because he or she can assist where the other members of the group have less skill or lack the necessary skills. Individuals with this power can achieve goals based on their abilities or training. For example, school counselors enjoy a high degree of expert power by virtue of their specialized training in areas such as consultation, counseling, data analysis, and collaboration. Counselors can capitalize on their expert power in order to benefit students by providing information to teachers, parents, and others on topics that support students in areas such as interventions for special needs students, e.g., underachievers, Attention Deficit Hyperactivity Disorder (ADHD) students, and aggressive students. The special education qualifying criteria, postsecondary admissions information, and academic advising are but a few examples of areas in which school counselors exercise expert or informational power. Providing parents, students, and teachers with critical, timely information furthers a school counselor's leadership stance.

These various power types can influence and support the direction that school counselors choose for leadership effectiveness. Like other educators, school counselors need to develop an effective leadership style. The higher the comfort level, the more school counselors will exercise leadership and increase their opportunities for positively impacting the lives of the students in their charge. The development of leadership means capitalizing on one's "natural power" in addition to the "groomed power" that school counselors have by virtue of training, professional development, and their penchant to be helpers.

School Counselors Developing Leadership Skills

Developing leadership skills is not an event or a one-time professional development opportunity, but a long and conscientious process in which you will continually reassess how your progress, gaps, victories, and deficits align with the leadership needs of your students. Over the years, it has been our observation that school counselors who are effective leaders developed their leadership skills through attention to four areas: self-awareness, facilitative communication, team development, and staff development.

Self-Awareness

Developing leadership skills starts with a personal analysis of your current strengths and weaknesses. From the self-knowledge gained, you can begin to develop a style of leadership that can grow and be enhanced. Leadership development is less daunting if you begin by focusing on your strengths. Working from a position of strengths will allow for creativity and excitement as you acquire greater self-knowledge and skills.

There are many techniques to help you understand your leadership strengths, such as examining your behavior in prior leadership roles and using feedback from colleagues and friends as an opportunity to grow. Examining prior leadership roles is a great place to start the self-awareness process. Follow these steps to help organize this effort.

1. Think back to a time when you were in any leadership role. The leadership role might have been large or small, professional or personal (professional usually refers to a paid position, and personal refers to a nonpaid position). An example of a personal leadership position would be taking charge of organizing your team's tennis matches, being your child's Girl Scout leader, or taking on the task

of leading the July 4 celebration in your neighborhood. This leadership position may have been an appointed one, such as Guidance Department chairperson; an elected one, such as a school board member; or one bestowed on you informally by others because of your ability to influence people.

2. Think about this leadership position and examine how you proceeded to make policy, shape behavior, organize work, and/or set and meet goals. In other words, examine your "way of work" in the leadership arena.

3. From this leadership experience, make a list of the skills, competencies, and dispositions you brought to the leadership role. Reflect on the approaches that were the strongest for you and the areas in which the comfort level was lowest and the success was weakest.

4. Turn some time and attention to the strong areas. Consider how these areas promoted success, and how the weak areas detracted from or hindered success. Consider what you would do differently in the future. Write a plan of action for a future leadership role that builds upon your successes and minimizes your weaknesses or grows them into strengths.

Facilitative Communication

Another approach to self-analysis of your leadership strengths is to reflect on any feedback you have been given by employers, coworkers, or people in your personal life regarding your interaction with others. Leadership depends on personal relationships, and informal and formal feedback can help illuminate areas of strengths and weaknesses.

Facilitative communication is valuable in developing a successful leadership style. Facilitative communication strengthens interactions with others by increased understanding and sending a message that you are listening and understanding what is being said to you. Facilitative communication involves the skills of reflecting, paraphrasing, clarifying, and questioning.

1. **Reflecting** means that the leader responds by capturing the meaning beyond the expressed words. Responding to the speaker with a high degree of sophistication lets the speaker know that he or she has not only been heard but, more important, has been understood, because the listener has reacted to unexpressed meanings or feelings. Sometimes the listener reacts and misses the intent of the speaker. This generally is not a major drawback, because the speaker knows that the listener is trying to understand the concerns or expressions of the speaker at a deeper level.

2. **Paraphrasing** means that the leader uses active listening to repeat in summary what was communicated. Paraphrasing can be a powerful communication tool

when used judiciously to reinforce to others that they have been heard. When a leader pays attention to verbal and nonverbal behavior and communicates this to others by paraphrasing, it is a relationship builder. The difference between reflecting and paraphrasing is that paraphrasing usually just captures the words and gives back to the speaker a succinct response that captures the main meaning. Reflecting captures the meaning and/or feelings behind the words.

3. **Clarifying** occurs when the leader helps others in the school bring ambiguous meaning into focus. Clarifying helps the speaker define and refine thoughts, motives, feelings, and actions through the carefully chosen words of the listener.

4. **Questioning** is gathering information by carefully choosing open-ended questions, which in turn gives the speaker the chance to convey such things as information, feelings, and understanding. Open-ended questioning invites the speaker to talk, whereas closed questions are less facilitative and reduce the speaker to answering "yes," "no," or responding with only a word or two.

To demonstrate the need for **facilitative responses** on the part of a school counselor, three examples of dialogues follow: (a) a teacher who is resisting a principal mandate that all teachers must seek consultation with the pre-referral assistance team before his or her students can be considered for a special education referral; (b) a consultation exchange between the school counselor and a mathematics teacher about Samantha, his student; and (c) an exchange between the school counselor and Samantha.

Facilitative Responses With a Resistant Teacher

As the school counselor, you have tried to explain to a resistant teacher the benefits and purpose of the pre-referral assistance team (a team that tries to help teachers with students instead of referring the student right to special education), but the teacher continues to resist using this team and insists on skipping over this step.

> *Teacher:* "I really think it is insulting that I have to go before a pre-referral team before Jim [her student] can be tested for special education. I have tried everything, and if I say Jim is not going to make it in regular education then I think that should be enough. I have been in the classroom for 32 years and I have never before had to beg my way into getting a student into special education. Who knows a student better than the classroom teacher?"
>
> *School Counselor:*
>
> Reflecting: "This change in SE procedure has you reeling."
>
> Paraphrasing: "You believe you should be able to make a recommendation for SE, as has always been the procedure."

Clarifying: "You are struggling to avoid what you believe is an unfair change in procedures."

Open-Ended Question: "Would you talk more about why this procedure is so offensive to you?"

Closed Question: "Would you give the Pre-referral Assistance Team a try?"

Interpreting/Analyzing: "You really think it is second-guessing and questioning a teacher's competence and judgment to insist that all students come before the Pre-referral Assistance Team."

Facilitative Responses in Teacher-Student Conflict

Mr. Jefferson, a seventh-grade mathematics teacher, and Samantha, one of his students, are at odds.

Teacher: "I have tried to work with Samantha, but her attitude makes it so difficult. She never turns in any assignments and she makes it impossible to help her or correct her on anything, as she will refuse to communicate when you try to talk to her. I really have tried but I am at the end of my rope with her. I don't know if she can do the math, as I never get any work from her. She may need a lower level math class."

School Counselor:

Reflecting: "You are really frustrated with Samantha."

Paraphrasing: "You are at a loss as to how to get Samantha to complete her work."

Clarifying: "There are two issues working here. You are stumped as to what to try next with Samantha and you are considering the possibility that the work may be too hard for her."

Open-Ended Question: "Can you describe a time when Samantha responded positively?"

Closed Question: "Do you want me to move her from your class?"

Interpreting/Analyzing: "I suspect the math class is too challenging and that Samantha needs to stay for afterschool tutoring."

Interpreting/Analyzing: "Samantha is a strong personality, and it is a well-known fact that you expect a great deal from your students. If you agree, we can have a three-way conversation to try to resolve the standoff between you and Samantha."

Student: "I want to try to succeed in that class, but Mr. Jefferson has it in for me and no matter what I do, he is going to make sure I fail. I really do try, but then I think why bother, it's no use. I was doing my work, but he wouldn't help me when I didn't understand, so I quit."

School Counselor:

Reflecting: "You are really discouraged about your math class."

Paraphrasing: "The conflict with your teacher has caused you to stop trying."

Clarifying: "You are struggling to figure out how to salvage your math class, but the answer is not apparent right now."

Open-Ended Question: "Can you describe the last incident of conflict between you and your teacher?"

Closed Question: "Are you asking to drop this class?"

Interpreting/Analyzing: "I think your troubles are only partly with your teacher, as I suspect you have found the subject matter too challenging."

Interpreting/Analyzing: "Both you and Mr. Jefferson are strong personalities. The trouble lies in the fact that you are having a test of wills and neither of you will budge an inch."

As is true in a counseling and consultation role, lower level questioning in the leadership role is best used sparingly or avoided. The facilitative responses outlined above are in hierarchical order from most facilitative, which encourage conversation and problem solving, to least facilitative. The first four facilitative skills encourage the student and teachers to continue to talk so that the school counselor can more successfully guide them toward a resolution. Interpreting and advising are low-level skills, as they often shut down communication, especially if the recipient feels that he or she is being judged or misunderstood. In the leadership role exercised by school counselors, interpreting and advising are sometimes necessary and appropriate. Facilitative communication skills have helped school counselors in their leadership role to become more effective communicators, which is an important asset for leaders of influence.

Team Development

Prior to becoming a school counselor, begin developing your team-building skills by practicing with a real team, perhaps on a class project. Whether for a class project or as a school counselor, the best place to start for team building is to tackle a project for which you have a passion, because this will fuel your energy and enthusiasm. For example, maybe you are interested in developing a bully-proofing program because you know that too many students are afraid while at school. The likelihood of success will be greater when you are working on something that you feel compelled to impact. Your enthusiasm is likely to be infectious to the rest of your team members. Develop your team with Hackman's (2002) principles in mind. Hackman found five areas of consideration that made for effective teams:

- Is the team a real team or a team in name only?
- Does the team have a compelling direction for its work?
- Is the structure of the team designed to enable rather than impede team-work?
- Does the team operate within a supportive environment?
- Does the team have expert coaching? (p.31)

Hackman (2002) advises that your team should contain no more than six members, and that bringing together only people who get along is not necessarily always best. Also, Hackman cautions that group leaders cannot assume that individual and group skills will evolve on their own, but will need grooming and attention. Your facilitative communication skills will be effective in supporting group cohesiveness. Start with a small project and carefully grow your skills and increase your leadership so that you can enjoy a high-profile, powerful role that makes a difference for your students.

Staff Development

School counselors who seize opportunities to stand before the faculty, parents, students, and community stakeholders to deliver presentations are exercising a particularly powerful leadership role. Learning to be comfortable with presentations is a matter of practicing. Presentation software, such as PowerPoint from Microsoft, is a great medium that is easy to learn and makes presenting more comfortable because you have an outline to cue your content. In Chapter 5, School Counselors as Advocates, the subject of staff development will be discussed in more detail.

The Impact of the School Counselor as Leader

In the remaining sections of this chapter, four specific areas demonstrate how school counselors behave as members of the school's leadership team. Examples illustrate how practicing school counselors and other stakeholders collaborate to demonstrate leadership and advocacy. You will "meet" school counselors who will help translate these leadership concepts into the day-to-day reality of school counseling. The four specific areas that follow are not all-inclusive; they provide just the tip of the iceberg with examples of opportunities to exercise a leadership role that can translate into greater opportunities for students. Operationalizing leadership means taking a closer look at (a) improving school climates, (b) successful instructional programs, (c) developing high aspirations in students, and (d) course enrollment and tracking patterns.

Improving School Climates

School counselors continually scan the school landscape, alert to recognizing an unhealthy school climate and promoting a safe environment that supports opportunities for all students to get a good education. A safe school environment and healthy climate will be a major topic of discussion in Chapter 13. However, in order to demonstrate advocacy in action and to operationalize how these skills play out, let us now examine how an elementary school counselor can advocate for change in an unsafe school climate. Mary Ann Dyal suspected that bullying was affecting students in her school. It has been shown that bullying adversely stratifies educational opportunities for students and establishes a hostile and dangerous climate for the bullied. Mary Ann, like countless other counselors, knew she needed to promote a safer, more inclusive school climate.

Counselors Making a Difference

Meet Mary Ann Dyal

A Leader in Changing School Climates

Mary Ann suspected that bullying was going on in her school and she tested her hypothesis by discussing discipline referrals with her principal and assistant principal. They confirmed her suspicions that the majority of referrals were due to conflicts, bullying, and aggressive behavior. Mary Ann regularly used various resources to help her deliver an effective school counseling program. With a population of more than 1,000 students, Mary Ann knew that she would have to once again bring in an army of resources in order to tackle the problem of bullying and conflict resolution. In her years as a school counselor, Mary Ann had orchestrated dozens of schoolwide programs that enabled her to meet the needs of all her students. Her experience told her that this program, more than any other, would require collaboration with every member of the internal and external school community. Mary Ann established a committee primarily comprised of members of the Parent Teacher Association (PTA), and they set as their goal a reduction in the number of discipline referrals that involved fighting, name-calling, verbal harassment, and other forms of bullying. Collaboration came from all areas. Classroom teachers followed through with activities suggested in the guidance lessons that Mary Ann delivered. The teachers also were consistent in implementing various conflict resolution strategies, such as teaching the students to identify bullying behavior and charting it as a class, until they extinguished the behavior. The principal provided leadership and support for all facets

(continued)

of the program. The navy base in the area provided mentors for students with a history of problems with anger management and for students identified as at-risk for dropping out of school. The art, music, and physical education teachers and the media specialist established lessons and activities in concert with schoolwide efforts to eliminate bullying. The media specialist, collaborating with Mary Ann, developed daily closed-circuit television clips that addressed bullying and its effects. One such skit had Mary Ann trying to return toothpaste to a large tube to illustrate that once hateful words are spoken, they cannot be taken back easily, just as toothpaste squeezed from a tube cannot be put back without much destruction of the tube. Local businesses provided volunteers as well as incentives for classes to reduce their bullying behavior.

Reprinted with permission by Maryann Dyal.

Successful Instructional Programs

The school counselor can successfully impact the instructional program through collaborative efforts with the principal and other key stakeholders. Conducting staff development for teachers and parents in such important areas as educational planning, motivation, student appraisal, interventions, and diversity issues are but a few examples of school counselors leading and teaming to play a unique role in fostering understanding and cooperation among the school community. Student leadership training, cooperative discipline, classroom management, study skills, and postsecondary admissions procedures are areas that have long been influenced by school counselors. The ultimate goal of staff development is to collaborate to provide support to teachers through information, interventions, modeling, and encouragement (Lewis & Bradley, 2000). The opportunities for impacting the instructional program are limitless.

One middle school counselor decided to try to address some student behavioral issues that frequently frustrated parents and teachers by organizing a Parent/Teacher Forum. She conducted a needs assessment and identified the most frequently occurring problems and concerns of educators and parents in her school, such as Attention Deficit Hyperactivity Disorder (ADHD), lack of study skills, underachievement, aggressive-defiant behavior, and substance abuse. Each year, this school counselor hosts a one-night fair in which parents and teachers are able to choose three different presentations by local experts.

Helping teachers understand and use tests to maximize learning for students is another area in which school counselors can impact the instructional program. Teachers receive critical information in the form of test results. Analyzing and interpreting these test results and sharing the results in such a way that they can be used to benefit the instructional process is a powerful way to support students. For example, if school counselors can help increase students' chances of doing well on the Preliminary Scholastic Achievement Test (PSAT), their future chances of being admitted to the college of their choice and to get scholarship dollars will soar. Much controversy surrounds high stakes standardized testing in this country, and it is understandable that school counselors may want to avoid involvement. However, standardized tests are a fact of life. It is through these tests that opportunities are advanced, such as determining who will have access to higher education and thus

Counselors Making a Difference

Meet Robert (Bob) Turba

Improving an Instructional Program

Bob, a high-school counselor in a college preparatory magnet school in Florida, established a relational database in the guidance office using information from the school's student information system. The guidance department ordered the Preliminary Scholastic Aptitude Test (PSAT) scores on disk and imported these scores, along with all information the students provided on the PSAT application, into the database. The students' biographical information and their PSAT scores were paired with the names of their mathematics and language arts teachers. Those teachers then received reports that contained their students' PSAT results on verbal, math, and writing scores, and the answers that the students gave for each question. The teachers also received the correct answers and a class set of unused PSAT booklets. The teachers reviewed the test questions and answers and then held sessions with the students to help them understand why their answers were incorrect. In this way, students (especially 10th graders) were able to understand more about the PSAT, its format, and how they could maximize their scores for both the Scholastic Aptitude Test (SAT) and their 11th-grade PSAT scores. This is an example of a counselor being able to impact the instructional program by providing teachers with critical information about their students. Because all students in this school system take the PSAT, all students' learning and instruction were impacted by this proactive approach.

It is ideal but not necessary that counselors know how to set up a relational database. If a counselor understands the power of data to inform teaching, he or she can find the person in the school district who can disaggregate the information so that teachers can receive information for their particular students. This approach to helping students gives considerable credibility to this counselor and helps students learn and acquire more scholarships. Bob is exercising the rule of parsimony, which means impacting the largest number of students with the most efficient investment of time. Bob's students earn considerable scholarship dollars for college due in no small part to Bob's leadership in helping students raise their PSAT and SAT scores.

Reprinted with permission by Mickie Stricker

benefit from the economic rewards that correlate with postsecondary education. Testing also impacts who will get college credit for a high-school course, and who will be promoted to the next grade, thus reducing the risk of becoming a dropout.

Developing High Aspirations in Students

School counselors can work with other key stakeholders to help students develop high aspirations rather than waiting for aspirations to emerge. Improving student motivation is an area in which school counselors can have tremendous influence. For example, by helping students understand their choices and the full meaning of those choices, school counselors can positively impact students' desire to stretch and strive academically (Stone, 1998). Students need to understand the logic and inter-relatedness of the curriculum, and the consequences of academic choices. Devising ways to clearly communicate to students and their parents that academic choices widen or narrow future options and opportunities is a central task of all school counseling programs (Carnevale & Desrochers, 2003; Daggett, 2003). The academic advising role includes informing students of appropriate courses to take that match their aspirations, helping them understand the interrelationship between curriculum choices and future economic success, and showing them that financing a higher education is possible.

In our world, knowledge is both the capital and the premier wealth-producing resource, making the process of education the ultimate supplier of power (Druker, 1989). Although over a decade old, Druker's thoughts have even more meaning today. The most basic and significant mission of schools is helping youth develop into productive adult citizens who will effectively contribute to society. Adults of tomorrow need adequate preparation to function intelligently in their social, civic, and work worlds. With rapid changes that are occurring in the work force, today's schools have a tremendous responsibility to prepare tomorrow's workers to be productive in an ever-increasing global economy (Carnevale & Desrochers, 2003). To this end, helping students understand the relationship between academic preparation and career development is paramount (Carnevale & Desrochers, 2003). This can be done by sharing statistics with students about the impact that education has on lifetime salaries (Hoyt & Wickwire, 2001). Sharing this information may encourage a higher degree of motivation and understanding of course relevancy. Giving specific up-to-date information about the jobs and accompanying skills and training that are required in the work force will in turn contribute to students' understanding of the interrelatedness between what they do in school and future economic opportunities. Employment statistics will serve as a blueprint for students who are trying to build a future or who need encouragement to do well in school. Students will realize that their success in school is connected to future opportunities available to them. This type of information sharing is something that can begin in elementary school and can continue as a regular part of the school counselor's

Counselors Making a Difference

Meet the High-School Counselors of Jacksonville, Florida

Developing High Student Aspirations

An example of school counselors taking a leadership role in helping students develop high aspirations can be found in the high schools in Jacksonville, Florida, where each student is informed about available financial aid and scholarship opportunities. The school counselors in this district annually collaborate with the supervisor of guidance to train and place approximately 100 volunteers into the 17 high schools of the district to deliver individual advising sessions about accessing financial aid and scholarships for postsecondary education. Harvey Harper, a volunteer, is one example of the many committed people who have helped countless students gain greater hope in financing a postsecondary education. Harvey has been volunteering each year in the program since its inception in 1991. A similar program, called Horizons, is conducted in the junior year and includes additional information about college entrance examinations (Stone, 1998). When students understand that financing a higher education is possible, they often gain hope and inspiration to do better in school.

role in career and educational planning leading to higher aspirations (Murrow-Taylor, Foltz, McDonald, Ellis, & Culbertson, 1999).

Course Enrollment and Tracking Patterns

School counselors, in collaboration with other members of the leadership team, are ideally situated to positively impact **course enrollment and tracking patterns.** School counselors can operate professionally as "door openers" when they understand how tracking and course-taking affect opportunities for the students in their schools. Course selection contributes to furthering or hindering educational opportunity; teachers, parents, administrators, students, and school counselors can choose course assignments that significantly narrow or widen future opportunities. Furthermore, students often make decisions that are inconsistent with their future goals. Hart and Jacobi found that by tenth grade, only half of the ninth graders who had said they were going to college were enrolled in courses that would qualify them for college entrance (Hart & Jacobi, 1992). School counselors can influence enrollment patterns and implement academic safety nets so that students can take courses commensurate with their future goals.

A study by Stone (1998) examined the mathematics placement of the ninth graders of one large urban school district. An analysis of the 1,611 ninth graders

Counselors Making a Difference

Meet Joni Shook

A Leader Who Impacted Enrollment Patterns

Joni Shook is a leader. She impacted her schools' program by possessing a leadership mindset in addition to holding a position of leadership as chairperson of the School Improvement Team. As was stressed earlier, though formal leadership in terms of the chairmanship of a committee, task force, or team is not necessary for effective leadership, a formal committee can provide a perfect vehicle for being a force for change.

The special education (SE) students in Joni's school were pulled out of their regular education classes for a portion of their day and placed into special education classes. Joni, an elementary school counselor and chair of the School Improvement Team, charged the members of her team with changing the enrollment patterns of special education students so that these children could stay in the regular classroom environment in an inclusion model. In an inclusion model, SE students remain in the regular education program. Special education teachers come to the classrooms and help the students rather than having the students leave class during part or all of the day to receive the SE intervention. As predicted, the inclusion model was met with significant resistance among teachers who were partial to the "pull out program" in which they could send students with identified handicaps under special education placement to other teachers for help. It seemed to these teachers as if the burden of educating students with learning disabilities and other handicaps was falling back in their laps. Through staff development in showing research that supports inclusion, highlighting individual successes at their school, and having each of the teachers experience how their own students benefited from the inclusion model, the School Improvement Team was able to change the teachers' viewpoint, resulting in the expansion of the inclusion program to include grades 1 through 4. Although Joni is now an administrator at the district level, the inclusion model has flourished. Students have more opportunities for success because Joni exercised a leadership role in which she was able to really change attitudes and beliefs about course enrollment patterns.

Reprinted with permission by Joni Shook.

who scored in the upper quartile on one of three mathematics subtests revealed that placement in higher level mathematics differed for upper quartile students depending on where the student went to school. In this school district, a student's future opportunities were stratified based on the course enrollment patterns exercised by the educators and community of each individual school (Stone, 1998).

School counselors also can find leadership opportunities in professional organizations. The American School Counselor Association (ASCA) is the national organization for school counselors. It is the opinion of the authors of this text that it is important for school counselors to become members of their local, state, and/or national professional organizations. Membership in professional organizations gives one a collective voice legislatively; provides a multitude of professional development opportunities, which include print materials, workshops, and conferences; and increases your enjoyment of your work as you build relationships with your fellow professionals. Professional stagnation is less likely when one challenges oneself by the most current and effective practices and information, brought to you by professional organizations.

Counselors Making a Difference

Meet Lou Nussbaum

Exercising Leadership Through Committee Membership

Lou is an elementary school counselor who is keenly aware that his school often used special education (SE) as a first-line intervention for students. Lou believed there was an overidentification of students for SE, and he began exploring ways to reduce the number of students going through these lengthy procedures. It is Lou's position that with appropriate intervention efforts, SE referrals can be reduced. Lou took the step that many counselors are taking across America: he established a pre-referral intervention team. Lou's team decided to study the SE data of the school to (a) identify the prevalence of the primary presenting problem for each child referred, (b) learn the success rate of the students placed in SE for the last two years, and (c) disaggregate the students referred by race, ethnicity, gender, referring teacher, and grade level. What emerged was the realization that a disproportionate number of students of color were being referred for SE and that boys were two times more likely to be referred for emotional concerns than were girls. Armed with this information, Lou and his team got busy and linked the school with greater available resources to support students and to reduce the number of students who needed SE. For example, acting-out behavior was the number one reason why boys were referred to SE for emotional problems. Mentors were assigned to each male who was brought before the Pre-referral and Intervention Assistance Team for acting-out behaviors. Tutors, parental involvement, consultation with agency personnel, and behavior management programs were but a few of the interventions that the team and the teachers collaborated upon to implement. In one year, Lou and his team were able to drop the SE placement rate by 20%! The team continues to set goals for reducing this number further. They plan to continue until they are certain they are using the most appropriate intervention.

Reprinted with permission by Lou Nussbaum.

Leadership: Rewarding but Difficult

Leadership is not easy. Hold firm in your leadership role, and in the words of Trish Hatch, co-author of the ASCA model (2003), "don't blink." Leaders are not always popular, and it is a given that with leadership comes the understanding that the decisions made and the positions advocated for naturally result with someone disagreeing. Hold steady and move carefully toward the goals of the school's mission and the school counseling program with conviction and a clear eye on what you are trying to accomplish for students. This will result in garnering respect and reducing resistance. Leadership is difficult but rewarding. Seize the challenge and embrace it as an opportunity to grow as you figure out how to negotiate the school terrain. Success will be yours. Refuse to fail.

> *Success*
>
> When we think of failure
> Failure will be ours.
> If we remain undecided
> Nothing will ever change.
> All we need to do
> Is want to achieve something great
> And then simply do it.
> Never think of failure
> For what we think,
> Will come about.
>
> — *Maharishi Mahesh Yogi*

TechTools

When you become a school counselor, use the power of technology to maximize the efficiency and effectiveness of your leadership.

- Query databases to answer questions about course enrollment patterns. Order computer generated information such as The College Board's report on PSAT results that Bernadette Willette used to try to initiate higher level academics for more students.
- Impact the instructional program by helping to provide student achievement data in a way that is most advantageous for students, such as the work Bob Turba did by disaggregating the PSAT scores by teacher.
- Use tech tools such as listservers, e-mail messages, and websites to increase communication and the exchange of critical and timely information. For ex-

ample, some counselors write weekly electronic newsletters, which are sent via e-mail. Counselors are increasingly collaborating via listservers.

- Regularly seek a spot on the faculty meeting agendas to deliver an 8- to 10-minute bullet point PowerPoint staff development presentation as part of your role as a member of the leadership team.
- Consider using spreadsheets to help you keep track of a number of important clusters, such as parent conferences, students who have completed a career plan, classes that have received classroom guidance, and so on. Spreadsheet programs have the capability of generating summary data and graphs, which you can include in your end-of-the-year report about your program's progress toward student outcomes.
- Establish electronic support groups and supervision groups with other counselors so that collaboration can help you more efficiently and effectively do your job.

School Counselor Casebook: *Voices From the Field*

The Scenario Reviewed

In your school district, large numbers of students are placed in special education. The school where you've just begun your school counselor position seems to be especially entrenched in the practice of testing and placing students in special education as a natural intervention for students struggling academically. It has become an automatic practice to test for special student education when a student is in danger of failing.

A Practitioner's Approach

Here's how a practicing school counselor responded to this school scenario:

Teachers and counselors always struggle with deciding what is the best way to help a child. Do we look for a classroom situation that will provide support, a slower pace of instruction, and a teacher especially trained in individual educational planning, or do we maintain the child in the regular education placement, where she or he is floundering, adding some accommodations and strategies to aid in learning? Special education may not be the answer, especially when students are already in high school. We need to look much further. Scenarios like these are a real dilemma.

If this were the situation in my school, I would present this challenge at the weekly Building Based Intervention Team meeting. This team is made up of an administrator, the school counselors and counseling supervisor, the student assistance coordinator, the school nurse, the school psychologist, and the learning consultant. The purpose of this committee is to be a pre-referral intervention for students not meeting with academic success. After meeting, strategizing, and sharing the outcomes with the student's teachers, a better view of the student's needs would be available. The team would begin by reviewing feedback sheets from each teacher who has this child in class. As the child's counselor, I would have already gathered all the pertinent information, including report cards, standardized test scores, and so on.

As the group brainstormed ideas, led by the school counselor, we might come up with a list of strategies that would be recommended to the child's teachers. These interventions must be put in place and evaluated before a child study team evaluation can occur. It is difficult to immediately determine the difference between the child who is a slow learner and one who has a learning disability. Often, by the time a child has reached high school, he or she has either learned to compensate for an undiagnosed learning disability or has failed before reaching ninth grade.

I would propose that we convene a meeting of all the student's teachers. Each teacher would have the opportunity to discuss the successes and failures he or she has had with the student. Any successes would be shared and other teachers would be encouraged to try that particular technique. I would hand out the list of strategies compiled by the Building Based Intervention Team and ask that all teachers incorporate them into their teaching with this student. Often these are strategies that work well with all students but may not always be used. One such technique that works well for reluctant learners is to break larger testing units into smaller pieces so that students are not forced to learn more than they can handle at one time. Another technique for children struggling with recall might be to give that child a word bank from which to choose the answer on a test or quiz.

We would also map out all of the resources that we have in the building to help slow learners and our students who are at risk of failing. We might assign a student tutor, or assign the student to a basic skills class in language arts or math, if appropriate. We could identify any gaps in our services that we may have and look at what could be added to help students to pass their courses. We could look at this from a twofold approach—how do we educate the faculty, and how do we encourage students to avail themselves of existing resources to help them succeed? Recognizing that there is a lot to be learned from data, we would also analyze the referrals, review placement decisions, determine which students access academic support services, and identify which clubs have a service component and could provide students volunteers to tutor. With a plan in hand, the school counselor would make an appointment to meet with the student's parents to see if there is any support that could be offered at home.

The school counselor would now be at the front and center of the intervention plan. The intervention team would reconvene in a month to review the student's progress. I would share reports from each teacher to see if progress had been made. If the student were still in danger of failing, a referral to the child study team would be appropriate.

Special education is an excellent education plan for some students, but we need to make sure we have explored all options and interventions to ensure that students first have the opportunity to succeed in the regular education program. Our data analysis revealed that the majority of the referrals did not result in special education services and many students were not participating in academic help programs.

It would be my hope that special education referrals are reduced with the help of a strong intervention team with membership from each significant area of the educational arena to add strategies to the regular education program. I would like to see many more students involved in academic support and interventions to help them succeed in their high-school classes.

Mickie Stricker has worked as a high-school counselor in New Jersey and is currently the supervisor of guidance and counseling at Kinnelon High School in New Jersey. Mickie has been actively involved in school-to-work and in developing student portfolios and career curriculum. She is a past president of the New Jersey School Counselor Association and is actively engaged in legislative initiatives in New Jersey to implement comprehensive national standards—based school counseling programs.

Chapter Summary

Collaborative Leadership for the 21st-Century School

Leadership is becoming an increasingly valued and shared phenomenon at the school level. Leadership in the school of the 21st century entails collaboration among multiple parties for the development, acceptance, and achievement of goals that lead to academic success for all students. A multiplicity of student needs requires all stakeholders to bring their skills and talents to bear in support of students' academic, career, and personal-social success. Leadership is group authority, responsibility, and expertise, and leadership teams change according to the activity or need.

School Counselors as Leaders

Leadership for the school counselor is fully participating as an integral part of the mission and function of schools, supporting each and every student to be a successful learner, and impacting the system to enable student success. Leadership for school counselors requires joining forces with other educators and the larger school community to positively impact the opportunities that students will have to be successful learners and to achieve high standards. Leadership means entering into partnerships to demonstrate commitment to help the principal and other internal and external stakeholders deliver all of the critically important tasks that need to be done to support student learning.

Developing Leadership Skills

Leadership development is less daunting when a counselor begins leadership building by starting with his or her personal strengths. Working from a position of strength will allow for creativity and excitement in the venture.

Facilitative Communication for Effective Learning

Good communication is a key ingredient in successful leadership. School counselors who use high-level facilitative skills such as reflecting, paraphrasing, and clarifying can capitalize on these skills and enhance their ability to influence others.

The Imperative to Move to a Leadership Role

The students we are educating today are different from the students we educated yesterday, and the students we educate tomorrow will be different from those of today. The implications for school counselors is that we cannot continue to hold on to just the traditional ways of practice when faced with the reality that students will be a more diverse group in the future. Educators are faced with the need to prepare all students for a society that will be unlike any that has come before us. The school counselor as part of the leadership team can join forces with others to ensure that all students have access to the information and experiences that will allow them to influence the society of the future. This type of leadership team is ideally situated to advocate for all students by providing the support and encouragement necessary for students to obtain the best possible education, which is the gateway to greater social and economic opportunities for their futures.

The Impact of the School Counselor as Leader

School counselors can become members of the leadership team formally, but this is not necessary. Leadership is a mindset and a way of work for school counselors, who will join forces with other educators to assume and exert leadership within their schools and communities. The school counselor as educational leader establishes a vision and belief in the development of every child. Opportunities for leadership are plentiful. School counselors can view themselves as natural allies with other educators of the school's leadership team and to look for opportunities to develop and implement their special leadership skills in order to maximize their effectiveness in the promotion of success for all students.

Key Terms

Caring power p. 97
Clarifying p. 101
Collaborative leadership p. 91
Connection power p. 97
Course enrollment and tracking
   patterns p. 109
Facilitative responses p. 101
Leadership mindset p. 94
Leadership team p. 93
Paraphrasing p. 100
Position or jurisdictional power p. 96

Power p. 96
Questioning p. 101
Referent or relationship power p. 96
Reflecting p. 100
Reward power p. 98
Stakeholders p. 94
Technical, information, or expert power
   p. 98
Transformational or developmental
   power p. 97

Learning Extensions

1. Which of the types of power described do you believe you most often use, and why? Which type of power do you least prefer, and why?

2. Using the points presented throughout the chapter, describe a leader whose style you admired and for whom you responded positively. Explain why you appreciated his or her leadership approach.

3. Find two counselors who have operationalized leadership in one or more of these areas: (a) changing attitudes and beliefs, (b) impacting the success of the instructional programs, (c) developing high aspirations, and (d) changing course enrollment and tracking patterns. Interview these counselors to gather the facts and then write up your findings. Include a brief description of what they did and your reaction as to whether or not their activities reached a large number of students. Was each activity an efficient use of time? Finally, what impact did each activity have on the success of the students?

4. Leadership opportunities for school counselors are all around us. Imagine that you are a practicing school counselor. How do you envision exercising a leadership role in your new school?

5. Describe your leadership style. What are your areas of strengths and weaknesses?

6. The principal is a key partner in enabling school counselors to exercise a leadership role and in delivering an effective school counseling program. Name six to eight strategies you will employ to develop a partnership with your principal.

7. How did Bob Turba change the instructional program for his school? Why was his approach effective?

8. Describe Joni's advocacy. What personal attributes and skills do you believe Joni needed in order to have the influence she did with the teachers of her school?

9. Discuss how the school counselors of Jacksonville, Florida, are raising aspirations rather than just attending to aspirations as they emerge.

Chapter 5

School Counselors as Advocates

Chapter Objectives

By the time you have completed this chapter, you should be able to:

- Describe how school counselors work as advocates and describe areas in which school counselors are having success as an advocate.
- Identify the personal-social consciousness skills needed for advocacy.
- Understand the ethical imperative for school counselors to behave as advocates.
- Begin the process of developing your own plan for behaving as an advocate.
- Describe research and accountability measures that reveal areas of inequities in schools and the need for school counselors to advocate.
- Understand how technology and staff development skills can help you in your advocacy.

School Counselor Casebook: Getting Started

The Scenario

You have just finished a session with the fifth student in your caseload who is in danger of failing the marking period because she was suspended for tardiness. The halls of your overcrowded school are almost impassable during the five-minute class changes. The school policy states that students who are late for class are locked out until they bring a tardy slip from the office. The line to get a tardy slip is very long, causing students to sometimes miss as much as the first 20 minutes of class. Additionally, seven total tardies in a grading period mean five days of after-school detention or suspension for two days. Many students are choosing suspension instead of detention because of their work obligations. You take a look at the discipline data and you are shocked to learn that 27% of the suspensions began as multiple tardies.

Thinking About Solutions

As you read this chapter, think about possible solutions. Is there a role for you in this situation? What would you do? When you come to the end of the chapter, you will have the opportunity to see how your ideas compare with a practicing school counselor's approach.

The Role of Social Advocacy in School Counseling

Advocacy in the counseling world involves "identifying groups of people who might benefit from increasing their own strength" (Lewis, Lewis, Daniels, & D'Andrea, 1998, p. 25). Groups of people for whom policy, procedures, and practices adversely stratify their opportunities have been referred to as "socially devalued populations" (Lewis et al., 1998). Because individuals in these socially devalued groups typically have limited power and little say about things that happen in their families, schools, workplaces, and/or communities, they frequently come to believe that they are not valued by others (D'Andrea & Daniels, 1999; Lee, 2001). "Social advocacy implies questioning the status quo, challenging the rules and regulations that deny student access, protesting changes . . . that decrease opportunities for the under-represented" (Osborne et al, 1998).

Problems that individuals face often can be traced to the system(s) in which they live, work, and play. Some examples of these systems are families, work environments, social agencies, the legal system, neighborhoods, educational institutions, and many others. The origins of problems and impediments to effective decision making often lie not in individuals but in an intolerant, restrictive, or unsafe environment (Lee & Walz, 1998; Lewis et al., 1998). The practice of counseling is more complete and effective when the counselor helps students and their families negotiate through the systems that impact their lives or when the counselor impacts a change in the system. Changing systems increases counselor effectiveness in multiple ways.

The School Counselor as Advocate

A school counselor as advocate is one who feels compelled to survey (scrutinize) the internal and external school landscape to identify the barriers that are impeding student success and to collaborate to impact the conditions necessary for all students to be successful in their academic, social, emotional, career, and personal development (Stone & Dahir, 2004). Educational reform and professional leaders are increasingly focusing on the school counselor as advocate and change agent (Ericksen, 1997; Hart & Jacobi, 1992; Lee & Walz, 1998; Osborne et al., 1998; Perusse, Goodnough, & Noel, 2001). School counselors are ideally situated to serve as conduits of information and practices to promote a **social justice agenda** (House, Martin, & Ward, 2002; Lewis et al., 1998). School counselors who have strong **personal-social consciousness skills** and understand equity issues are contributing to a global society in which students who have not traditionally been served well in the past have a chance to acquire the skills necessary to unconditionally participate in a 21st-century economy (Stone & Clark, 2001).

School counselors help members of a school family become inspired to consider greater possibilities for their students and to usher students toward these possibilities

(Dahir & Stone, 2003; Galassi & Akos, 2004; Sears, 1999). Advocacy for the school counselor is helping all students realize the American dream of an optimum and quality education (Lee, 2001; Toporek, 2000). Because counselors care about students a great deal, they motivate other critical stakeholders to build systems that widen students' opportunities. Conversely, school counselors look for those systems that impede success, and then inspire, instruct, and incite others to eliminate these obstacles. School counselors have been engaged in advocacy for years, especially with individual students, but their role is expanding to include advocating for social justice and challenging oppression on a wider scale (Lewis & Bradley, 2000).

Counselors who understand issues impacting equity and opportunity are changing systems that continue to adversely stratify opportunities, influencing attitudes and beliefs regarding equitable practices, providing attention to equity and access issues, and securing resources designed to improve opportunities (Dahir & Stone, 2003). Counselors bring expertise to strategically challenge the status quo in systems where inequities impede students' success. School counselors are specialists in helping change human behavior. For example, the preparation that school counselors receive in communication skills and interpersonal relationship development is needed to change the school climate from a potentially hostile one to a productive learning environment for every student (Martin, 1998; Sears, 1999; Stone, 1998).

Advocacy and the Achievement Gap

A primary focus for the school counselor as advocate is to become the voice for those students for whom educational opportunity has traditionally been adversely stratified, especially low socioeconomic students and minority students of color (Lee, 2001; Martin, 2004). For students who do not have equal access to a quality education it is a "grave educational injustice" (Lee, 2001). The school counselor as advocate raises aspirations, nurtures dreams, and empowers students to become their own advocates. School counselors have a critical role to play in supporting brighter futures for all students, especially for those traditionally underserved, such as minorities, those in lower socioeconomic groupings, and those persecuted because of their sexual orientation (House et al., 2002).

Empowerment

Learned helplessness or situational helplessness can be impacted when counselors work with individuals in helping them feel empowered. McWhirter (1997) defined this empowerment:

> . . . the process by which people, organizations, or groups who are powerless or marginalized (a) become aware of the power dynamics at work in their life context,

(b) develop the skills and capacity for gaining reasonable control over their lives, (c) which they exercise, (d) without infringing on the rights of others, and (e) which coincides with actively supporting the empowerment of others in their community. (p. 12)

The concepts of empowerment and advocacy provide the basis for the role of counselor as a social **change agent**. Empowerment is a complex process that encompasses self-reflection and action; awareness of environmental power dynamics that may impact upon psychosocial development; and the development of skills to promote community enhancement (McWhirter, 1997). Any counselor with a belief in the possibility of a better world develops a sense of social responsibility. Part of such a counselor's philosophy should be a commitment to the idea of social change within a larger context beyond schools and his or her role as a catalyst for such change (Lee & Walz, 1998).

Characteristics of an Effective Advocate

Interpersonal skills, communication, empowerment, leadership, and advocacy skills are areas in which many counselors excel, and they are the critical skills needed to address social and economic issues that challenge our global society. Although advocates first need heart and a passion to help students, they also need the skills that are examined in this section.

School counselors are willing to listen, a quality that makes strong advocates. Advocacy for all students requires a high level of caring for students, parents, and fellow educators. Generally speaking, these qualities are often present in people who seek the school counseling profession. School counselors by and large do not like to see students' opportunities limited and want to create a shared vision of the possibilities that are beyond the students' current realities. It is good that school counselors generally come to the profession with the personal quality of caring, because according to Kottler (2000), preparation programs in counseling, law, and medicine cannot possibly do justice to the development of caring and compassion.

School counseling candidates usually have strong **personal-social consciousness** and a desire to be a voice for students who are underrepresented or not considered part of the mainstream. School counseling students often are risk takers, as advocacy involves sometimes having to take an unpopular position.

Qualities appreciated in school counselors are sensitivity to the needs of students, genuine positive regard for others, compassion, flexibility, understanding, empathy, insightfulness, and emotional stability. Can one be taught to be a passionate advocate? "Each of us can be encouraged to access that part of us that is most compassionate and caring" (Kottler, 2000, p. 3). It is not enough to know how to use technology for advocacy, to have skills to disaggregate and aggregate data, to understand

Counselors Making a Difference

Meet Kerri Ann Jannotte

A Heart for Advocacy

Kerri is a school counseling student and a self-contained special education teacher in upstate New York. Kerri, like many teachers, has a propensity to advocate on behalf of her students. Kerri will make an amazing school counselor because she fights to widen opportunities for her students. For four years, Kerri's request to take her self-contained special education students to the Museum of Natural History was denied with the explanation that her students would not benefit. Kerri knew how much her students were interested in the subjects that they would find explained in the museum, and she was convinced that this would be a life-changing experience for her students, most of whom had never been 10 miles from their home. Kerri learned that the science club had been granted permission to go to the museum, so with her encouragement, her students all joined the club. Ten of her students boarded the bus with the other science club members for the trip to New York City. Kerri said she spent the day fighting back tears as she watched her students' faces while they relished each moment of the bus ride, museum, and restaurant.

Reprinted with permission by Kerri Ann Jannotte.

how to negotiate the political landscape, to recognize inequities, and to establish connections in order to influence change. Without deeply held beliefs about students and their need for a voice, and without a willingness to be a passionate advocate, the profession will not move in the right direction. Skills alone are not enough. The school counselor of the 21st century must negotiate bureaucratic systems and be willing to be labeled an idealist.

School counselor advocates are risk takers, sometimes taking on causes to the displeasure of colleagues or others (Chen-Hayes, 2001; Lee, 2001). The role of advocate can be uncomfortable, because it sometimes carries controversy, conflict, and personal risk. However, advocacy also is a rewarding role that school counselors embrace because it calls on them to champion the causes of equity, justice, and inclusion. To maintain their effectiveness and influence, school counselors exercise caution and political astuteness by negotiating the pitfalls and landmines in the political landscape. Conversely, fear of falling into disfavor does not paralyze the school counselor from fully exercising an advocacy role. School counselors often are the voice of advocacy when no one else will take that responsibility.

There was a simple job that Everybody wanted done
and Anybody could do.
But Everybody thought Somebody should do what Nobody would.

So Nobody did what Everybody wanted, and thought Somebody should, even though Anybody could.

— *Author unknown*

School counselors benefit from giving themselves permission to be idealists and optimists. The school counselor/optimist, far from being the proverbial "Pollyanna" who just relies on goodness, puts effort and skill behind the idealism. The optimists who bring skills to the fight for systemic change and believe in students and their abilities will sometimes have to steady themselves before the cynics, who will quickly point out that "we have tried that before," and "your ideas won't work." The dispirited cynics are found everywhere, insisting that students are hopeless and the situation is dire; fortunately, tenacity most often allows school counselors to stay focused. The cynics may have been spirited fighters for students at one time. Acknowledge them, respect them, work with them, or if need be, work around them, but don't succumb to the negativity. The cynics may even respect you for all you do for students and wish they still had the will.

The Ethics of Advocacy

Advocacy is an ethical imperative for school counselors. ASCA's *Ethical Standards for School Counselors* (2004) states in A.1.b., "The professional school counselor is concerned with the educational, career, personal, and social needs and encourages the maximum development of every student."

Advocacy is also a legal imperative. Chapter 11 covers court cases that give legal muscle to counselors to advocate on behalf of their students (e.g., *Davis v. Monroe County Board of Education*; *Sain v. Cedar Rapids Community School District*; and *Eisel v. Montgomery County Board of Education*).

The ethical obligation that school counselors have to advocate for their students is complex and not without controversy as to whether or not advocacy is an ethical imperative. Kitchener's Five Moral Principles (1986)—beneficence, nonmaleficence, loyalty, autonomy, and justice—are most often applied by counselors when in the throes of an ethical dilemma. However, we believe that the moral principles also provide a fitting lens through which to view the concept of advocacy as an ethical obligation. The moral principles are presented here in the context of social advocacy as an ethical imperative.

Beneficence, or to "do good," means to continually seek ways to groom opportunities for student success. Exercising an advocacy role is one of the most ethical behaviors in which a school counselor can engage. This concept is examined in greater detail later in this chapter.

Nonmaleficence, or "above all do no harm," implores school counselors to consider the impact of their action or lack of action to determine if potential harm will result. If a school counselor cannot be certain that an action will "do good," at least one is to be confident in the knowledge that it will "do no harm." Nonmaleficence requires that one is vigilant as to motives, biases, and prejudices that one may know-ingly or unwittingly allow to guide individual behaviors.

Loyalty in advocacy means remaining steadfast in the efforts to make systemic change and change for individuals and groups of students. Loyalty means trying to make an impact for all students, not just the top 5% or those who are most at risk. School counselors can figuratively "wrap their arms" around all students through ad-vocacy by implementing a systemic change that involves every student. If there is a bullying problem in your school that impacts more than 70% of the students, and de-spite resistance you are able to team with others to deliver an effective prevention program, then you are being loyal to your students and advocating on their behalf.

Promoting **autonomy** is a delicate balancing act for school counselors, because students are minors and also are in a school setting. This combination requires loy-alty to the minor, but also the school counselor's loyalty extends beyond the student to the parents or caregivers. The advocacy role can help us promote autonomy in many ways. For example, the goal of a career guidance program should be to em-power each and every child to become his or her own advocate. Career counseling for all students closes the **information gap.** The existence of that gap enables some students to make informed decisions while others wander aimlessly through their school experience never understanding the connection between academics and their future. School counselors can work to promote students' autonomy, under-stand and apply childhood development principles to help them, and equip them with as much "armor" as possible to support their full development.

Justice means treating equals equally and treating unequals unequally, but in di-rect proportion to their relevant differences (Kitchener, 1986). In other words, we avoid a one-size-fits-all educational system; we look at each individual and his or her unique needs. Justice means that when we treat students differently we need to be able to justify to ourselves and to others why we acted as we did. Why did we choose to ad-vocate for some students in certain situations and not for other students who appear to have the same circumstances? To put it another way, what differences are there among these students or their circumstances that allow us to be there for one individual or group of individuals and not for another? Did one group need us more because they have had fewer advocates in the past? Did one group need us more because we knew that their voices were really weaker than others who, on the surface, may appear to have an equal voice? School counselors have to wisely choose their advocacy battles, and this sometimes means making tough decisions about which causes we tackle.

The Impact of Advocacy on Students, the School, and the Community

School counselor advocacy contributes to furthering educational opportunity. The school counselor as advocate is ideally situated to impact important areas, such as helping students to access and succeed in rigorous academics, creating a safer school climate, and helping students and families understand and widen their opportunities

Advocating for Systemic Change

What does **systemic change** mean? Systemic refers to the organizational policies, procedures and/or practices of either a school or school district. The literature on systemic change frequently cites critical principles of change, such as a shared vision to guide change; leadership capable of driving the change; research upon which to build change; professional development and other opportunities for learning to implement and sustain the change; organizational arrangements to support change; and strategies to implement change (Raelin, 2004).

As participants of the leadership team's effort to drive change, school counselors think systemically by examining the institutions in which they work to identify both those practices that negatively impact students and should be eliminated and those systems that positively impact students and should be replicated or expanded. Through systemic change school counselors reach many more students (Keys & Lockhart, 1999). With systemic change, school counselors look beyond developing their school counseling program as an isolated entity of the school to that of understanding the context in which their program is embedded. For example, does your school have a policy that automatically fails students if they are absent a set number of days? This policy has an adverse effect if implemented without considering individual students' circumstances. The counselor can advocate for a change in this policy or, in other words, impact systemic change.

Poor learning is frequently explained by enumerating the barriers such as poverty, crime-ridden neighborhoods, lack of parental support, and lack of motivation that students bring to school rather than examining the **systemic barriers** that schools and districts place before students (Haycock, 2001). Educators are turning attention toward the system and the damage done there. "We take the children who have less to begin with, and then systematically give them less in school, too. In fact we give these children less of everything that we know makes a difference" (Haycock, 2001, p. 1). In order to become a school counselor/advocate, it is important to study the systems, practices, and ideologies that negatively and positively impact student success so that you have the knowledge to assist in adapting or replicating those systems.

School counselors are infusing principles and practices that are being used in school reform into school counseling, and connecting their programs to the school's mission for the purpose of supporting students to be successful (Burnham & Jackson, 2000). The role of the school counselor as advocate involves looking at the individual student but also examining the systemwide inequities and practices.

Educational reform and societal changes are compelling reasons for school counselors to join forces with other educators and use their influence to eradicate systems and ideologies that have the potential to impact negatively upon students (House & Martin, 1998; Lee & Walz, 1998; Stone & Turba, 1999). Helping to examine institutional and environmental barriers so that these obstacles can be eliminated will in turn create alternatives and opportunities for the people who have not enjoyed the full advantage of an equal opportunity education. There are communitywide, districtwide, and school site–based systems and practices that stratify opportunities for students; the results are reflected in the data presented in Chapter 1. School counselors, collaborating with other educators, can take action to identify, eradicate, and/or replace those policies and practices that have marginalized groups in our society (Lee, 2001; Lee & Walz, 1998).

What are some of the systems that impede student success? The following list poses just a few policies, practices, and procedures that on the surface or on closer inspection may reveal that they are hindering students. Think about what you can add to this list of possible systemic barriers:

- giving the best teachers to the most capable students in the most rigorous courses in the most affluent schools
- tracking students into course work based on test scores
- focusing most of the school counseling program goals on the top 5% of the students or the 10% of students most at risk for failure
- shifting unsatisfactory educators to the schools with the least parental involvement
- encouraging only select students in certain categories to take the Preliminary Scholastic Achievement Test (PSAT)
- expecting teachers who have poor classroom management skills to improve in absence of support
- supporting students with career and academic advising only when they seek the counselor's help
- having a 27% average absenteeism rate without a strategic plan to address the problem
- having a 42% failure rate for the ninth graders without safety nets such as alternative schedules, summer school, and tutoring
- automatically assessing students for special education when they fail a grade
- having a 36% failure rate in algebra without academic safety nets
- focusing on the demands of the most vocal parents while ignoring the needs of the silent majority
- not placing students into higher level academics based on a brief scheduling contact in which the student says that he or she does not want to be in the higher level academics

Bernadette Willette, a high-school counselor in Maine, broke down a systemic barrier by skillfully changing her school's practice of not offering Advanced Placement courses. This practice was born of the attitude and belief that the stu-

Counselors Making a Difference

Meet Bernadette Willette

A Systemic Change Agent Who Impacts Attitudes and Beliefs

Advanced Placement (AP) courses are important to students at all schools. Students who take AP courses are actually taking college-level courses in high school if at the end of the course, a student takes the AP exam and scores the college's required score for credit. The consensus at Bernadette's school was that AP offerings were not necessary because the students were not aspiring to go to college. Bernadette decided to tackle this belief by arming herself with data from the College Board, which is the organization that administers the AP program. With data and research, Bernadette demonstrated to teachers the correlation between the PSAT scores of many of their current and former students and the students' predicted success in AP courses. Faced with the fact that many of their students' PSAT scores predicted success and the realization that these students would now graduate without ever having the opportunity to take AP courses, these teachers made the commitment to offer AP courses in the future. In her leadership role, Bernadette Willette identified attitudes and beliefs that were adversely stratifying students' opportunities and advocated with facts in hand. She made a systemic change that will benefit many students in the future; her school now offers three AP courses with plans for two more. This collaborative leader changed attitudes and beliefs (Stone, 2003)!

dents in this school did not need higher level academics. Bernadette felt that the status quo adversely stratified opportunities for the students in her school. She quietly and respectfully went about changing attitudes and beliefs, considerably widening opportunities for these rural, low-socioeconomic students, who had traditionally accessed postsecondary opportunities in dismal numbers.

Another example of systemic change comes from Paul, a high-school counselor who has watched with dismay as large numbers of his ninth graders are retained. Paul observed that there were no significant interventions for students between their first year as ninth graders and the year they repeated ninth grade. Paul gathered data on all the interventions and learned that they were few, infrequent, and disjointed. Armed with the information he collected, Paul mobilized other educators to implement a tracking system for these students and to provide summer interventions for each student, to include mentoring, tutoring, and contacts by school officials. Paul's advocacy skills enabled him to implement a systemwide change that included safety nets for the students of his school.

Changing Attitudes and Beliefs

A leadership effort among school counselors, principals, teachers, other educators, and community members is particularly crucial in changing attitudes and beliefs about student success and students' abilities to learn. School counselors as human relations experts can impact the beliefs and attitudes of teachers and administrators regarding widening opportunities for students.

The school counselor collaborating with other educators can help foster a vision and belief in the development of high aspirations in every child. The school counselor, who believes that all children should be supported to be successful in rigorous academic course work, will act in ways that demonstrate this belief, influencing other educators (Stone & Clark, 2001). For example, if a school counselor advocates for students to have access to rigorous course work and then helps to establish safety nets such as tutoring and mentoring to support the success of these students, then the counselor has acted in a way that demonstrates a belief that all students can be supported to be successful.

The preparation that school counselors receive in communication skills, interpersonal relationships, problem solving, and conflict resolution gives them a vantage point in promoting collaboration among colleagues. In a collaborative leadership model, the roles of principals, teachers, and school counselors are interchangeable, allowing them to work together to impact attitudes and beliefs in each student's ability to learn and also to improve instruction and provide support in the classroom.

Advocating for Individual Students

Advocacy for early prevention and systemic interventions should focus on all students. Changing the system to meet the needs of individuals rather than trying to make the round peg fit into a square hole is a large part of advocacy. We impact systems to make a difference for every individual in that system. Advocacy requires us to give some individual students more help to right an injustice against them, improve their condition, or provide an opportunity.

Advocating for Your School Counseling Program

School counselors who know how to advocate for their program are less likely to be saddled with responsibilities that are extraneous to the goals of school counseling. Behaving as an advocate demonstrates that school counselors can carry out a program curriculum just as the English, mathematics, and science teachers are implementing their curriculum. Having a plan in mind assists school counselors to assess

Counselors Making a Difference

Meet Sejal Parikh

An Advocate for Individual Students

An example of changing systems while also working with individuals can be found in the work of Sejal Parikh, an urban elementary school counselor. Sejal suspected that there was an inordinate number of discipline referrals in fourth grade. She tested her observations by gathering school data on the referrals. She found that for the previous year, discipline referrals increased each month, until finally there were 30 suspensions for the month of May. Sejal took this information to the administration of the school, who gave her time on the next faculty meeting agenda to discuss the information. In a presentation, Sejal used charts and graphs to demonstrate the discipline and suspension rates for each month. The teachers were alarmed; they had no idea so many students were out of school on a daily basis. During the next hour, the teachers, administrators, and Sejal brainstormed and strategized to find ways of reducing or eliminating suspensions and the attendance problem. Sejal established a new goal for her school counseling program: to deliver classroom guidance lessons on conflict resolution and to work with individual students who were most in danger of being suspended. Sejal brought her skills and her programs' objectives to bear on changing discipline and suspension rates by establishing a behavior management program, which included a brief daily contact to check on progress, for the students most at risk of suspension. This is an example of a counselor identifying a problem through observation, corroborating her observations with real data, developing a plan with the faculty and other stakeholders, and implementing that plan with good results. The discipline referrals for fourth grade went from 19 in February to 7 in April.

Reprinted with permission by Sejal Parikh.

the needs of the school and develop program strategies around those needs. This is vitally important to the success of the school counseling program. Advocacy requires placing a schedule on the office door which demonstrates that taking assignments such as hall monitoring means that some vital contact time with students will be lost. If extraneous duties are suggested, then the school counselor can present the schedule and ask for help with solving the problem of what to take out to comply with their request. Advocacy is educating legislators, school board members, parents, administrators, and teachers about the school counseling program. Advocacy for the school counseling program is joining a professional organization that provides school counselors with a legislative voice.

Advocating for Social Action in the Wider Context of Community

Families and Institutions of Society

Counselors can be agents of social change in the wider community by helping students and families develop the strength and the strategies needed to advocate for themselves in relationship to other institutions in society. For example, counselors can provide information and resources or teach families how to

- use legal aid to get delinquent child support for their families;
- negotiate city hall to force their landlord to make needed repairs on their dwelling;
- file for financial aid assistance so they can go back to school;
- get job training;
- find free medical help;
- find counseling services for their children;
- get special services for their academically challenged child;
- find mentors and tutors for their children;
- access social services for elderly parents.

A counselor who is an agent of social change can rally families to write legislators to push for changes in laws that adversely impact them and to lobby lawmakers for their rights. Political action, voicing their concerns, overcoming reticence to advocate for themselves, and other such proactive steps usually result in families who are better able to shake helplessness and exercise more control over their own destiny (Lee & Walz, 1998).

Service Learning

School counselors can encourage involvement of students in service learning and also address some of the social problems, issues, and injustices of their larger community. The tragedy of September 11 resulted in many school counselors taking the time to advocate for tolerance and cultural acceptance while advocating against labeling our Muslim neighbors as dangerous.

Advocacy Skills

Advocacy to support students involves specific skills, not just a philosophical orientation to function as an advocate. It is important that counselors learn how to bring about change. Simply suggesting that counselors be change agents without helping them grow in acquiring the specific skills needed for educational advocacy is unlikely to produce positive effects on students, schools, or counselors.

Use of Technology for Advocacy

One of the most powerful skills acquired in school counselor preparation and in-service programs is technology. School counselors use technology advances to offer better services to students, and with a concerted effort have enhanced and changed forever the way they support teachers and foster student development (Tyler & Sabella, 2003).

Martin (1998) described technology as a critical tool in advocacy, explaining that counselors must learn to use technology in monitoring student progress, student career planning, and in acquiring and accessing the data needed to inform the decision making of individual students and of the entire school. School counselors who understand equity issues and have the technological skills to aggregate and disaggregate student information have critical, powerful skills that allow them to act as advocates in identifying and eliminating school practices that deter equitable access and in providing opportunities for student success in higher level academics. Through the use of technology, the school counselor/advocate can identify broad systemwide practices that deter access to rigorous course work and also can uncover inequitable situations for individual students. Using school district data obtained from a school's student information management system, school counselors can manage and monitor patterns of enrollment and student success.

Technological skills are needed by school counselors in their role of social advocates in order to support students' academic achievement. Technology enhances the counselor's role in advocacy, and in certain situations, such as looking at course enrollment patterns, the advocacy task can only be accomplished through the use of technology. "Today's students have changed the way they learn and today's counselors must change the way they communicate on behalf of student academic success. . . . If learner outcomes can be better achieved through technology, it is incumbent that counselors adapt their strategies accordingly" (Casey, 1995, p. 34).

Many school counselors have student information management systems or databases available within their schools or districts. These databases are extremely useful when working with students because the systems contain student biographical information as well as data regarding scheduling, attendance, discipline, current grades, past academic performance, test scores, test history, and so on. The information in these systems can be exported to relational databases to provide more flexibility and increased accessibility to more student information. Student data management systems can be accessed with varying degrees of ease depending on the school system. Some school systems go so far as to give laptops to administrators; at the touch of a finger, the administrators are able to access data that others wait weeks to acquire. However, when advocating for the needed information, know what to ask for and go after this information with a steady insistence. If the information is not available, ask for a program to be written to provide you with the data necessary to make informed decisions for your students. Assurances that no student will be left out of the picture are built into the student information management

Counselors Making a Difference

Meet Bob Turba, Penny Studstill, and Nan Worsowicz

Three Counselors Who Use Technology As an Advocacy Tool to Close the Information Gap

Lack of access to school counseling services means that academic counseling at critical junctures will be weak or nonexistent, which is a travesty for our students! School counselors are helping to close the information gap despite high caseloads. Here you will meet three counselors who represent the hundreds of school counselors who are exercising advocacy by offering their academic and career counseling to more students through technology. Shawna, a 12th-grader, is seeking advice on careers. She starts her search with the help of the school counselor, who assists her in completing a career inventory on the computer in the school counseling office. Shawna receives immediate feedback linking her results to national organizations, where she gets up-to-date information about possible careers and discovers trends in employment, salary, and other useful information. An example can be found at Career Mosaic (http://www.careermosaic.com/). After narrowing her choices of careers, Shawna conducts a college search by linking her career choices to college majors. Shawna compiles a list of colleges that interest her and decides to apply to four of the colleges that she discovered with her search. She applies online, searches the virtual college catalogs for all information about the schools, and even interfaces with students attending the colleges and majoring in the same field! Shawna applies online for all of the state scholarships, and also searches for other financial assistance. Shawna was able to use her parents' financial information to complete an online financial need estimation form that indicated the expected family contribution for a year of college expenses. An example of a site where this can be done is The Financial Aid Information Page (http://www.finaid.org). An example of a scholarship search site can be found at FastWeb (http://www.fastweb.com). Finally, Shawna linked to the Free Application For Federal Student Aid (FAFSA) website and completed an online FAFSA, receiving her results in 48 hours. With a little help from her counselor, Shawna began and finished a search for a career, college, scholarship application, and financial aid without leaving the computer (adapted from Stone & Turba, 1999).

From "School Counselors Using Technology for Advocacy," The Journal of Technology in Counseling, 1 (1) 1999. Retrieved from http://jtc.colstate.edu/vol1_1/advocacy.htm. The strategies were contributed by Bob Turba, Penny Studstill, and Nan Worsowicz, high-school counselors.

Reprinted with permission by Nan Worsowicz.

system. This provides equity in analysis as well as in access to opportunities, and also guarantees that no group of students will be left out of calculations.

Advocacy Through Staff Development

One of the principles of systemic change in education is to advocate for opportunities for staff to practice new skills, gather new information, or learn new behaviors. School counselors can have a significant role in this by contributing to staff development opportunities. The best educational practices or changes will not become daily practice if the faculty has not been properly educated and equipped.

Challenges exist in delivering staff development, but there are strategies that will help the counselor ensure success and gain support from administrators, teachers, parents, and other stakeholders. Getting the input of teachers before planning a staff development activity is a smart approach; top-down planning is rarely welcomed by participants. Collaborative planning is the optimum way to proceed because it brings greater commitment on the part of teachers as stakeholders. Collaborative planning is time-consuming, but the results are worth the investment when the staff development activity proposed has the potential for impacting students.

Counselors Making a Difference

Meet Chris Bryan

A Counselor Who Uses Technology to Increase Professional Development

High-school counselor Chris Bryan believes in the value of technology to help him do his work. He has developed four websites, primarily to promote his professional development and that of his colleagues. Chris graduated from the University of North Florida school counseling program called SOAR (School Counselors: Supporters of Academic Rigor) and has for the last three years kept a website of PowerPoint presentations, journal articles, and other materials created by his professors and all SOAR students. That website (http://www.crb9000.com), which is the first one he developed, is a valued tool for helping counseling candidates and graduates share their talent, creativity, and ideas. Chris says, "I hope this site will help future counselors become more comfortable with technology as it relates to school counseling so that they are prepared to utilize it as a medium to advocate for their students and faculty."

(continued)

Chris created another website, found at http://www.jaxcollegefair.com, in his work as a member of the National Association for College Admission Counseling (NACAC) college fair committee (his first year as a counselor!). Again, this is a valued resource for his colleagues' professional development. His third site, which is at http://www.educationcentral.org/rhs, is the site for his high school. Chris maintains the site, and he says, "Although this work has cost me some time, I feel that it has been worth it, as I have been able to develop and disperse tools that are tailored to empower students and parents to make well-informed decisions concerning [the students'] current academic careers and their life after high school. I am also able to use the communication and public relations skills I learned in the SOAR program to help bring Ribault High School and the community together in a positive and productive way. For instance, I recently added an alumni page that I feel will help us recruit volunteers and possibly help us network with business partners."

Chris's fourth and last website is the district guidance site for Duval County Public Schools in Jacksonville, Florida (http://www.duvalguidance.com). The supervisor of guidance, Judy Cromartie, asked Chris about collaborating with her and the other district staff to create the site. The result of this collaboration is a website that "contains pretty much everything the district staff, other counselors, and I know about school counseling and using the Internet for advocacy for students, and [it] includes all of the latest and greatest resources and information available. I am also especially proud of the counselor's corner section, dedicated to helping the counselors of the DCPS with professional development and resources. I could go on for pages about all the reasons I love this site, but I kind of hope that it speaks for itself."

Because of Chris's advocacy through technology work, the district school counseling program has been promised "favorable consideration" for the guidance site in the new website design that's due out shortly. Also, Chris reports, "the extra work I do at the school to help out with technology issues has allowed me to do certain things I may not otherwise have been able to do. I have procured two new computers for student use in the guidance office for college and career preparation, whereas before there was no computer access for students in guidance. I have been able to advocate for students and teachers to have not only technology, but the proper support and training needed to make the technology work properly. I believe that, in general, I have more of a voice in the school, and am perceived as more of a leader than I would be without my dedication to technology."

Reprinted with permission by Chris Bryan.

Seven Recommended Steps When Advocating for Change

Here is a set of seven steps you can use to approach any advocacy situation, regardless of the change you are attempting to effect.

1. *Identify the problem.*   Informally identify a situation in your school that you believe to be an obstacle or problem. Test your hypothesis by gathering data to illuminate the problem. Is the problem multidimensional? In other words, what is the scope of the problem? Who is affected by the problem?

2. *Gather additional information.*   Determine what additional information one needs to know in examining the problem. How will this information be gathered? Can you gather the information through informal conversations, formal interviews, surveys, and/or tapping into the student-information management system?

3. *Identify the stakeholders.*   Who needs to be involved in addressing this problem? Who are the stakeholders that need to come together to address the problem? Is there already a vehicle or forum in place, such as the school improvement team, to help address the problem? With the help of the stakeholders, identify the internal and external community members who must be involved in addressing the problem.

4. *Research the advocacy history of the problem.*   What has already been done by others in your school to address the problem? What can you learn from these previous efforts? Is there any research you can find from other school sites on strategies to address the problem?

5. *Identify the institutional and/or environmental barriers contributing to the problem.* Analyze the barriers. Are the barriers systemic in nature, easy to remove, complicated? Identify those who would bring conflict or resistance to efforts to implement the strategies the collaborators have identified as needed. From where does the resistance originate? Should you tackle trying to change the resistance, or in this situation should you just move through, around, or over it?

6. *Develop an action plan.*   In concert with the other principal stakeholders, develop an action plan to address the problem. The action plan consists of stakeholders identifying proven strategies that they would feel qualified to implement. A timeline for completion of strategies and for an interim check of progress would be a helpful part of the action plan.

7. *Set goals and develop accountability measures.*   How will you evaluate the effectiveness of your advocacy program? Does the program have a timeline? Determine the goal of the program and set interim targets that you will aspire to reach as you steadily move toward improvement. Decide in advance how you will measure achievement of those goals.

Advocacy in Action

You can best learn the steps to advocacy by working through an exercise using a hypothetical example. We will provide the story line of the example and insert information at various points in the exercise. Use what you have learned so far—and some imagination—to fill in the information we have left blank.

In this example you are using data to advocate for students and your school counseling program. As a member of the leadership team of the school, you are in step with the mission of your school to impact the academic achievement of your students. You want to be another set of "eyes" and "ears," ferreting out problem areas and addressing them. You continually hear from teachers that there is an attendance problem but none of them are able to give you specific information about the problem.

1. *Identify the problem.*   Using Step 1, you have identified attendance as a problem area for your school. Your data gathering has revealed that

   32% of absences of the school are for fifth graders;

   71% of these students are boys;

   51% of the absences happen on the first day back after a weekend or holiday.

2. *Gather additional information.*   After additional research using Step 2, you have found that bullying is a serious problem in fifth grade and that many students are avoiding coming to school because they are being bullied. On Mondays the rate of absence is aggravated by bus delays, parents and children who have problems getting started on Mondays, and so on.

3. *Identify the stakeholders.*   Who needs to be involved in addressing the problem of bullying? How might they be brought to the table?

   _____

   _____

   _____

4. *Research the advocacy history of the problem.*   What may already have been done by others to address the problem of bullying? What can be learned from these previous efforts? Is there any research on addressing the problem?

   _____

   _____

   _____

5. *Identify the institutional and/or environmental barriers contributing to the problem.* What institutional and environmental factors might constitute barriers to solving the problem of bullying at this school?

_____

_____

_____

6. *Develop an action plan.* What will be the specific strategies of your school counseling program to reduce bullying, and therefore absenteeism, for the fifth-grade boys?

_____

_____

_____

7. *Set goals and develop accountability measures.* How will you evaluate the effectiveness of your school counseling program to reduce bullying, and therefore absenteeism, for the fifth-grade boys? Does the goal have an interim target that you are aspiring to reach as you steadily move toward improvement? Does the target have a timeline?

_____

_____

_____

Guiding Principles of Effective Advocacy

1. Be a risk taker; that is, be a calculated risk taker. You must be politically astute to live to "play the game" another day, but at the same time, being too conservative or paralyzed by the fear of possibly bringing disfavor on yourself or being overly concerned about protecting yourself will keep you from exercising an advocacy role to the extent to which you are capable. Your students need you to be their voice when no one else will.

2. Believe you can make a difference as you relentlessly, respectfully, and collaboratively pursue your advocacy role. Just as it is the salesperson's responsibility to make a sale, the CEO's responsibility to monitor the profit margin, and the nurse's responsibility to make certain the right medicine is administered, it is your responsibility to act as advocate for your students. Make it happen.

3. Believe in your students. Don't allow yourself or others to sidetrack your efforts at advocacy with the "bless their hearts" syndrome. Students need our empathy, not our sympathy, which only serves to hinder us from challenging and causing students to better their situation. Empathy will help us empower students and support them to achieve despite their sometimes dismal options.

4. Advocacy is difficult, and we should be willing to take advantage of opportunities to be kind to ourselves and to celebrate our successes, however small.

5. Stay the course. Don't accept failure. As school counselors we must believe we can effect change. *"Those who entertain the possibility of losing are only a doubt away from its reality."* (Author unknown.)

TechTools

When you become a school counselor, use the power of technology to maximize the efficiency and effectiveness of your advocacy.

- Use technology to help you develop four-year career plans for students. Help students become their own advocates for their future career plans by helping them learn to use the Internet for career tasks such as interest inventories, identifying job clusters, and finding higher education institutions that offer preparation in the job clusters or specific jobs in which they are interested.
- Using technology, identify school practices that deter equitable access and opportunities for student success. For example, find out who has access to the higher level classes.
- Provide staff development using PowerPoint presentations so that teachers and administrators can acquire new skills, gather new information, or learn new behaviors. A 10-minute presentation during weekly faculty meetings can strengthen your position as a member of the leadership team.
- Set up computer conferences for your students who are experiencing personal, social, or emotional problems.
- Set up videoconferencing so that students who do not have the benefit of visiting college campuses can virtually tour campuses and meet with the admissions people.
- Develop listservers for parents, students, and school counselors to exchange information needed to advocate for students.
- Develop e-mail mentoring or tutoring programs so that older students, business partners, and community agency members can encourage or assist students. For example, if the absenteeism for chronic offenders happens on Mondays, have your e-mail mentoring on Mondays.

- Have computers in the school counseling office for mentorship, career advising, and other such activities. Find businesses and community members to donate them and help them stay up and running.
- Benefit from collaborating with fellow counselors who have established websites that offer critical, timely information about student issues ranging from scholarship resources to eating disorders. Some examples of sites are http://wisemantech.com/guidance and http://www.cyberguidance.net.
- Build the potential of students to participate in the 21st-century economy by helping all students have access to technology.

School Counselor Casebook: *Voices From the Field*

The Scenario Reviewed

You have just finished a session with the fifth student in your caseload, who is in danger of failing the marking period because she was suspended for tardiness. The halls of your overcrowded school are almost impassable during the five-minute class changes. The school policy states that students who are late for class are locked out until they bring a tardy slip from the office. The line to get a tardy slip is very long, causing students to sometimes miss as much as the first 20 minutes of class. Additionally, seven total tardies in a grading period mean five days of after-school detention or suspension for two days. Many students are choosing suspension instead of detention because of their work obligations. You take a look at the discipline data and you are shocked to learn that 27% of the suspensions began as multiple tardies.

A Practitioner's Approach

Here's how a practicing school counselor responded to this school scenario:

After observing the lengthy tardy lines, I checked with data processing to confirm the scope of the problem and indeed, the number of tardies is troubling. Using this data, I identified my students who are accruing significant numbers of tardies. I interviewed them as to why they are late for classes. They said consistently, "Mr. Katz, the distance between our classes is way too long for us to get through these crowded halls in time and if we are even 30 seconds late the teachers will not admit us!"

Armed with data to support the seriousness of the problem and feeling confident that my students' reasons for being late are valid, I set up a time to meet with the administration. They stated that there is plenty of time for the students to get from any point in the building to any other point in the building during the five-minute passing period and that they supported the teachers not admitting the students who are late. I acknowledged that many students do dawdle in the halls; however, I was not sure that it is possible for some students to make it from the east end of the first floor in the old building to the west end of the third floor in the new building in only five minutes. After a brief discussion, we decided that a teacher and I, along with the assistant principal, will follow the schedule of a student traveling from the farthest extremes of the building. We soon discovered that this trip from classroom to classroom takes us between 5 minutes and 20 seconds to 6 full minutes with not a second to stop!

With input from the teachers, we decided to issue a color-coded ID to the students who must make these long passages, and their teachers consented to admit them if they are less than two minutes late to class.

Eric D. Katz, MSAC, is a New York State Certified School Counselor working at Newburgh Free Academy, a public high school in Newburgh, New York. Mr. Katz is a member of the College Board's National Faculty for the Equity and Excellence Program and has conducted counselor trainings across the United States. In addition, he has served as the vice president for secondary level school counselors for The New York State School Counselor Association. Reprinted with permission by Eric D. Katz.

Chapter Summary

The Role of Social Advocacy in Counseling

School counselors who understand issues impacting equity of opportunity can help change systems that continue to adversely stratify students' opportunities. The school counselor who behaves as a social change agent plays a high-profile, powerful role and increases his or her effectiveness in multiple ways.

School Counselors As Advocates

The preparation that school counselors receive in communication skills and interpersonal relationship development facilitates their effectiveness in advocacy for both individual students and for systemic change. Social action and social intervention are readily available roles, because counseling is generally perceived by administrators, parents, and teachers to be a natural fit for advocacy.

Personal-Social Consciousness for the School Counselor As Advocate

School counselors do not merely master the nuts and bolts of counseling, but have the heart and soul needed to advocate for their students. School counselors who serve as social activists are risk takers with a sensitivity to the needs of students, genuine positive regard for others, compassion, flexibility, understanding, empathy, insightfulness, and emotional stability.

The Ethics of Advocacy

Advocacy is both a legal obligation and an ethical imperative for school counselors. The Five Moral Principles of beneficence, nonmaleficence, loyalty, and the promotion of autonomy and justice serve as a context for framing ethical behavior.

Advocacy Impacts Students, School Climates, Systems, the School Counseling Program, and Communities

Counselors as systemic change agents are able to impact all students in their caseloads when they change or improve the policies, procedures, or practices in the school that are hindering students. School counselors as advocates examine and intervene in the environment to promote an emotionally and physically safe school that supports equal opportunities for all students to get a good education. Other systems in which students have to move, such as home and the wider community, are also of concern to school counselors.

Advocating for Social Action in the Wider Context of Community

School counselors who have a strong sense of social responsibility often seek to be agents of social change in the wider community by helping students and families develop the strength and the strategies needed to advocate for themselves. School counselors are encouraging involvement of students in service learning and are also addressing some of the social problems, issues, and injustices of their larger community.

Skills for Advocacy

A philosophical orientation to function as an advocate is important but is of little use in isolation of the specific skills needed by advocates. Using technology and providing staff development are two of the advocacy skills examined throughout this textbook.

Key Terms

Advocacy p. 121

Autonomy p. 126

Beneficence p. 125

Change agent p. 123

Information gap p. 126

Justice p. 126

Loyalty p. 126
Nonmaleficence p. 125
Personal-social consciousness p. 123
Personal-social consciousness skills p. 121

Social justice agenda p. 121
Systemic barriers p. 127
Systemic change p. 127

Learning Extensions

1. Interview a practicing counselor about three or four systemic practices, policies, or procedures that he or she believes enhance students' ability to be successful, and three or four systemic barriers to students' success. Discuss how you would try to address these barriers.

2. Think about your time as a student in a school, or your work with any school. Can you describe the course assignment or tracking procedures of the school? In other words, who decided which procedures were used for determining who gets in the blue bird or the red bird group, Spanish I, or AP calculus? What data were used in making these decisions?

3. If you were given 15 minutes at the next faculty meeting for a staff development presentation, what topic would you like to deliver that would make a difference for students? What data would you use? How would you use technology to deliver this topic?

4. Your principal is desperately trying to raise the dismal 70% daily attendance rate, which is one of the areas of accountability for principals in the district. Devise a plan to help effect this change by applying the seven steps to advocacy.

5. Chose four of the following topics and write a two-paragraph response explaining what the topic means to you in your future role as a school counselor.
   - Collaborating with Stakeholders to Make Systemic Change
   - Using Data As an Advocacy Tool
   - Connecting School Counseling to School Reform
   - Achieving Access and Equity for All Students
   - Surviving Financial Crises Through Accountability
   - Building Multicultural and Diversity Skills for All School Personnel
   - Creating a Climate Sensitive to Diversity and Cultural Differences
   - Challenging and Changing Attitudes and Beliefs
   - Using Technology to Support your Advocacy Role

6. Discuss all the ways you can think of in which Bernadette Willette impacted her school's students, parents, teachers, administration, and community. Why was her approach effective?

Chapter 6

School Counselors as Consultants

Chapter Objectives

By the time you have completed this chapter, you should be able to:

- Define consultation and apply models of consultation.
- Explain the role of the school counselor as a consultant.
- Understand the power of collaborative facilitation and how to use the model.
- Define the relationship between the consultant and parent as consultee and teacher as consultee.
- Describe effective parent conferences.
- Describe the four Ds of the consultation process.
- Develop a collaborative action plan.

School Counselor Casebook: Getting Started

The Scenario

Currently there are 22 students who have been referred to you because they are underachievers, capable but not completing work. You have limited time to work individually with these students but you want to impact their progress. In the past you have had a good success rate in working with underachievers individually in behavior management programs. As your success rate climbs, more teachers are referring underachievers to you.

Thinking About Solutions

As you read this chapter, think about possible solutions. Describe the consultation role you might exercise in helping these 22 students and other underachievers. Consider whether the consultation role might be preferable to just working with these students individually. When you come to the end of the chapter, you will have the opportunity to see how your ideas compare with a practicing school counselor's approach.

The Effectiveness of Consultation in the Schools

Research supports consultation as an effective method of service delivery in a school setting (Wilkinson, 2003). **Consultation** in schools is described by authors in many different ways, but is commonly described as a problem-solving approach with the adults in the student's life that are in a position to impact positive change (Friend & Cook, 2003; Kampwirth, 2003; Zins, Kratochwill, & Elliott, 1993). The consultant brings expertise to another professional or parent in this triadic relationship to benefit the third party, the student or the system (DeBoer, 1995; Friend & Cook, 2003). Consultation is a specialized problem-solving process in which one professional who has particular expertise assists another professional (or parent) who needs the benefit of that expertise (DeBoer, 1995).

In the **triadic-dependent model,** the consultant is viewed as an expert in child behavior. The consultant advises as to the origins and causes of problems and makes recommendations as to how to alleviate the difficulties the student is facing (Kratochwill & Bergan, 1990). In this model, the immediate goal of the consultant as expert is to increase the skills, knowledge, and objectivity of the consultee so that the consultee can more successfully help the consultant implement an intervention plan (Delaney & Kaiser, 2001). Kampwirth (2003) defines consultation as a collaborative process in which the consultant and consultee share responsibility for designing and implementing interventions that are in the best educational interests of their students.

Kampwirth (2003) provides a critical viewpoint for school counselors to consider when developing their role as consultants. While others in the helping field speak of the differentiated responsibilities for decisions and accountability for outcomes (Friend & Cook, 2003), Kampwirth (2003) discusses a shared responsibility with regard to decisions and outcomes. Kampwirth's spirit of collaboration is an excellent fit for the school counselor/consultant because it maintains an equal partnership among all parties involved, including shared responsibility for outcomes and accountability.

In the past, collaboration and consultation were viewed as discrete skills, with consultation requiring an expert. This view implied a differentiation of power. Collaboration had little to do with the consultation process, but was considered a valued skill among educators in their roles as team players and committee members. **Collaborative consultation** is now a consultation model for the school setting (Kampwirth, 2003). There is consensus among many authors of consultation texts that in schools the expert model is far less effective than is the collaborative model, because in schools people are more likely to implement change if they are involved in discussing and creating the solutions (Dettmer, Thurston, & Dyck, 2001; Friend & Cook, 2003).

For example, teachers have a tough job, and when they reach out for help it can be frustrating if the school counselor as "expert" comes in and, without collaboration, offers solutions that the teacher feels miss the mark because the counselor is unaware of the interpersonal dynamics, concerns, or issues involved in the teacher's daily struggles. In the collaborative approach, the synergy generated by an interchange of ideas will lead to relationship building and increases the potential for success. The remainder of this chapter will emphasize a collaborative consultation approach, placing attention on relationship building, communication skills, problem-solving approaches, and accountability for results.

The American School Counselor Association (ASCA) position statement entitled *The Professional School Counselor and Comprehensive School Counseling Programs* requires school counselors to deliver consultation services as a member of the educational team (1997). "Professional school counselors are indispensable partners with the instructional staff in the development of contributing members of society" (ASCA, 1997, p.1). Consultation and collaboration with teachers, administrators and families helps students be successful academically, vocationally and personally (ASCA, 1997).

Consultation as a Powerful Tool

Consultation is valued by school counselors as a powerful tool that allows them to have a far-reaching, lasting impact on the school's internal community members, such as students, teachers, administrators, and paraprofessionals, and on the external community members, such as parents and counseling agencies (Fitch & Marshall, 2004; Gysbers & Henderson, 2001; Kahn, 2000; Myrick, 2003a).

The school counselor as consultant extends his or her reach to more students by working collaboratively with the adults in a student's life who can make a major impact on the student's academic, career, and social-emotional life (Fitch & Marshall, 2004; Kahn, 2000).

School counselors behaving as skilled consultants are key contributors toward helping give students the gift of becoming successful in school (Fitch, Newby, Ballestero, & Marshall, 2001; Stone & Clark, 2001). There are many **unalterable factors** that school counselors are powerless to impact, such as whether or not a student has at least one loving parent and comes to school fed and ready to learn (Kenny, 2003). However, there are alterable factors over which school counselors wield tremendous influence when, as consultants, they work with parents, teachers, and administrators to benefit a student, or to remove a barrier that is impeding progress for a student.

Consultation as an Effective Use of Time

Parsimony refers to an efficient use of time described as advocating that school counselors spend their time where they can impact the most students (Myrick, 2003). When working in partnership with an administrator or teacher to develop strategies to positively impact one student, the consultee can go on to apply those skills, knowledge bases, and resources to many more students. Even though counselor-to-student ratios are often too high, consultation helps meet the needs of many more students through the **rule of parsimony**. The impact of consultation is exponential as the consultee and the school counselor together learn intervention strategies for future application. In a successful consultation, knowledge gained is transferred to new situations, ideas germinate into plans that benefit many more students, and highly skilled professionals emerge. Direct service delivery, such as individual counseling, reaches one student at a time, while consultation indirectly impacts the student by working with the other adults in the student's life (Gysbers & Henderson, 2001; Myrick, 2003a).

There will always be a place for individual work with students; however, "there is evidence that consultation enables practitioners to lend assistance to larger numbers of children in a more timely manner than approaches used in the past" (Zins et al., 1993, p. 5).

The Consultant as Facilitator

The complex problems of children in schools often go beyond the expertise of even the most seasoned and skilled school counselor. Equal collaboration avoids having the unilateral onus of fixing problems. The simple gesture of admitting that no one person has all the answers (no school counselor does) helps ease the burden on school counselors to magically solve students' problems and in many cases promotes a partnership when the counselor is clear that only a collaborative effort can adequately address a student's problem. Conveying that you don't have all the answers will at times encourage consultees to voice their ideas and opinions and also communicates to consultees that they are needed and valued players.

Consultation should focus on an equal partnership, but there will be many occasions when the school counselor will have greater knowledge and a larger contribution to the problem solving required in the partnership. The point of an equal partnership in consultation is to focus on the facilitative role rather than accepting the burden of acting as an "expert" in all the problems that students and families face. School counselors who understand the developmental issues and academic and personal-social concerns will often bring more expertise to the consultation partnership. Consultation is a process of problem solving; it is not an imbalance of power with the need to possess all the answers. In school consultation, the power comes from the consultation partnership, in which equal problem solving is expected and helping others feel empowered is one of the goals (Friend & Cook, 2003; Kampwirth, 2003). Differentiation of power or lack of some of the basic tenets of relationship building complicates the work and unduly burdens counselors to carry the load. A skilled consultant knows that an equal partnership better prepares consultees to handle their next crisis or obstacle. The school counselor's power comes not from being the child development expert, but rather from possessing strong interpersonal skills and a willingness to be engaged with the consultee.

We have observed that effective school counselor/consultants bring commitment, skill, resources, and knowledge to the consulting relationship. The counselor/consultant is resourceful, working to find answers, solutions, strategies, and resources; effective in interpersonal skills; and committed to collaboration. Textbook knowledge about causes of and solutions to students' and system problems will not translate into an effective consultant.

Consultees may include internal members of the school, such as a classroom teacher, administrator, media specialist, special education teacher, or school nurse. The **external consultee** may be a parent, agency personnel, mentor, tutor, community health care provider, or any other member of the larger community who has an interest in student success but is not regularly housed in a school setting. School counselors as consultants will use both their internal and external resources to try to help their students.

Your primary consultees will be teachers, parents, and the system. The remainder of this chapter will focus on the consultation role with these three consultees.

Consulting With Teachers

Teachers will seek you in the halls, the lounge, through e-mail, and through notes in your mailbox, and they also will appear at your office door. Teachers as consultees will be as varied as the myriad problems that students face. In our experience, teachers as consultants generally fall into one of five categories: confident, questioning, dependent, absentee, or dominating.

1. *The confident teacher.* Highly skilled teachers who have sound ideas will collaborate with the school counselor to validate and confirm that the approach they plan to use with a student is the right one. The confident consultee is the teacher who has a history of being successful with students, and she or he reaches out to the school counselor to serve as a resource for agencies, tutors, mentors, materials, and as a sounding board. The confident consultee generally supports even your smallest effort and appreciates the fact that you have listened and offered thoughtful comments and ideas.

2. *The questioning teacher.* These teachers come to the consultant because they have tried and failed to effect change in students; they need a new voice and new strategies. These skilled teachers only ask for shared responsibility in trying to help their students. Questioning consultees are rewarding to work with because they exercise a good-faith effort to follow through and to take responsibility for implementing the strategies that were generated through your partnership.

3. *The dependent teacher.* Some teacher/consultees will demand immediate results. These teachers often are less skilled at behavior and classroom management and are struggling or overwhelmed. These teachers have unrealistic expectations of counselors and maintain a "take these students and fix them and send them back cured by sixth period" approach. Rather than falling into the trap of unrealistic demands, the consultant must spend time and energy reframing these teachers' requests that the consultant be in the "fix it" business and skillfully coax a collaborative effort that will examine the strategies that the

teacher has tried in the past and develop interventions and resources for the future. Dependency on the consultant may develop if the counselor as consultant acts as the expert and takes on the problems as his or hers to solve.

4. *The absentee teacher.*   Certain teachers will never call on you, either because they feel that they should be able to solve all problems in their class or because they refuse to admit that any problems exist. There are ways to groom a collaborative relationship with the absentee consultee through other areas, such as jointly planning classroom guidance lessons. Assisting in this way will place you in a positive light and help grow the working relationship between the teacher and counselor.

5. *The dominating teacher.*   The fifth type of teacher as consultee is the one who will try to monopolize your time. Unfettered, this teacher will deplete your energy and time. It is necessary to set boundaries to combat the teacher who behaves as if she or he is your only consultee, demanding your undivided attention. Setting and keeping specified appointment times, collaboratively developing action plans, and establishing one or two weekly check-in times for action plan evaluation may help to reduce the dominator's demands on you.

No one teacher/consultee falls neatly into these categories, but will display combinations or variations of these. With patience, flexibility, and interpersonal skills, you are acquiring what West and Idol (1987) refer to as the art of consultation. Strong collaborative communication and negotiation skills will move teachers along the continuum to the questioning or confident consultee.

PREPARE for Effective Consultation With Teachers

To help you remember the key concepts, best practices, and pitfalls of effective consultation, we have developed **PREPARE**—an acronym for Philosophy, Relationships, Equity of power, Professional development, Accessibility, Resources, Evaluate.

Philosophy

School counselors establish a philosophy of consultation that matches the mission of their schools. The mission of the school counseling program aligns with and follows the mission of every school in America: to support all students to be successful learners and productive citizens.

Relationships

Relationship building is vital to each role you will perform as a school counselor, but never more so than in the consultation role, in which interpersonal skills can spell the difference between success and failure. Other chapters have addressed relationship building, but this section focuses specifically on the importance of relationship building in the consultation role. Here are some guiding principles for building a reputation and interpersonal relationships with teachers:

- Appreciate and understand how demanding and difficult it is to be a teacher.
- Avoid absolutes, blame, and judgment. It is not a function of the consultation relationship to assign guilt or blame or to categorize.
- Avoid absolute statements such as "her classroom is chaos" or "he could care less about teaching"; rarely are they true. Consultants usually cannot hide a judgmental attitude. Facial expressions, tone of voice, and choice of words will convey true feelings. Consultees sense and react to a judgmental attitude by raising their defenses, which in turn lowers their willingness to cooperate (Gable, Mostert, & Tonelson, 2004; Staton & Gilligan, 2003).
- Follow through on commitments made to consultees. This is essential to achieve credibility.
- Identify teachers and parents who are open to working with you and use that as a starting point in your consultation role to build your confidence before moving on to more challenging consultees.
- Recognize the irrevocable harm to your role if you are viewed as untrustworthy. For example, avoid reporting a colleague to the administration unless you are certain it will be handled skillfully. Once it is known that you deliver information to the administration, you have diminished your capacity to be effective. Work through other channels to help teachers bring resolution to their problems before taking the drastic step of reporting. A good relationship with the administration will help you forward the consultation role without risking being viewed by the faculty as being against them.
- Provide a welcoming atmosphere and demeanor. Personable individuals tend to be more successful in school consultation. "People are more willing to work with affable, outgoing, friendly people than with people who aren't" (Kampwirth, 2003, p. 143).
- Practice genuine respect and a belief that the consultee can effect change and contribute to the consultation process. Search your consciousness and truly believe in the inherent dignity and worth of each consultee (even those whose actions offend you). Beliefs determine actions (Martin, 2004). **Positive self-talk** before each work session about the potential of the consultee to make progress will translate to positive interactions.

Equity of Power

A critical factor of "a collaborative approach to consultation is that of egalitarianism, or a non-hierarchical relationship between the consultant and the consultee" (Kampwirth, 2003, p. 145). There is much wisdom in helping your consultee feel empowered to be an equal partner or dominant force in solving problems. Reframe discussions when the consultee wants to place the burden on you to solve the problem. A carefully worded request, such as "let's sit down and brainstorm some strategies," emphasizes the need for a partnership. Treating consultees with patience, avoiding a condescending tone or behavior, listening authentically, soliciting their suggestions, and showing that you value their input by incorporating their ideas into the plan promotes **equity of power.**

Professional Development

Grow your body of knowledge and expertise while fostering the professional development of potential consultees. Professional development is two-pronged: it enhances your own skills and delivers staff development to support the growth and development of faculty members and administrators.

Professional organizations, literature, conferences, and in-services will contribute to your professional development. Observations of other counselors or teachers who are most effective in meeting the needs of difficult or troubled students can help you grow your skills.

Position yourself as a vital resource to teachers and raise your profile by making staff development a routine part of your work. A 10-minute staff development workshop at each faculty meeting in which you convey information to help all faculty and staff places you in a favorable light as a willing respondent to teachers' and students' needs. Arrange for speakers or present important topics such as special education eligibility, eating disorders, Attention Deficit Hyperactivity Disorder (ADHD), suicidal ideation, or bullying. Other mediums for staff development would be grade level or departmental meetings, the school newsletter, PTA meetings, and parent workshops. Grant writing might help to provide the funds you need to bring in resources in the form of people and materials. Secure speakers by swapping places with another counselor so that each of you can present to the other's faculty. Without promoting unhealthy competition, find a way to focus on your teachers' best practices so as to replicate areas such as good classroom or behavior management.

Accessibility

Being accessible, professionally available, and approachable will further your efforts to be taken seriously as a consultant and to be considered a partner in the educational process. These guiding principles will assure your accessibility:

- Be visible in the halls, cafeteria, and classrooms consulting with teachers.
- Provide teachers and other potential consultees with a note that tells them you are there to help them and a list of the different types of consultation services you can deliver.
- Post your daily, weekly, and monthly schedule on your door with time for consultation clearly marked. Be flexible, and if at all possible, accommodate people who come in unannounced for consultation.

- Let it be known through various media that you are an advocate for students, parents, and teachers. Publicize consultation activities that extend beyond the traditional role of helping with troubled students to areas such as helping teachers with resources to support their classroom management, or finding tutors and mentors for students.
- Be part of the mainstream of the faculty, attending functions, socializing, and exchanging pleasantries. Avoid setting yourself apart, as this will impact your ability to be an effective consultant to help the students in your school.

Resources

Brokering and managing resources, both human and material, increases the effectiveness of the consultation role and allows you to widen your realm of influence. By becoming a manager of human resources, you extend your reach without overextending yourself. A consultant who brokers resources brings in as many agencies, business partners, parents, and other resources as possible to deliver strategies such as mentoring and tutoring. Just one eager trustworthy volunteer, under your direction, can set the wheels in motion to garner support from a variety of sources to help you with specific needs. The chapters on coordination of resources and accountability offer extensive information on potential stakeholders and resources to bring into your program. Groom a relationship with community agencies so that you can have contact information when you need to refer parents and others to outside resources. Some agencies will reposition support personnel into your school if you provide them with facilities.

- Develop a library of resources that address the issues and special needs of your student population. Use other media for your consultation role to supplement face-to-face conversations. Create a newsletter that features critical, timely information. Make computers available with important websites earmarked for parents and educators to use in searches.
- Provide teachers and administrators with resource materials. When you find a valuable free resource, order one for everyone in the school, and advocate for money when you need to purchase vital resources. For example, the U.S. Department of Education, at http://www.ed.gov/index.jsp, has online guides, programs, and the latest research to assist teachers and administrators.

Evaluate

Evaluate your effectiveness as a consultant by establishing baseline data, collaboratively implementing strategies, and then looking at the results in the form of impact data to see if the student improved in troublesome areas, such as attendance, grade point average, or promotion. Refer to Chapter 9 to learn how to evaluate your work through a six-step framework called MEASURE.

Consulting With Parents

Outcomes of educational consultation are likely to be more successful when there is an effective parent-educator partnership (Delaney & Kaiser, 2001; Epstein & Sheldon, 2002; Sanders, 2000). Student success is not only home or school, teacher or student, but the dynamic relationships between them; learning takes place where there are productive relationships among all participants in the educational process (Epstein & Sheldon, 2002; Sanders, 2000). It is a well-documented fact that student performance is enhanced by a strong relationship between parents and the school (Adelman & Taylor, 2003; Bemak, 2000; Epstein, 1988, 2001; Porter, Epp, & Bryant, 2000; Taylor, 2000).

Positive effects of parent involvement on student achievement are apparent across grade levels and for all socioeconomic status (SES) levels (Sanders, 2000; Sheldon & Epstein, 2002). When parents are involved, we know that students show improvement in grades, test scores, attitudes, and behavior; complete more homework; are more engaged in classroom learning activities; and have higher attendance rates and a reduction in suspension rates.

PARTNER for Effective Conferences With Parents

PARTNER is an acronym to help you remember a seven-step approach in facilitating the success of conferences with parents or guardians: Planning for success, Acknowledging parents as partners, Rapport building, Teaming to identify the problem, Negotiating a plan of action, Ending effectively, Regrouping. The school counselor as consultant can provide ongoing staff development to teachers and other educators about communicating effectively with parents and also facilitate the exchange of tips for conducting parent conferences and managing parent visits. Counselors acting as advocates can collaboratively create ground rules about how to conduct parent visits and help to establish a climate of acceptance, openness, and trust that will promote goodwill between the school and community (Anderson-Butcher & Ashton, 2004a; Keys, 2000; Sheldon & Epstein, 2002).

It is dangerous to assume that everyone understands the basic do's and don'ts of communication. Be an advocate for all members of the school community by helping teachers understand the tenets of positive written and verbal communication. By conducting staff development you can place the school in a better light, reduce the gossip and naysaying about the school, and minimize some of the problems that teachers have with parents. When parents visit the school for a parent conference, school counselors and teachers have the opportunity to develop an ally or a foe (Keys, 2000; Sheldon & Epstein, 2002). It is in everyone's best interest, but most important, in the best interest of the student, to try to maximize the school visit (Staton & Gilligan, 2003). These very basic, simple PARTNER skills will facilitate the parent conference:

Planning for Success

Prior to a teacher/parent conference, school counselors can help teachers plan for success. In advance of the conferences, help the teachers to:

- Recognize that they will be talking to parents about their child, someone for whom parents would give their lives. Helping teachers keep this thought in the forefront of their minds will reduce the defensiveness and frustrations that teachers feel when parents cannot be objective about their child's problems.
- Be prepared to hear angry words, accusations, and unfair statements, with the realization that to respond in kind is not an option. Parent's defense mechanisms may mean that they will behave badly. Teachers can learn to react all the more kindly under these circumstances.
- Think positive thoughts about the student. Remember, beliefs and attitudes are conveyed in our faces, tone, words, and actions.
- Recognize that for parents to come to school is sometimes intimidating or embarrassing. Create a pleasant physical environment where parents feel welcomed. If possible, offer them coffee, water, or a soft drink.
- Provide for an interpreter and/or someone to be present from the culture of the family if the teacher believes it will put parents more at ease.
- Keep the number of people in the room to a minimum. It is sometimes intimidating when a parent has to come into a room full of people with titles such as school psychologist and social worker. If possible, spend some time with the parent(s) alone to discuss confidentiality, to work on relationship building, to increase parents' comfort level, to explain to them who will be in the meeting and why, and if necessary, to help them understand you are an ally before plunging parents into a room full of people.
- Dress professionally, but in a way that helps parents identify with you. This approach may require professional dress that is more understated.

Acknowledging Parents as Partners

School counselors can help teachers increase the likelihood of a successful conference if they can help the teacher validate and acknowledge parents as true partners in the problem-solving arena. Help the teachers to:

- Understand that parents are doing the best they can or know how to do. They love their children, and should not be dismissed just because they do not respond the way we believe they should.
- Convey confidence in having the parent as a partner. By having parents feel empowered to be a partner, teachers reduce the likelihood of one-upmanship

that can drive a wedge between teachers and parents and places the burden on each party to solve the problem alone.

- Recognize and value the parents' rights to be the guiding voice in their child's life and really listen to what their needs are for their child.

Rapport Building

School counselors can help teachers build rapport with parents by helping the teachers to:

- Use facilitative skills to defuse anger and to let the parents know that in the teacher resides a genuine listener. Ask genuine questions of the parents. Show an interest in their answers. Reflect and paraphrase. Avoid acronyms and educational jargon that leaves parents confused. Check for clarity and understanding often.
- Begin with positives about the student. It may seem like a cliché, but make some positive comments about the child rather than launching into a list of problems. You can build on the positives to impact problem areas.
- Avoid absolute statements such as "your child is out of his seat *all* the time," or "*never* does his work," or "*always* picks a fight on the playground." These statements usually give parents nowhere to go but on the defensive.

Teaming to Identify the Problem

School counselors can help teachers build a team mentality with parents by helping the teachers to:

- Encourage parents to talk about how they see their child's progress in school. This should come before a list of concerns from the teacher.
- Collaborate with the parent to recognize and acknowledge the shared goal of removing barriers so that the student can be a successful learner. Identifying common goals helps the teacher/parent/counselor partnership pinpoint the problem (Scott, DeSimone, Fowler, & Webb, 2000). Accurate problem identification starts with common goals for the student's behavior and academic work (Scott et al., 2000). Discuss the parents' and teachers' perspectives of desired performance on the part of the student early on in the meeting.
- Avoid fixed ideas about how the problem should be solved. Be open to the possibility that parents may really have the best ideas for addressing the issue or that a completely different approach may be needed. The agenda should be flexible and receptive to really hearing what a parent has to say with an urgency to accomplish preset goals.

With parental input, prioritize concerns and settle on the area(s) of concern that warrant the greatest effort and attention (Scott et al., 2000). Ideally, this will be an area that impacts the child's ability to be a successful learner. Avoid trying to tackle all of the problems at once; improvement in one area will hopefully impact others. Have resource material and agency referrals available to address the issues you plan to discuss.

Negotiating a Plan of Action

School counselors can help negotiate a plan of action by helping the teacher to:

- Search for congruence with the parents in defining the problem to be addressed and the plan of action to be implemented.
- Develop the plan of action in measurable goals, not in the form of problems. For example, say that "John will complete 75% of his work the first week." As you will learn in Chapter 9, MEASURE is a good tool for framing a plan of action.

Ending Effectively

School counselors can further the success of the parent/teacher collaboration by ending the conference on a positive and productive note. The counselor can achieve an effective end to the conference by helping the teacher to:

- Summarize the conference, and check for understanding and the willingness of everyone to work together. If in doubt about the acceptability of the action plan, then speak up and raise the issue.
- Process what was said in the conference. A recap of the content of the conference can help further understanding and avoid confusion down the road.
- End with affirmations about the potential for making a difference and the 100% commitment that all parties plan to give in working together.
- Acknowledge and respect parents by thanking them for their time, presence, and for demonstrating a commitment to be in partnership with the school for the greater good of their child's education.

Regroup

School counselors can further the effectiveness of the action plan by working along with the teacher to analyze the effectiveness of the strategies and regroup and revise depending on the results, to help the teacher to:

- Monitor the interventions during the designated allotted time and adjust the interventions as needed. Be prepared for the possibility that all partners will need to return to the table and start anew on a different plan. Accentuate and expand what worked. The plan of action may not be successful the first time around. Be willing to try alternative interventions without jumping to more restrictive classroom settings, such as special education placement.

• Accentuate and expand on stategies that worked.

The Action Plan

The action plan is the heart and soul of the consultation process. The mechanics or steps in developing and delivering an action plan are presented as The Four Ds to serve as a memory aid: (a) **D**ata gathering, (b) **D**evising the action plan, (c) **D**elivering the action plan, and (d) **D**ebriefing.

The first step, in collaboration with others, is to gather the facts through one or more of a variety of data gathering methods. In this chapter, we discuss 10 basic approaches to gathering information:

1. Educational record review

2. Interviewing the teacher

3. Interviewing the parent

4. Interviewing other educators

5. Interviewing the student(s)

6. Interviewing other helping professionals

7. Student observation

8. Systems observation

9. Educational assessment

10. Psychological assessment

Data collection helps participants in the consultation process make better decisions by accurately identifying the problem and narrowing the focus of the interventions so that the resources and energy brought to the table are really addressing the critical issues.

After the facts have been collected by all parties involved to accurately determine the student's (or students') need, the consultant and consultees will start devising an action plan. Delivering the action plan will require all stakeholders to set timelines and strategies that they will implement. The next and final step is the debriefing. This is the time to determine whether the action plan was effective and what revisions, if any, are necessary.

Application of The Four Ds in the Case of Susan

Application of The Four Ds will be presented here in the context of a most prevalent teacher complaint: underachievement. The case of Susan will serve as the context to learn how to develop an action plan. Imagine yourself as the school counselor in this case.

Ms. Lawrence comes to you and tells you that one of her students, Susan, "has not completed any work the entire year." Ms. Lawrence explains to you that she has "tried everything" and would like your help in trying to determine what to do next. Where will you start?

Data Gathering in the Case of Susan

Data gathering is the first step in the consultation process. Here you will find some data gathering steps in this hypothetical case, along with some possible outcomes. You will usually not have the time, resources, or the need to complete all of these steps for one student. The steps and the sequence will vary according to the specifics of each situation, and rarely would you attend to all of the steps. However, as an introduction and in order to learn the application of the data gathering methods, all of the methods will be applied to the case of Susan.

Educational Record Review

A review of the student's educational record is usually a good place to start the data gathering process. Critical information is kept in the educational record and differs by school district according to policy. Typical information includes attendance, screening results for vision and hearing, cumulative grades and test records, and entry and withdrawal information. Cumulative information can determine patterns that may reveal the sudden onset of problems or chronic issues. Did the problem have roots in years earlier? Were there early or recent indicators that this student was going to have difficulty? Are there records of interventions already applied to the problem?

Examination of Susan's educational record reveals a pattern of low marks and teacher comments regarding Susan's failure to complete work and her lack of motivation. Other discoveries added to the cause for concern. In the five years Susan has been in school, her grades and test scores were consistently just below the average range, but her reading comprehension had never been above the 20th percentile. On the positive side, her attendance has always been good.

Interviewing the Teacher

Probably the most powerful tool in terms of information gathering for the school counselor as consultant is the interview, especially the interview with the teacher. Good teaching matters, and what happens between the student and teacher can spell the difference between a student who is academically successful and one who gets left behind. Using a face-to-face interview to question, gather, and probe, a school counselor can put together information that will get to the heart of the issue and help clarify, define, and focus the work of the consultant and consultee. The interview helps to set the stage so that the work of all stakeholders can be rendered more effective. Good interviews eliminate false starts, unnecessary struggles, and trial and error in trying to get at the issues.

Interviews can yield anecdotal information. Allowing a teacher or parent to just talk about the student can provide information about areas that you as an interviewer may not even think to explore. Anecdotal information is an opportunity to learn about the strengths of a student and to discover some positive information from which to build, especially in terms of establishing rapport when you start to interview the student or parent. Anecdotal information gives you a stronger sense of the student as a person and begins to round out one's perspective of the student rather than compartmentalizing her or him as "the student who has a problem finishing work."

An interview can determine the scope of the problem and help to prioritize which issues should be the foci. Baseline data can be collected, goals set, and a timeline established. (See Chapter 9 for information about establishing baseline and outcome data.)

In your interview with Ms. Lawrence, she says that Susan has not done any work all year. As is often the case with absolutes, you know that the word "any" is a blanket statement made out of frustration. So you gently focus on what is really meant by "all year" and you learn that Susan's work is uneven but not completely nonexistent.

You are able to get an accurate description of the problem with probing questions, such as "Are there subjects in which Susan will complete work?" and "What percentage of Susan's math problems go unsolved?" "Is there a difference in Susan's response if the problems are given all at once or a few at a time?" "Does Susan work better when collaborating on work with other students, such as peer helpers?" "Does Susan participate in art, music, physical education?" "Does Susan respond better when she is isolated to do her work?"

Questioning and listening helps you to pinpoint that Susan's problem occurs most often when she is left alone to complete work. With carefully worded questions, you also learn what interventions have not been tried in the past. Together you and Ms. Lawrence generate ideas for interventions. Because it is a team effort, Ms. Lawrence is more willing to take ownership. For example, by asking about peer helpers, you have encouraged Ms. Lawrence to try this approach to keep Susan on task.

The school counselor in this scenario was careful to avoid making the consultee feel that she was being subjected to the third degree. Interviewing is not just about questioning but about effective listening as well. Skilled interviews can plant ideas that the consultee can implement.

Interviewing the Parent

A partnership with parents is powerful. "A positive home-school partnership is almost always the basis for improvement in behavior and learning problems, and this is true from preschool through adolescence" (Kampwirth, 2003, p. 191). Parent interviews can provide rich information, but these interviews often are fraught with landmines. "The idea that an outsider (an individual representing the school) is asking to get involved in a family's life may have threatening connotations, especially for families that may already be somewhat dysfunctional or confused about how to deal with their child's school-related problems" (Kampwirth, 2003, p. 132). In his 1996 work, Maital (as cited in Kampwirth, 2003, p. 133) noted, "parents may seek, and at the same time build defenses against, information and advice that they find uncomfortable." Later in this chapter, we address partnerships with parents.

When you interviewed Mr. Kurtz, Susan's dad, he talked about his daughter's successes and challenges, and described what he had tried in the past to help Susan, such as rewarding good grades with money. Mr. Kurtz said he did not have the money to pay for a tutor and that he could not help with homework because his job required long hours. Because he is a single parent, Mr. Kurtz said he relied on Susan's older siblings to care for her, admittedly a poor plan because the older siblings had problems doing their own schoolwork. Mr. Kurtz said the house was often chaotic with teenagers everywhere and loud music. He expressed a determination to try to improve the situation so that Susan could study. Mr. Kurtz seemed genuinely interested in trying to help Susan be more successful academically. He was very willing to cooperate on an action plan and to set a time to meet again to discuss progress.

Interviewing Other Educators

Often it is appropriate to interview other educators and support personnel. Examining how the student behaves with other teachers can lend insight. If the student displays acting-out behavior, identify what the paraprofessionals observe while working with the student in the classroom or on cafeteria duty. Ask the administration about their opinions and observations regarding this student and his or her problems.

Mr. Mott, Susan's teacher from the previous year, was very willing to describe interventions that he had tried with Susan. Mr. Mott said he had his greatest success with Susan during the three weeks before Christmas break. Susan's mother had promised to visit Susan and her brothers at Christmas. Mr. Mott said that Susan talked about the upcoming visit constantly and that he encouraged her to write letters to her mother during English class, draw pictures for her mother, and receive free time in the art corner to make presents for her mother in exchange for completing her work. Mr. Mott said he was able to get Susan to work really hard by putting her work in a portfolio in anticipation of showing her mother her work. Susan's work was still below grade level, but her efforts were yielding results. Mr. Mott said sadly, "I think Susan thought that if she

*could show her mother that she could be really good that her mother would come home."
Mr. Mott says he never got the entire story, but he believes the Christmas visit was not the happy
occasion Susan had anticipated. Susan came back from Christmas break more erratic in her performance than ever, and it was a constant struggle to find ways to motivate her. Mr. Mott said
he occasionally had success by pairing Susan with an older student who would come to tutor
Susan two times a week.*

Seek out other educators who have had success with students with like problems. Gather ideas and interventions from these teachers and seek their input in developing an action plan. For example, an elementary counselor who enrolled a
student with autism arranged to have an Exceptional Student Education (ESE) specialist come to his school to help the current ESE teacher as well as the rest of the
school develop strategies for working with this student, as they all lacked experience
with autistic students.

Interviewing the Student

Oftentimes it is appropriate to interview a student or conduct an individual counseling session to get the student's perspective about the problem. From listening to
the student's perspective, the school counselor can often learn what motivates the
student and then initiate strategies that will boost the student's success. Students of
all ages can take part in problem solving, but the older the student, the more necessary his or her involvement becomes in order to ensure and increase the likelihood
of success.

*You meet with Susan three times over the course of two weeks. She tells you that she feels she is
dumb and that no matter how hard she tries, she will never be able to understand what the
teacher is telling the class. Susan talks about her family, but she paints a far better picture than
what was described by her father and Mr. Mott. Susan talks about a family that does "great stuff
together, like go out to eat." She describes brothers who take her places, a father who gives her
things, and a mother who has a very important job. Susan can't name anything that she likes
about school, but she does talk about Mr. Mott and how much she liked being in his class last year.*

Interviewing Other Helping Professionals

Reaching out to other members of the helping profession can provide resources that
the school would not otherwise be able to offer. Whether internal to the school,
such as a school psychologist or school social worker, or external to the school, such
as agency or community mental health providers, helping professionals may also
offer experience or expertise to support internal school members.

*In Susan's case, you are becoming concerned about issues of abandonment. With the permission
of Susan's father, you consult with an agency counselor to get some information that you can pass*

along to him. The discussion helps you understand that Susan may indeed be experiencing adverse effects from abandonment. Abandonment, or "withdrawal of support," involves rejection and/or being left behind by an important figure in one's life (Hyperdictionary, n.d.). Susan's limited contact with her mother may mean that Susan has abandonment issues (Zide & Gray, 2001). Without a formal diagnosis, yet with the observable behavior that Susan is struggling, you encourage Susan's father to seek counseling for her at an agency that offers a sliding fee scale and secures volunteers who will bring children to their counseling sessions when transportation is a problem.

Student Observation

Observation can be done by any qualified, certificated educator in the building and can take many forms. Sometimes a counselor will sit and work an educational game with a student to observe the student's thought and problem-solving processes, behavior, and social skills and capture these in a written summary afterwards. An observation can take the form of recording the student's actions by positioning yourself out of the direct line of vision of the student. Observations are best when they begin by recording overt information; that is, those behaviors that are observed without interpretation, such as "the student moves the chair from under the table, sits down, immediately leans over and whispers something to the student sitting next to him, and then shares a laugh with the student." The observer then follows up the recording of overt behavior with the subjective part of the observation, which is an interpretation and opinion of what the observer believes is the meaning of the overt behaviors. Many observers skip the recording of overt behaviors and just report the meaning of what they observed. Observers will need to train themselves to record what the eye sees; that requires the observer to focus and therefore not miss important messages by trying to interpret or bring meaning to the observations prematurely. The observation should not confirm preconceived ideas about what is believed to be the issue but identify how the student functions in the school environment. Train yourself to record objective information and then connect the dots to form your opinions about the meaning of the information. Following is an observation of a reading lesson in which the teacher is checking for comprehension following a silent reading assignment.

With the agreement of the teacher, you observe Susan in class. The students, including Susan, do not know why you are sitting in the back of the classroom and soon forget that you are there. Following is just the first 8 minutes of the 25 minutes of the observation, and a partial interpretation.

Systems Observation

Don't forget the system in which Susan is functioning. Observing and gathering information about how the system has added value or stratified Susan's opportunities is critical in order to help her and other students' progress.

Student Observation

Student: Susan
Time: 8:52 to 9:17
Place: Room 224
Activity: Reading

Susan traces the pattern on the tile floor with her toe. She intently watches her toe as she carefully tries to remain within the lines of the pattern. She goes outside the line. She stops moving her foot, gets a distressed look on her face, and then she starts all over from where she began tracing. She repeats this pattern several times.

(The teacher asks a student next to Susan a question, and the student responds).

Susan appears startled at the sound of her neighbor's voice. She stops the movement of her foot and stares intently at the student answering the question. She raises the front legs of her desk off the ground and balances on the back two legs. She lifts her feet and the desk slams down. Susan twirls her hair into tight coils and pulls the hair straight out from her head and parallel to the floor. Susan continues to play intently with her hair for the next two minutes, bringing her hair around to cover her eyes, selecting strands to put in her mouth, and studying the ends by bringing them around close to her eyes.

(The teacher continues to ask closed questions so that all the students can respond in unison, e.g., "What was the name of Kindra's dog?")

The sound of her classmates responding in unison brings a puzzled look to Susan's face. She lays her head in her hands and gently rocks herself back and forth and back and forth. This movement continues for two minutes until the teacher switches from having the students respond in unison.

(The teacher asks the students to stand behind their desks and act out the part of the story where the main character had to crouch behind a table.)

Susan appears startled when she sees each of the students crouching behind their desks. She looks around as if to copy the other students but tentatively crouches and then stands and then crouches again. She smiles big and then laughs out loud.

(The teacher asks the students to sit, and shifts into asking for individual responses again.)

Susan watches the other students take their seats and then after everyone is seated, she takes her seat too.

Interpretation: Throughout the lesson Susan was not engaged except to copy other students who crouched behind their desks, apparently unaware of the purpose of the crouch. Susan's affect led me to believe she felt sad, lonely, and disconnected from the rest of the class. Susan's face transformed when she was doing what all the other students were doing (crouching). It is as if Susan rarely is able to follow along and feels left behind most of the time. Being able to be part of the group seemed to be very important to Susan and brought a light to her face, animated movements, and laughter, the only sound I heard from Susan.

When looking at the educational institution in which Susan is functioning, several stratifiers are found. Susan has been missing school at least three days a month because the bus came early. Additionally, you find that Susan often is not allowed to eat breakfast on the days her bus arrives late, because the cafeteria has closed. Susan depends on the breakfast provided at school, because her home life does not include a morning ritual of breakfast. In addition, Susan has been missing reading class not only when she is absent, but also when her bus is late, because she has had to wait in line at the office to get her re-admittance pass, and this cuts into the morning reading time. You have also learned that the special reading support is no longer being offered to Susan because a student must demonstrate progress to remain in the program. Last year Susan was not able to demonstrate progress, so this year she was not assigned to the program. Additionally, the school has a special Saturday tutoring program for students who have a B average. You never paid attention to the requirements for the tutoring program or the special support reading program, but it has become apparent to you that maybe students who need the most support in reading are really given the least, a systemic problem that you can advocate to have changed.

Educational Assessment

What assessment instruments do you have at your disposal to understand the reading problems and other academic problems that Susan is suffering? An educational evaluation, such as the Woodcock-Johnson Tests of Achievement III (Woodcock, McGrew, & Mather, 2001) can identify areas of strengths and weakness for Susan so that strategies can be brought to bear on those areas. For example, the Woodcock-Johnson III provides information about general intellectual ability, specific cognitive ability, oral language, and academic achievement. This assessment then provides an extensive measure of achievement and ability (Blackwell, 2001). Data analyses of other test results that are part of the student's educational record can be used in lieu of or in addition to an individual educational assessment such as the Woodcock-Johnson.

You have decided to give Susan the Woodcock-Johnson III as a measure of her achievement. The results of her assessment reveal that her standard scores are close to the mean for her age in all areas, with reading comprehension slightly lower than the other scores. The results of the test helped pinpoint where Susan's academic functioning is and can help provide guidance in how to address those deficits.

The Psychological Assessment

Sometimes a student may need to be referred for a battery of tests called a psychological assessment, which may include an intelligence quotient (*IQ*), a personality assessment, and projective evaluations, among other possibilities. A school psychologist usually administers this battery. In many school districts this step would be taken only if it were believed that the student might need special education placement.

For Susan it was determined that classroom and home interventions were adequate at this time and that Susan would not be referred for Special Education nor for consideration for a full psychological assessment.

The information gleaned from your data gathering provides the basic information for you and the consultees to start devising an action plan for Susan. The data gathering stage may include one or more of the data gathering approaches listed earlier in this chapter and/or other data approaches not described. For example, it may be determined that a developmental history is needed, or a medical evaluation, or a visit by a social worker.

Devising an Action Plan in the Case of Susan

The second step of the consultation process is to organize the data and take it to the consultee(s) so that an action plan can be devised, complete with strategies and stakeholders' responsibilities for implementing each strategy. This is also the time to establish your baseline data so that after the interventions are put into place, you can track Susan's progress on her reading comprehension scores. The data will allow all participants to know if progress is really being made and whether certain interventions are more effective than others, as well as which interventions should be replicated and which should be eliminated. Devising an action plan means that you and the consultees identify stakeholders to help you make progress with Susan's academic success, especially her reading comprehension skills.

School counselor as Stakeholder could:

- Assist in the preliminary data gathering and collaborate on developing strategies.
- Administer or access a qualified educator to give the Woodcock-Johnson III Tests of Achievement or another assessment instrument to determine current level of performance.
- Help Ms. Lawrence (the teacher) and Mr. Kurtz (Susan's father) establish a behavior management program.

Teacher as stakeholder could:

- Give work in small chunks rather than the complete assignment.
- Assign a buddy to the student to help her stay on task.
- Tape instructions and lessons, and then allow Susan and her buddy to replay the tape as needed.
- Provide older students to peer tutor with Susan.
- Send home a daily assignment book to be signed by Mr. Kurtz.

Mr. Kurtz as stakeholder could:

- Check and sign the daily assignment book.
- Provide a quiet study environment.
- Get the older siblings to work with Susan on her homework.

Administration as stakeholder could:

- Change the breakfast policy so that food is always available for late arrivals.
- Change the tardy policy so that student's re-admittance does not depend on waiting in lines.
- Change the criteria for admissions into special programs and tutoring programs so that students who need the most help can get it.

Big Brothers and Big Sisters and Boys & Girls' Club as Stakeholders could:

- Help Susan develop confidence and academic skills by: (a) involving her in sports, (b) giving her time and attention, (c) orchestrating opportunities for Susan to develop friendships, and (d) providing her with tutoring.

Delivering the Action Plan in the Case of Susan

The teacher, parent, and school counselor connect the other stakeholders to the effort of delivering the action plan. The Big Brothers Big Sisters organization and Boys and Girls' Club are contacted. Stakeholders have agreed to deliver their component of the action plan, a timeline is established for completion and an interim check of progress, and a date is set for the next meeting.

Debriefing and Accountability

At the close of the time period set for the action plan, the stakeholders meet to answer the following questions: Did Susan's reading comprehension scores increase, her behavior improve, and her completion of work increase? Which part of the action plan worked and therefore should be enlarged upon or replicated? If no progress was made, which strategies of the action plan did not work and therefore need to be adjusted slightly, altered significantly, or discarded? These are the questions that the consultees and all the stakeholders wrestle with during the debriefing stage. This is the time to look at the data (reading scores) to see if progress is being made and to reanalyze and refocus. A consultant who checks his or her progress by looking at the baseline data and impact data is a consultant who does not have to guess whether the strategies that he or she suggested and is helping to implement have any value to the student. In the case of Susan, her reading scores have gone up 14 percentile points. She scored at the 28th percentile in reading comprehension by the end of the school year. All the hard work of the consultants is paying off! It is the savvy consultant who knows where they are (baseline data), where they are going (strategies), and if they ever got there (impact data) (MacGregor, 2004).

Reanalyzing

Restate the baseline data. Where is the data after the action plan? Did the strategies have a positive impact on the data?

Susan's baseline data: 14th percentile
Data after action plan: 28th percentile

Systemic Changes Made

How did the action plan contribute to systemic change? Each action plan will in some way change a school, home, or community system to enhance student learning.

In the case of Susan, three policies were changed:

1. *food is now available in the cafeteria for late arrivals;*
2. *the tardy policy changed so that the student's re-admittance did not depend on waiting in lines;*
3. *the criteria for admissions into special programs and tutoring programs changed so that students who need the most help can get it.*

Special Education (SE) and Consultation

What if all strategies failed and Susan were in danger of repeating for the third time? It might then be time to consider a Special Education placement. Let's take a look at Public Law 94-142.

In 1975, Public Law (PL) 94-142 was passed (renamed the Individuals with Disabilities Education Act [IDEA]), which resulted in many students who had disabilities receiving educational support. Under the provisions of IDEA, regular education teachers are responsible for teaching SE students mainstreamed into their classroom and are entitled to receive additional help (Dettmer, Thurston, & Dyck, 2005). The school counselor as consultant can be one of the contributors to the support team for regular education teachers who have SE students.

There are some students whose behavior challenges the normal solutions to behavioral problems. In 1997, IDEA was amended to include the use of functional behavior assessments to develop intervention plans for the behavior problems that prevented students from learning. Functional behavior assessment is a problem-solving process that uses a variety of techniques and strategies to help the Individual Education Plan team identify social, affective, cognitive, and environmental behavior and use the assessment results to develop an intervention plan. The intervention plan must address short-term prevention, teaching of alternative skills, responses to problem behaviors, and long-term prevention (Dettmer et al., 2005).

There is no doubt that IDEA has tremendously increased services for needy children; however, the downside is that large numbers of students are being placed in SE who, with appropriate interventions, could be very successful in the regular education classroom. A benefit to effective collaboration is a reduction in referrals for SE. When effective consultation is in place to help teachers with appropriate interventions and strategies, then SE referrals can be reduced. It is hoped that in all but the most severe cases, SE will be considered only after a serious action plan, such as the one described for Susan, has been put into place to try to help the student be successful in the regular education program. "It follows that ancillary personnel, such as those engaged in consultative responsibilities, should not search for intrachild deficits and treat them somewhere else but find ways of modifying and improving the regular program to enhance educational opportunities for these students" (Kampwirth, 2003, p. 18).

The consultation role in SE referrals has taken a giant step forward with the advent of the pre-referral team (Lane, Mahdavi, & Borthwick-Duffy, 2003; McEachern, 2003; Ormsbee, 2001). Many states and school districts are now requiring Pre-referral Teams or Student Support Teams, which provide consultation and collaboration regarding a student's problem for the purpose of eliminating overidentification of students into SE and to ensure that when a student is referred for SE, the referral is an appropriate one (McEachern, 2003; Ormsbee, 2001). Pre-referral team members discuss a student's academic, personal, and social-emotional needs and pose strategies, deliver interventions, and establish timelines to try to address the problem in the regular education program. If the problem is such that more intensive services are needed, then a direct referral for SE testing may be made.

Parent Education

In addition to parent consultation, school counselors educate parents by providing training opportunities, programs, and materials. Parent education can take many forms, such as workshops, trainings, written material, or one-on-one interactions via a phone call or meeting. Parent education designed by a school counselor has the purpose of helping parents achieve better parent-child communication, teach useful information that parents need in order to support and work with their child on academic issues, and/or to strengthen the home and school partnership. In a school setting, parent education is usually directed toward helping parents change specific behaviors in their child that are interfering with the educational process, such as acting-out behavior, but it can also include general information, such as how to help your child prepare for tests. Parent education may take a formal approach, such as providing newsletters or a predetermined number of sessions on specific topics (for example, "Helping Your Child Prepare for Postsecondary Education"), or a more informal approach such as a phone call and discussion as a topic emerges.

Parent education programs have been around for a number of years, and many of the early programs continue to exist. Parent Effectiveness Training (PET) (Gordon, 1977) and Systematic Training for Effective Parenting (STEP) (1997) are two long-standing, popular programs that attempt to help parents understand child development and behavior management. The intent of these programs is to help parents learn about motivation for behavior, reinforcement, and how to reward and extinguish certain behaviors. Other resources frequently used by school counselors are the Center for the Improvement of Child Caring (CICC), found at http://www.ciccparenting.org, and Parent Project, found at http://www.parentproject.com.

Research results are mixed on the effectiveness of parent education programs, but generally speaking, research on parent education and training programs that have a behavior modification component have received the greatest amount of attention and positive results (Fitch & Marshall, 2004; Friend & Cook, 2003; Kaiser & Hancock, 2003).

TechTools

- Consider developing an electronic self-help library with links that will take parents and students to websites that inform them about specific issues.
- Using word processing (or a spreadsheet program if you are more technologically astute), develop a directory of all agencies, their phone numbers, and the services they offer for specific problems found in children and adolescents. Have this information printed and distributed in administrators' offices, the front office, and other appropriate locations. By using a word processing program, you can easily update the information regularly.
- Find and publicize databases such as PubMed (http://www4.ncbi.nlm.nih.gov/PubMed/) that can help parents with information about Attention Deficit Hyperactivity Disorder, school phobia, and other health issues.
- Technology can help parents link with other parents through focus groups, support groups, and/or learning teams. Provide information for parents in the form of websites and chat rooms.
- Use technology to help you improve communication. For example, send home the letters of concern, letters of praise, and so on more easily by developing a bank of letters that are appropriate for the different grade levels

in your school. These letters can then be stored electronically, retrieved, and personalized.

- Provide teachers with a bank of letters and written approaches, such as templates for newsletters to keep parents informed. Paraprofessionals can tailor letters to the grade level or situation. For example, if you have letters congratulating the eighth graders on being on the honor roll, paraprofessionals can easily personalize the letters.
- Deliver PowerPoint presentations to teachers on effective consultation skills, parent-teacher conferences, and topics concerning special needs children.

School Counselor Casebook: Voices From the Field

The Scenario Reviewed

Currently there are 22 students who have been referred to you because they are underachievers, capable but not completing work. You have limited time to work individually with these students but you want to impact their progress. In the past you have had a good success rate in working with underachievers individually in behavior management programs. As your success rate climbs, more teachers are referring underachievers to you.

A Practitioner's Approach

Here's how a practicing school counselor responded to this school scenario:

My colleagues and I know that sharing information and strategies is the most effective way of improving our students' success in school. As a school counselor, I have already developed a solid working relationship with classroom teachers, and this in turn has garnered me much support from my department chair and the administration. The teachers and I know that we all have knowledge and skills that will help us to get our students on track. I can use my consultation skills to help my teachers learn new strategies for our students who are not achieving to their ability.

I asked my building principal if I could have a time slot at the faculty meeting to give a brief presentation about working with underachievers. I will put together a booklet of materials collected from conferences (i.e., American School Counselor Association [ASCA] summer conference), articles from professional journals, and materials from other resources related to the topic, and will give it to the faculty members. At the end of the presentation I will ask for volunteers to work with me on a committee to develop more materials and an action plan that could be implemented in each class. This committee can also help us to investigate how our state's academic standards and ASCA's national standards in academic development could be intertwined to result in a successful plan. We will also offer our staff members ongoing support in student behavior strategies, learning styles, and in motivating underachieving students.

Other staff members and I can co-lead an underachievers group to meet two to four sessions per quarter. I would ask teachers for names of students they believe would benefit from such a group. I would develop a parent permission form explaining the purposes of the group, meeting times, and number of sessions. Each participating student would take it home, get it signed, and return it to me. This would allow us the opportunity to work with a group of up to 20 different students each quarter. We would have various handouts for the students, having them actively participate in each group session. At our high school, I would seek the principal's permission to rotate sessions by class period.

The teachers at my school know that I am always available to them to put our heads together to develop strategies to help our students achieve at the expected level of success. If we set goals and work together, our students will be more successful in passing their classes.

Lin Roy is a 30-year veteran counselor who serves her 9th through 12th graders in all three domains, academic, career, and personal-social, at Lincoln Way Central High School in Illinois. She is a past president of the Illinois School Counselor Association and has served as the chair of the ASCA Committee for Children. Lin has received the American Counseling Association Humanitarian and Caring Person Counselor of the Year award and has been honored for her advocacy work on behalf of children. Reprinted with permission by Lin Roy.

Chapter Summary

Consultation in the Schools

Consultation gathers "experts" together, be they teachers, parents, or community-based professionals, in order to bring their collective knowledge to bear on resolving a situation for an individual child or group of children.

The School Counselor as Consultant

Consultation extends the school counselor's reach by allowing the counselor to work collaboratively with the adults in a student's life who can make a major impact on the student's academic, career, and social-emotional life. The consultation role is becoming more and more important because consultation is effective and efficient in removing obstacles to implementing a standards-based educational system, in challenging low expectations, and in promoting access and success in rigorous academics.

Consultation follows the rule of parsimony because with each successful consultation you are helping a teacher, parent, or other adult gain the knowledge that they can use with other children in the years to come. In a successful consultation scenario, both the teacher and counselor are learning intervention strategies for application to future problems; ideas germinate into plans that spill over to benefit more people.

Teachers, Parents, and the System as Consultees

Your consultees will include many people, agencies, and institutions, but your primary consultees will include teachers, parents, and the system—meaning the school district and your individual school. Student outcomes of educational consultation are likely to be more successful when there is an effective parent-educator partnership. Although it is easier for counselors to concentrate on individual student needs and not look at the system, systemic consultation impacts many more lives.

Consultation as a problem-solving process sometimes involves an expert teaching knowledge and skills to a consultee. The definition that this textbook promotes is that of collaborative consultation or shared responsibility with regard to decisions and outcomes, which relies on maintaining an equal partnership among all parties involved.

Teachers as Consultees

Teachers as consultees vary widely in skills and confidence, with some needing very little support while others place unrealistic demands on the consultant to own the problem and fix it. A skillful consultant must be able to work with all teachers on the continuum, and for this reason relationship building considerably facilitates the consultant's role. PREPARE is an acronym for **P**hilosophy, **R**elationships, **E**quity of power, **P**rofessional development, **A**ccessibility, **R**esources, **E**valuate—key elements of effective consultation with teachers.

Parents as Consultees

Parental involvement yields positive effects on student achievement. We know that when parents are involved, students show improvement in all areas of academic and social achievement. PARTNER is an acronym for steps to effective conferences with parents. PARTNER stands for **P**lanning for success, **A**cknowledging parents, **R**apport building, **T**eaming, **N**egotiating a plan of action, **E**nding effectively, and **R**egrouping. The school counselor as consultant has a wonderful opportunity to provide staff development to teachers and other educators about effective communication with parents as well as tips for conducting parent conferences and managing parent visits.

The Four Ds of the Action Plan

Data gathering, Devising the action plan, Delivering the action plan, and Debriefing are the four steps in the consultation process. After completing the Data gathering and fact collecting to determine the student's need, the consultant and consultees will start Devising the action plan. Delivering the action plan will require all stakeholders to set timelines and strategies that they will be implementing. The final step is the Debriefing. This is the time to determine whether the action plan was effective and what revisions, if any, are necessary.

There are 10 basic approaches to gathering information: educational record review, interviewing the teacher, interviewing the parent, interviewing other educators, interviewing the student(s), interviewing other helping professionals, student observation, systems observation, educational assessment, and psychological assessment.

Data collection helps participants in the consultation process make better decisions by accurately identifying the problem and narrowing the focus of the interventions so that the resources and energy brought to the table are really addressing the critical issues.

Key Terms

Collaborative consultation p. 147
Consultation p. 146
Equity of power p. 153
External consultee p. 150
PARTNER p. 155
Positive self-talk p. 152

PREPARE p. 151
Rule of parsimony p. 148
Systems observation p. 164
Triadic-dependant model p. 147
Unalterable factors p. 148

Learning Extensions

1. Thinking about the power types described in Chapter 4, which are (a) position power or jurisdictional power; (b) referent power or relationship power; (c) caring power; (d) transformational power or developmental power; (e) connection power; (f) reward power; and (g) technical, information, or expert power (French & Raven, 1959), apply each to ways in which it can be used in the consultation process, and discuss the benefits of each.

2. Kampwirth (2003) provides a unique standpoint describing the collaborative nature of consultation. While others speak of the expert role of a consultant, Kampwirth discusses a shared responsibility for decisions and outcomes. Consider the continuum of consultation with *expertise* on one end of the continuum and Kampwirth's *collaborative problem-solving* idea at the other end. Where are you on the continuum? Do you believe you tend toward needing to be an expert in behavioral issues, or do you lean toward the collaborative problem-solving approach? Discuss the merits of your position on the continuum in relation to your role as an effective consultant.

3. The authors' definition of consultation stresses a partnership. Consultation is a partnership that the school counselor enters into with other adults in the internal or external school community for the express purpose of collaboratively problem solving and supporting the implementation of strategies designed to increase a student's opportunity to be a successful learner. Rewrite the definition in an attempt to add your own opinion about the definition of consultation. Defend the merits of your definition.

4. PARTNER is an acronym for **P**lanning for success, **A**cknowledging parents, **R**apport building, **T**eaming, **N**egotiating a plan of action, **E**nding effectively, and **R**egrouping. Consider the last time you worked with another adult in any consultation capacity. This occasion could have been a consultation outside the realm of an educational setting, such as problem solving with a friend about how to lose weight, or it may have been a complicated consultation about a student who was underachieving. Thinking back to your role as consultant, describe how you behaved in this real consultation and what you would do differently as a result of reading about the PARTNER process.

5. Debate with your classmates your opinion of the merits of the following recommendation. "Dress professionally but in a way that will help parents identify with you. This approach may require professional dress that is more understated."

6. Revisit data gathering and the 10 basic approaches to gathering information. Contact a school counselor and discuss with him or her your willingness to assist in gathering information regarding a student in need. In collaboration with the counselor, implement three of the nine data gathering areas and deliver the information you glean to the teacher, parent, and/or counselor. Be certain to get written permission from the child's parents before you start gathering information.

7. Develop and deliver a PowerPoint presentation to the faculty on effective parent conferences. The presentation should be 8 to 10 minutes long. Create a written feedback form so that you can grow your presentation effectiveness.

Chapter 7

School Counselors as Coordinators, Collaborators, and Managers of Resources

Barriers to Collaboration and Management of Resources

Collegiality: Taking Collaboration to a Higher Level

Application of CASTT in Building a Safe and Respectful School Climate

Chapter Objectives

By the time you have completed this chapter, you should be able to:

- Explain the role of the school counselor in coordinating a school counseling program.
- Discuss the benefits, barriers, and limitations of collaborating and partnering for student success.
- Describe the skills needed to collaborate and partner.
- Describe the benefits, barriers, and limitations of managing resources to deliver services to students.
- Take a problem that impacts student academic success and delineate strategies you would use to bring support and resolution to the problem through coordination, collaboration, partnering, and managing resources.
- Explain the power of technology to considerably enhance your school counseling program.

School Counselor Casebook: Getting Started

The Scenario

For the second consecutive year your school has been placed on the Critically Low Performing Schools list, which means that if test scores do not improve over the next two years, the state will take over the school. You believe that as a member of the leadership team, instructional success and student achievement are as much your job as they are that of the principal, teachers, and other critical stakeholders. Your principal does not assign you extraneous duties, and you have a comprehensive developmental school counseling program that is very solid and meaningful and already supports the achievement of students; yet, like everyone else in the school, you feel pressure from the possible state takeover. You want to extend your reach to support more students' academic success, but your day is already packed with very important tasks that you do not want to relinquish.

Thinking About Solutions

As you read this chapter, think about how you might extend your reach to support more students' academic success without relinquishing the important functions you already perform. When you come to the end of the chapter, you will have the opportunity to see how your ideas compare with a practicing school counselor's approach.

Coordination, Collaboration, and Management of Resources

Coordination of services, collaboration, and management of resources—three terms that are used interchangeably—are the mechanics or the "how" in delivering a school counseling program. In practice, these three terms have very unique aspects. The distinctiveness of coordination, collaboration, and managing resources as well as their interlocking components all work to the advantage of the school counseling program. The common denominator of the three is the power they have to extend the influence of the school counseling program to enhance the personal and academic success of each student in the counselor's charge. Coordination of school counseling means prioritizing, organizing, and delivering the components of the program, such as individual or group counseling, classroom guidance lessons, consultation services, career and academic advising, and systemic support. Collaboration is a process of partnering and teaming with other educators, individuals, and groups of the internal community (the school site) and the external community (outside the school site) to deliver the components of the school counseling program. Working collaboratively with the administration, the teachers, the community, and agency programs in overarching, interlocking commonalities strengthens the impact of the school counseling program by collectively focusing on common goals. Managing resources means extending the school counselor program beyond what just the counselor could do by bringing in human and material resources such as parents, students, teachers, administrators, community members, business partners, and technology. Resource management requires minimal or no additional funds to add support and redistribute some of the duties of the school counseling program.

> A teacher stood in front of his group of high-powered overachieving students and said, "Okay, time for a quiz." He pulled out a one-gallon, wide-mouth jar and a dozen fist-sized rocks, which he carefully placed into the jar. When no more rocks

would fit inside, he asked, "Is this jar full?" Everyone in the class said "Yes." He reached under the table and pulled out a bucket of gravel. Then he dumped some gravel in and shook the jar, causing pieces of gravel to work themselves down into the spaces between the big rocks. Then he asked the group once more, "Is the jar full?" By this time the class was on to him. "Probably not," one student answered. "Good!" he replied. He reached under the table, brought out a bucket of sand, and poured the sand into the jar, filling up the spaces that were left between the rocks and the gravel. Once more he asked the question, "Is this jar full?" "No!" the class shouted. Then he grabbed a pitcher of water and began to pour it until the jar was filled to the brim. Then he looked at the class and said, "the point is if you don't put the big rocks in first, you'll never get them in at all."

— Adapted from Covey, 1990

What are the "big rocks" in your school counseling program? The big rocks are the components of your school counseling program that need to be in place first, before everything else spills over into the school counseling office. Once these important rocks or components are firmly anchored, you have a solid framework in place and you can better protect your time and program when the flood of "other duties as designated" comes your way. Your role as **coordinator** requires that you determine the components of your program and then collaborate with others to fulfill an optimum educational opportunity for students. Managing resources allows for an extended reach.

Through coordination, collaboration, and managing resources, school counselors are able to deliver a comprehensive program that reaches just a few select students to benefit 100% of the students—each and every student in the school. Now we have a high-profile, powerful school counseling program. The "jar" in your program is full and heavy, yet, stable. You are not lugging around a container that is losing water, sand, and gravel as contents spill and you do damage control. Rather, you can be proactive and have a program that has set components, collaborating and brokering resources to see that the components are fulfilled.

Coordination

Coordination of services means prioritizing, organizing, and delivering the components of the school counseling program, including individual or group counseling, classroom guidance lessons, consultation services, career and academic advising, and systemic support, so that you increase the likelihood that the program will successfully impact the personal-social, career, and academic outcomes of each and every student in the school (Gysbers & Henderson, 2000; Haycock, 2001; Isaacs, 2003; Myrick, 2003b). In the coordination role the school counselor sets short-term targets and long-term goals.

The school counselor as coordinator determines the goals of the school counseling program and identifies the mechanisms and resources needed to carry out those goals. The coordinator role of school counseling requires putting into place a program that reaches each student through both direct service delivery and, more important, indirect service delivery through the brokering of resources. The coordination role has become one of the most important roles a school counselor can perfect (Bryan & Holcomb-McCoy, 2004; Staley & Carey, 1997). School counselors will more and more come to rely on the expertise and services of others in order to deliver optimum programs. You will become much more familiar with the four components of the comprehensive school counseling program in Chapter 8, which addresses the ASCA National Model (2003). Briefly, the four components are:

1. Guidance curriculum (e.g., structured groups, classroom guidance);

2. Individual planning with students (e.g., advising; assessment; placement; academic, career, and personal-social goal setting; and follow-up);

3. Responsive services (e.g., individual and group counseling; consultation; and referral);

4. System support (e.g., program management, coordination of services, community outreach, and public relations) (ASCA, 2003; Gysbers & Henderson, 2000).

This chapter focuses on one of the four components, system support.

Begin your system support role by answering these questions:

"Are the goals of the school counseling program aligned with the mission of the school?"

"What will be the priorities of the school counseling program for the year?"

"What data elements will the school counselor collaborate with others on to make positive change?" (See Chapter 9 for information about data elements.)

"Who in the internal and external community is working toward the same goals as that of the school counsel?"

"Which components of my school counseling program must I deliver and for which can I broker resources so that others can help me?"

"How can the school counseling program intersect with the other programs and resources to collaborate and partner to meet these goals?"

Setting Priorities

There will never be enough school counselors to meet all the needs of students; furthermore, counselors must work within the limits of time, resources, and their abilities (Gysbers & Henderson, 2000; Myrick, 2003b). *Developmental guidance and counseling: A practical handbook.*

With too many demands on their time, school counselors establish priorities by first identifying the guidance needs of the school. This can be accomplished by speaking with administrators and teachers to assess what they believe to be the pressing issues impacting students. Students and teachers can participate in establishing the needs by responding to a questionnaire and giving their perspectives on schoolwide problems, areas of concern, their needs, and so on. The guidance committee may also be helpful in setting priorities (Myrick, 2003a). The PTA can survey parents and report their findings back to the guidance committee. State and community reports may also shed some light on issues being faced by students, such as a rising drug problem or an increase in teenage suicides (Myrick, 2003b). However, critically important to determining the priorities of your program should be needs of your school as determined by the gaps and glaring problems revealed by the school report card data (Stone & Dahir, 2004).

Time Management

Time management is an important aspect of priority setting (Myrick, 2003a). One way to prioritize time and energy is to decide how much time you will spend with different types of interventions. For example, you may decide that you will only do small groups for 10 sessions per week, or 2 sessions per day. By scheduling time for each of your interventions, you are better able to achieve a balanced program. Develop a weekly schedule broken down into blocks of time, and display the times that you are available and the times that you have interventions scheduled.

Getting Organized

In organizing the school counseling program, the phases are: (a) planning, (b) designing, (c) implementing, and (d) evaluating (Gysbers & Henderson, 2000, 2001).

Planning

In the planning phase, desired student outcomes have been identified and the current school program has been scrutinized to determine what can be kept and what needs to change. Program goals are set in the planning phase based on the needs that were identified when priorities were set. School counseling programs in the past have rarely utilized student information data to try to establish program goals (Stone & Dahir, 2004). It is the school counselor of the 21st century who starts setting program goals by looking at the academic data for his or her students and asking questions such as "Where are students' deficits? Who is being left out of the academic success picture?" (Stone & Dahir, 2004). School counselors who start their program goals by looking at the identified needs of their students through hard data, not just needs assessments, will avoid running down rabbit trails and implementing services that are not needed and do not make a difference in students' lives (Stone & Dahir, 2004). Data tell you where your students are, where you need to help them go, and whether your program's strategies helped you realize your goals (Lapan, 2001; MacGregor, 2004).

Designing

Once planning and priorities have been set, the designing phase becomes the focus. At this point, the strategies needed to achieve the goals of the school counseling program are identified (see The Six Steps of MEASURE in Chapter 9 for more information). Then the components of the program should be assigned, and school personnel should be assessed for their abilities (Gysbers & Henderson, 2000). Myrick states that all school personnel should be included in order to accomplish program goals (Myrick, 2003a, 2003b).

The final task in the designing phase is to provide staff development, to inform them about changes and the new goals of the school counseling program.

Implement and Evaluate

The counselor starts to implement and evaluate the program to see if it is an accountable, data-driven program. The school counselor must collect data on the efficacy of program components (Gysbers & Henderson, 2000; Johnson & Johnson, 2001; Stone & Dahir, 2004). The data must then be analyzed and a report should be prepared to provide a better idea of how the program contributed to desired student outcomes. Chapter 9 provides considerable detail about evaluating the effectiveness of the school counseling program.

Collaboration and Management of Resources

You stand staring at a stack of 450 educational records, each representing a student in your caseload. Every student has career, academic, and personal-social needs. How do you get your arms literally and figuratively around all these students so that you can close the gaps in their information, support their social development, and widen their opportunities to fully participate in the U.S. economy? Stiffer standards, shrinking education dollars, and increased social stresses demand that educators—especially school counselors, who have always had demanding student-to-counselor ratios—collaborate with each other to optimally prepare students. Linkages within and among administrators, teachers, businesses, and community agencies, properly initiated and carefully nurtured, will improve school counseling programs and promote student success (Herr, 2001; Martin, 2002; Morgan, 2003; Schmidt, 2000; Stone & Clark, 2001).

Collaboration

Requirements for effective collaboration begin with a sincere need to make collaboration work, a commitment to the time and energy required to develop relationships, articulated common goals, and supportive key players who can smooth the way, such as principals and assistant principals for curriculum. Effective collaboration requires a willingness to share credit, blame, rewards, and penalties. Fairly healthy organizations are invaluable. In a climate for collaboration, the leadership provides mechanisms for collaboration, such as site-based teams and shared decision-making teams (Conley & Muncey, 1999; Doyle, 2004; Stickel, 1996).

Communication and problem solving among individuals are critical as the individuals are introduced to new ways of doing things (Doyle, 2004; Edwards, 1994). School counselors usually have an advantage in collaboration because they generally have a facilitative leadership style, good communication skills, an understanding of the nature and function of schools, and the "sink or swim" imperative to make collaboration work!

Collaboration is not for the faint of heart; it involves risk, relationship building, personal interaction skills that are above the norm, a spirit of cooperation, leadership ability, mediation skills, a thorough understanding of the nature and function of schools, likeableness, the ability to think on your feet, flexibility, a willingness to compromise, confidence, and an attitude and sincere belief that you can and will make a difference regardless of the attestations of the naysayers.

Management of Resources

Management of resources means implementing outreach efforts to get human, monetary, and technological resources from the internal and external communities. Grabbing and utilizing internal and external community members allows the school counselor to better deliver strategies to enhance student success.

School counselor service delivery is widening its impact from a direct service deliverer to a coordinator of resources, from individual focus to a systemic focus, from a small percentage of the population to a program focusing on all students (Stone & Hanson, 2002). The dilemma that many school counselors face today is how to adequately perform the varied roles that teachers, students, and parents demand of them without diluting their effectiveness (Stone & Hanson, 2002). If school counselors are going to be able to meet the needs of their heavy caseloads, efficient time management will be a constant priority. Student service personnel partnering with regular education teachers and parents to collaboratively solve problems can positively impact many more students than direct services allow (Anderson-Butcher & Ashton, 2004a; Idol & Baran, 1992; Myrick, 2003b).

Beyond reducing student-to-counselor ratios, which has been largely unsuccessful, what approach can school counselors employ in order to meet the needs of so many students? A delivery system is needed that places the school counselor at the hub of managing different stakeholders and resources to help the efforts of the school counseling program. This model requires that the school counselor must be comfortable being a leader and motivator to get others to be part of the school counseling program (Lieberman, 2004). A school counseling program comprised of many resources besides the school counselor is critical if all students (with "all" being defined as each and every student in the school) are going to be supported by the school counseling program.

The comprehensive school counseling program that reaches beyond the school counseling office to bring in resources such as parents, students, teachers, technology, school-based administrators, central administration, the larger community, and the business community redistributes duties so that counselors not only provide direct services, but also manage other resources and utilize other approaches to get the job done. When the school counselor is the direct deliverer, purveyor, and implementer of all activities, then it is impossible to provide a school counseling program that impacts all students. "All" is not possible in an overburdened model in which the school counselor protects the school counseling domain as a one-person operation. Educators and others already employed by the school system are primary resources to tap and can assist in many ways with minimal or no additional funds (Stone & Hanson, 2002). Outside resources are especially welcome and can be an incredible boost to the school counseling program and student success (Anderson-Butcher & Ashton, 2004a; Idol & Baran, 1992; Myrick, 2003b).

Resource brokering is an aspect of the school counselor's role that is only limited by the counselor's tenacity, creativity, and initiative. It is the school counselor who can determine the extent and variety of brokering efforts, which can increase the resources of the school counseling program. It is impossible to adequately describe all the wonderful, available resources that are out there, sometimes just for the asking, such as businesses (some of whom never get approached to help), senior citizen clubs, the military, agencies, and parents.

CASTT a Wider Net Through Partnering

CASTT is an acronym for Community, Administrators, Students, Teachers, and Technology. School counselors who have built a high-profile, powerful, resource-rich school counseling program have *CASTT a wider net* by involving community members, administrators, students, teachers, and technology in the daily work of their school counseling programs. Collaboration results in capacity building so that future work can be redistributed and the school counseling program can cast a wider net in a more efficient manner with minimum duplication of services. The payoff to collaboration and team building is a resource-rich program with an increased commitment to the school counseling program.

CASTT a Wider Net in the Community

External community members, such as agencies, businesses, organizations, civic groups, and other community members, are more and more feeling the responsibility of helping educators deliver the daunting task of educating our citizenry (Anderson-Butcher & Ashton, 2004a; Arriaza, 2004; Moore, 2003). Increasingly, schools are receiving public support in meeting the complex demands of a student population that continues to become more diverse. Educators are realizing that it is implausible to try to meet the needs of students in isolation of our larger communities (Morgan, 2003). Collaboration and partnership building with the community bolsters public faith in our schools but, more important, supports the efforts of educators.

Community volunteers, the greatest untapped resource, can come from churches, postsecondary institutions, the military, businesses—essentially, from all walks of life. Community members can serve individually or collectively on school improvement teams, citizen advisory committees, and/or **neighborhood associations** to impact the likelihood that students will be successful. This section will discuss just a few community resources to partner with your school counseling program: (a) parents, (b) human services agency members, (c) neighborhood associations and groups, (d) businesses, (e) colleges, universities, and other postsecondary institutions; (f) alumni.

Partnering With Parents

Parent-teacher associations or individual parents can serve as partners in the school counseling program. There are many ways in which parents can volunteer, such as sponsoring field trips, getting students involved in community service, serving as mentors and tutors, participating in advisory groups, and participating in telephone trees for emergencies and to advertise school events.

Counselors Making a Difference

Meet Cindy Funkhouser

Parent Volunteer and Full Partner of the School Counseling Program

Cindy Funkhouser, Parent Teacher Association (PTA) president, was a solid partner to Mary Ann Dyal, school counselor, in the following ways:

1. *Bully-Proofing Program*   Under Cindy's guidance, the PTA assisted mightily in implementing a school-wide bully-proofing program. Through provision of resources, financial assistance, manpower, time, energy, faculty trainings, school counseling lessons, and an essay/poster contest, this program impacted every student as well as every faculty and staff member.

2. *Mentoring*   This program was developed for at-risk boys in the fourth grade. Here, Cindy and Mary Ann reached out to a helicopter squadron of the U.S. Navy to provide role models for their at-risk students. The mentors had lunch with the students one day per week over a one-year period. The PTA, under Cindy's leadership, provided lunch for the participants, and teachers were included to reinforce the program's goals. The PTA also provided events such as ice-cream sundae parties for the participants. This program partnered not only the PTA but teachers, students, and businesses as well.

3. *Tutoring*   Cindy and the PTA helped recruit volunteers from the USS *Kennedy* aircraft carrier. This program provided a safety net for those students who were struggling academically.

4. *Parent Fair*   Parents were not attending functions, so the PTA provided the financial backing to offer dinner for the families before meetings began, as well as entertainment for the children while the parents were attending sessions on parenting skills. Some examples of the entertainment were movies, science experiments, and P.E. activities. Cindy and the PTA helped the school counselor pull in community agencies to provide valuable information to the parents.

5. *Character Education*   With the urging of the PTA, a business partner purchased a character education program for the school (it was so successful that the company branched out to other schools to provide the program). The business partner provides all the materials for each month's program, and Cindy helps coordinate the effort. For example, one month's character theme was "Respect." The PTA placed a table card with the word "respect" on it at each seat in the cafeteria. The students were encouraged to take the cards home and place them on their own dining room tables for family discussions about respect (adapted from Stone, 2003b).

Partnering With Human Services Agencies

Both public schools and human services are being challenged to rethink and re-design their efforts to educate, socialize, and intervene in the problems of children and their families (Atkins, Graczyk, Frazier, & Abdul-Adil, 2003; Peebles-Wilkins, 2003). School counselors and other members of the human services profession are searching for increased coordination and collaboration among disciplines to better serve students and their families (Paisley & McMahon, 2001). Many proponents of these changes point out that schools are a natural place for human services activi-ties because they provide maximum access to the majority of children and families (Morgan, 2003).

School counselors can tap community agencies to work in the schools as part of an outreach effort. For example, full-service schools collaborate with the agencies that serve the school community and move those resources onto the school grounds. This easy access helps a greater number of students, but the biggest payoff is the collaboration between agencies and educators, who are in a position to see the daily struggles of the student. Bringing agencies into the school facilitates the ex-amination of the multiple and interrelated etiologies of children's problems and reduces isolated treatment of the family situation, medical concerns, academic achievement, and emotional health. Even without full-service schools, counseling agencies can be repositioned onto the school campus. Seeking alternative ways of delivering family and individual counseling services is especially important given the student-to-counselor ratios, complex psychological issues, and the amount of con-tact hours needed by families. Agencies that can help provide counseling services to students will be a tremendous boost to the school counseling program as, out of necessity, this area usually catches a small percentage of the school population. Current reform efforts are placing renewed emphasis on the linkage of public schools and Human Services Agencies to address significant social problems (Morgan, 2003). School counselors, social workers, school nurses, and others who provide stu-dent support services can form the nucleus around which a collaborative service de-livery system can be built to help children and their families. The complexities and relatedness of student issues reinforce the need for school counselors to partner with agencies in an interdisciplinary manner (Anderson-Butcher & Ashton, 2004a; Gysbers & Henderson, 2001; Paisley & McMahon, 2001).

Partnering With Neighborhood Associations and Groups

Neighborhood associations generally are interested in education, housing, recreation, and community improvements. These groups offer another community resource, as they have a vested interest in making certain the schools of the neighborhood sur-vive and thrive (Langhout, Rappaport, & Simmons, 2002; Vigoda, 2002). Often real estate prices are tied to the success rate of schools. Potential volunteers are real es-tate agents, builders, and others with a vested interest in real estate prices who can come in to help with student needs. Even informal neighborhood groups can be an asset. An El Paso, Texas principal succeeded in stopping the nightly graffiti spraying of his school walls. This smart principal started to talk to the gang members who came to the school in the evenings to play basketball. In working with the gang members he learned that they could and would protect the school if they were allowed to play basketball later into the night. Gangs do not usually have the distinction of being neighborhood associations, but they can be more powerful than a formal group. The point is that all neighborhood groups, including those we generally feel are disenfranchised, can bring support to the school (Lopez, 2004).

Partnering With Businesses

School counselors usually can cite numerous ways in which business partners have helped the school with person-power and financial backing. Start tapping into this resource to support elements of your program that will lend themselves to business support, such as asking businesses to provide mentors and tutors, securing funding for T-shirts for the most improved student citizens, and getting restaurants to provide food for your parent fair. There is an endless list of opportunities for businesses to be part of the school counseling program.

Partnering With Colleges, Universities, and Other Postsecondary Institutions

Counselor educators, particularly those who teach the school counseling and career courses, can provide school counseling or mental health counseling candidates for brief experiences, practicum, or for full-time internships. Ask counselor educators to deliver professional development to programs for your school or for the school district. Counselor educators can be involved in your school counseling program in research projects, such as measuring the impact that your program or particular service delivery has on student outcomes. Consider asking to be a professional development school or a place where counseling candidates are prepared.

Partnering With Alumni

Universities have long courted alumni as a resource for economic support and status. Secondary education has not tapped this resource, which is a gold mine of potential volunteers. Many times alumni feel a sentimental attachment to the school and would love to be asked to contribute to their former institution. When you take a position as a school counselor, why not invite alumni to participate in a school counseling program event? For example, alumni probably represent many varied professions, and you could invite them to present at your career fair. You may find allies who have talents and interests that they want to lend to your program; for example, there may be former students who are mental health therapists, graphic artists, costume designers, writers, firemen, professional athletes, politicians, or photographers. If you groom a relationship with alumni, the possibilities of benefiting from their time and talents will be endless. To get your alumni involved, take some lessons from higher education: feature graduates in school newsletters, honor their achievements, feature them at career fairs, and have annual alumni events. When you are trying to find people who will bring a real commitment and sense of responsibility to the school counseling program, look for alumni.

CASTT a Wider Net With Administrators

Collaborating with administrators can strengthen the leadership team of the school. Counselors and administrators evolved from strikingly different origins but are practically indispensable to each other in a necessary partnership representing contiguous services for students (Wesley, 2001). The relationship between counselor and administrator can enhance or exhaust a school's ability to meet the needs of its students (Wesley, 2001). When school counselors view themselves as partners on the leadership team, their credibility, visibility, and power to effect change is strengthened, and their principals have extra sets of "eyes and ears" to help them impact student success.

Partnering with administrators is powerful. Counselors and administrators no longer think of administration as unconnected to the school counselors' work; rather, counselors and administrators are inseparable partners. "The relationship between counselor and administrator can enhance or exhaust a school's ability to meet the needs of its students. We are married in a tight, necessary partnership representing contiguous services for our students. As in a good marriage, we need to think of ourselves as both individuals and a single unit. Our positions may have evolved from strikingly different origins, but at present, we are practically indispensable to each other" (Wesley, 2001, p. 60). Counselor and administrator partnership activities include

- supporting the school counseling program in spirit and in funding and personnel support;
- keeping each other informed (for example, forewarning about a phone call from an angry parent, or consulting and debriefing on a change in policy);
- sharing critical data elements needed to develop a data-driven school counseling program and highlighting the successes of the school counseling program;
- providing input on evolving district policy;
- supporting a school climate conducive to success;
- working together to support classroom management programs and alternatives to ineffective discipline;

- sharing the burden of crisis intervention so that the counselor can count on delivering a program that reaches beyond crisis intervention to program implementation;
- building confidence that comes from a commitment to one another.

CASTT a Wider Net With Students

Students can be an extension of your school counseling program, serving as allies for students who are being bullied and as sounding boards for students who need another peer to talk to about personal issues. They also can bring talent and skills to serve as tutors, mentors, mediators, aides, speakers, and developers of materials. Students are accessible, willing, and can sometimes be instrumental in influencing their peers when adults cannot.

Peer helpers or peer facilitators are defined as students who assist other students in exploring ideas or feelings about a situation, look for alternatives, and make responsible decisions (Myrick, 2003b). The terms *peer helper, peer facilitator, peer mediator, peer tutor,* and *peer supporter* often are used interchangeably. Students can learn to be peer facilitators by learning basic skills to help others with academic and personal issues. Those who participate in comprehensive peer facilitator programs will be especially helpful in their interactions with others. Peers can have quite an impact on preventing social problems and can help other students gain positive experiences from school.

Peer mediators help resolve conflicts. Here they act as peacekeepers and work closely with administration to develop a set of procedures in handling student conflict. For example, two boys were found fighting in the cafeteria. After the boys were escorted to the mediation conference room, the mediation process was explained to them. Once the boys agreed to participate, the mediators clarified the events that led to the conflict, asked questions, and helped the boys discuss how they were feeling. Finally, they discussed how they might resolve this conflict and avoid any conflicts in the future. Peer mediation reduces discipline referrals and increases a positive attitude toward the school because students are no longer handed referrals or suspension without being able to tell their side of the story (Myrick, 2003b).

Peer tutors are used in all subject areas. With training, peer tutors not only assist students who are struggling academically; they also build relationships with the students. This in turn allows them to identify problems that impact students' study habits, as well as pinpoint other classroom issues that may be distracting. Students often feel embarrassed to ask for extra help and may worry about what their friends might think; however, peer tutors are responsive to these feelings and increase a student's ability to access extra help (Myrick, 2003b).

Peer facilitator training also has a positive impact on the work of student assistants (Myrick, 2003b), and this role is one of indirect assistance to peers. Students as aides or student assistants provide help to teachers and counselors by working in offices, helping with bulletin boards, distributing materials, or assisting with planning activities.

CASTT a Wider Net With Teachers and Other Staff Members

Teachers and other educators, such as teacher assistants (also called paraprofessionals or guidance assistants), special education teachers, school psychologists, and social workers, are accessible and vital partners.

Partnering With Teachers

Teaming school counselors with teachers can strengthen classroom management, bring attention to learning styles, provide safety nets for students, promote programs such as cooperative discipline, and deliver schoolwide programs such as character education to improve the school climate. Teachers can considerably promote and spread the influence of the school counseling program. Through teachers we get support for classroom guidance lessons, mentoring and tutoring programs, and interventions for special needs students. Teachers can instruct school counselors in how to disseminate effective instructional techniques to other teachers. Teachers can help develop schoolwide interventions such as behavior management programs, awards programs, and staff development.

Special education (SE) teachers must use many of the same skills in their jobs that counselors do, albeit to differing degrees. The two professionals are prepared in separate programs to assess student needs, pose appropriate developmental interventions, and consult with parents and teachers to analyze situations and generate possible alternatives for resolving them. School counselors and SE teachers are required to collaborate on teams when developing Individual Education Plans (IEP). Special education teachers and school counselors are natural allies in performing the sophisticated, demanding function of consulting effectively (Dettmer, Thurston, & Dyck, 2002). School counselors and SE teachers can greatly impact students when working together on teams to gather information and explore alternatives to help parents and teachers, who control so much of the physical, affective, and cognitive environment in which the child lives (Bergin & Bergin, 2000). Helping parents and teachers with their immediate problems improves their future functioning (McEachern, 2003).

Special education teachers can help further the goals of the school counseling program by

- assisting with remediation and prevention;
- developing strategies to assist many students with academic and social problems, not just special education students;
- offering consultation services to regular education teachers;
- closely monitoring students' progress;
- enabling the prevention of some problems as well as the remediation of others;

- reducing special education placements and the time students will spend in an SE placement;
- establishing, staffing, and supporting a **pre-referral team.** (This strategy has been adapted nationwide to provide more comprehensive consultation services before SE is considered.)

Pre-referral intervention assistance teams have emerged due to (a) excessive numbers of students inappropriately referred to and declared eligible for special education, (b) the need for greater levels of consultation and collaboration, and (c) the need to support teachers who have too many students and are struggling to accommodate special learning needs (Burns, 1999; Lane, Mahdavi, & Borthwick-Duffy, 2003; Zins, 2004). Special education teachers can serve as the backbone of pre-referral work, which will considerably reduce the work that school counselors have to do to get children through the child study team process in preparation for SE.

Partnering With Other Educators/Staff Members

Schools have tried to soften the grip of poverty and respond to student needs by providing lunch programs, health clinics, and a full range of services. A wide range of professionals, including social workers, nurses, and school psychologists, provide information in areas such as personal health, safety, and sex education, and they also serve as a critical link between the school, home, and community (Allen-Meares, Washington, & Welsh, 2004; Anderson-Butcher & Ashton, 2004a).

These same educators can be brought into the school counseling effort. For example, school psychologists or social workers can serve on SE pre-referral teams, can serve as a resource for interventions, and can help set up behavior management programs for teachers. Social workers also can help set up a parent night or parent fair. Attendance teachers can identify absentees and help to provide the interventions to get these students back in school; for example, the attendance teacher can alert others and seek help if they learn a student has been absent due to circumstances such as bullying, a bus schedule that does not work, or homelessness. Occupational specialists can help with career programs. The point is that school counselors can creatively and assertively look to each employee of the school district as a potential partner in the school counseling program. The teacher assistants, the custodian, the cafeteria workers, and the computer, music, art, and physical education teachers all can be extensions of the school counseling program.

CASTT a Wider Net With Technology

Technology has great potential for increasing school counselors' efficiency and requires little upfront expense compared to the valuable time saved. Computers have been considered a tool for expediting tedious, repetitive tasks, but computers'

potential for enhancing the roles, responsibilities, and effectiveness of school counselors is being expanded (Tyler & Sabella, 2004). Turba (1998) described the technology skills needed for the school counselor/advocate to perform his or her job
functions adequately:

- basic computer literacy skills
- knowledge of Internet resources
- ability to use software that relates to school counseling
- comfort level with virtual activities such as chatrooms, discussion groups, and listservers
- virtual guidance offices that help students access Internet resources (p.10)

Chris Bryan, Ribault High School counselor in Jacksonville, Florida, says it best,
"I believe that in the not-too-distant future, technology itself will be the biggest advocate for our teachers, students, and parents. Technology is all about communication, information, and potentially, the truth. The types of experiences technology
can provide are becoming more and more immediate with audio and visual Internet
connections. These connections have the potential to make education a much more
transparent process than it is today. Right now our classrooms are windowless
rooms. Parents can't see in. Teachers can't see out. Some school districts already
have systems in place in which direct Internet communication, including information about students' attendance, behavior, and grades, takes place among parents,
school counselors, and teachers." The speed with which counselors are now able to
get information ideally positions us to use technology to our advantage in our advocacy role.

Barriers to Collaboration and Management of Resources

Barriers to partnerships usually occur in the form of time, space, and personnel, all
of which are usually in short supply in schools. Other barriers, such as weak interpersonal skills, can prevent educators from establishing and maintaining collaborative efforts. An atmosphere of **collegiality** starts with an administration that
encourages collaborative efforts. Without administrative support, the collaboration
can become an arduous chore. Collegiality models shared decision making and mul-
tifaceted/multidisciplinary efforts, and reacts with enthusiasm to new ideas.

External members are harder to manage because services are often fragmented,
and the logistics of managing resources can eat up large chunks of precious time,
albeit time well spent as you meet the needs of more students. Rules and regulations of agencies, businesses, and civic organizations can severely limit the work that
can be accomplished. In addition, services cannot always be repositioned into the
school, and this means families may have to find transportation and finances for
services.

Parental involvement for some schools seems impossible to obtain. It can be very frustrating when parents do not respond, even when it is a matter of importance to their child's future. Herculean efforts to secure parental involvement can sometimes go unrewarded. For example, during the 2003–2004 school year the University of North Florida's (UNF) 18 school counseling candidates worked in an internship at a critical needs school. The school had low parental involvement, high dropout rates, low rates of students going on to postsecondary institutions, such as college or vocational/technical training, and was designated by the state as a failing school (students were offered waivers to go elsewhere). The school counseling interns made more than 900 phone calls to the parents of 320 students over the course of four months, in an effort to get the parents to participate in a joint career and academic advising session with their children. Information about the sessions was also communicated during visits to the local faith community and in written information disseminated to students and parents at the school, at sporting events, and through the mail. Parents were offered sessions at their convenience, including Saturdays, daytime, and nighttime. The results were disappointing; only eleven parents participated in a face-to-face advising session. However, the counselors did not feel it was without payoff, because during the 900 phone contacts, parents were given critical career and academic information. Later evidence revealed that the seeds planted bore fruit in the form of an increase in test scores for the 320 students who received career and academic advising. The school counseling interns regrouped and doubled their efforts to give students assignments and information to take home to discuss with their parents, and they turned to the faith community as a vehicle to reach parents. Research clearly indicates that children perform better, both academically and socially, if parents are involved in their children's education (Lewis & Forman, 2002; Menning, 2002). The connection between home and school is vital but sometimes impossible to realize in the traditional sense of parents coming to the school for PTA meetings or advising sessions. Rather than lament and sit on their hands, the UNF interns looked for alternate ways of reaching parents.

Collegiality: Taking Collaboration to a Higher Level

When schools have a climate of collegiality, much is gained. The benefits must be substantial for educators to put aside other activities in order to work with colleagues, for the principal to promote and organize such work, for superintendents to endorse it, and for the school boards to pay for this work (Doyle, 2004; Lieberman, 2004; Woods & Weasmer, 2004 this is the Lieberman reference). The perceived benefits must be great enough that the time educators spend together can compete with time spent in other ways, on other priorities that are equally compelling or more immediate (Everett, Tichenor, & Heins, 2003). School counselors can contribute mightily to an environment of collegiality. Collaboration is critical, but collegiality is collaboration at a different, deeper, and more professionally satisfying level. You can collaborate with other educators and not feel you have been collegial with them. Collegiality means the educator grows as a professional intellectually, personally, and in stature and standing. Collegiality means greater job satisfaction, and it attracts able and talented candidates by affording them work that is stimulating, meaningful, economically rewarding, and well regarded in the larger community (Lieberman, 2004). Collegiality results in a school that taps the collective talents, experience, and energy of its professional staff (Doyle, 2004; Edwards, Green, & Lyons, 2002). The achievement of strong collegial relations is a remarkable accomplishment; it is not the rule, but the rare, often fragile exception (Conley & Muncey, 1999). Most teachers can point to a treasured colleague, but few work in schools where cooperative work is a condition of employment. Many teachers are satisfied with their peer relationships, but few claim that those relationships make their way into the classroom (Conley & Muncey, 1999). Many schools offer congenial work environments, but few offer a professional environment that makes the school as educative for teachers as for students (Edwards et al., 2002; Everett et al., 2003; Doyle, 2004). Collegiality increases the social aspect of schools. Social interactions with other adults, especially one's peers, can increase job satisfaction, and negate the loneliness and stress some educators feel (Woods & Weasmer, 2004; Black, 2004).

Teachers who have worked together closely over a period of years celebrate their accomplishments by pointing to gains in the achievement, behavior, and attitude of students (O'Day, 2002). What are the implications for school counselors? As we work on systemic change, as we collaborate and partner, and as we manage human resources, we will want to concentrate on collegiality as a central focus and not just a happenstance byproduct of good collaboration.

Application of CASTT in Building a Safe and Respectful School Climate

Using a typical example in our schools, let's look at how school counselors can broker resources to impact the No Child Left Behind (2001) goal of a safer, more respectful school climate for all students.

The climate at your school is dangerous for gay, lesbian, and bisexual students. You want to try to promote a safer, more inclusive school climate for this at-risk minority. How will you and the other members of the school's leadership team coordinate, collaborate, partner, and manage resources to help create a safer, more respectful school climate for this vulnerable student population? Who will be your stakeholders and resources? What strategies will you use? The following discussion gives examples of how to address the problem and answer the questions.

1. *Community Resources*   Gay, lesbian, and bisexual students often are isolated from the normal family support that is vital for successful identity development. Parents who have already been through the revelation that their child is gay, lesbian, or bisexual can offer support to families of students who are in the throes of trying to learn how to support their child who is wrestling with sexual identity issues.

   Agency counselors who work often with gay, lesbian, and bisexual youth can provide information about the best way to support these students. The local chapter of Parents and Friends of Lesbians and Gays (PFLAG), an international support group, can serve as a resource for information about local resources and support groups to assist students and their parents. Lambda Legal Defense and Education Fund (e-mail lambda@lambdalegal.org) can deliver professional development on *Davis v. Monroe County Board of Education* so that teachers will understand the implications of the Supreme Court's decision on school safety and management of harassment.

   Community groups can work to reduce hate crimes and heighten understanding among all citizens. For example, two weeks after Matthew Shepard was killed in what was at the time determined to be a gay hate crime, 17 school and community groups, composed of straight, gay, lesbian, and bisexual students as well as parents, teachers, and counselors joined together in Rockland County, Massachusetts, to develop strategies aimed at reducing hate crimes. Supported by GLSEN-Hudson Valley, participants left with action plans to attack one area of prejudice in their school or community (GLSENTalk, 1998).

   Faculty, staff, and students from postsecondary institutions can provide speakers, money, facilities, and materials to help school counselors and others toward a safe and respectful school climate for gay, lesbian, and bisexual youth.

2. *Administrative Resources*   Administrators can promote the implementation of a policy protecting all students against sexual harassment to include a clause that expressly mentions sexual orientation. Elements of an effective sexual harassment policy should include the applicable laws, a zero tolerance statement, and due process procedures to address complaints. The last ten years have been defined by disturbing research demonstrating that gay, lesbian, and bisexual students are at greater risk for physical and emotional abuse in schools than are their peers, yet this research has had minimal influence on changing school systems (Garcia, Adams, Friedman, & East, 2002; Keeling, 2001; Keeling, 2002; Stone, 2003e).

   Students hear anti-gay remarks 25 times per day (PFLAG, 2004). The dropout rate for gay students is estimated at three times the national average (Bart, 1998). Administrators can lead the charge to implement violence prevention activities that involve the students helping to solve the problem. Too many times, violence prevention looks at installing more surveillance equipment or increasing security. These measures may be very vital for a given school, but nothing can take the place of getting the students involved in tackling the problem.

Administrators can support an assembly on diversity and tolerance and include a speaker like Corey Johnson, the co-captain of his high-school football team, who came out in his junior year (Lipsyte, 2000). Administrators can allow written information on bulletin boards advertising support groups and community activities for all minority groups, to include gay, lesbian, or bisexual students. It is less threatening to school officials to have a bulletin board that gives referral resources in the community for support groups for a number of minority groups; gay, lesbian, and bisexual groups then are just one more minority group in the information exchange.

3. *Student Resources*   Students can establish the role of heterosexual allies and call for systemic reform. Students can promote bully-proofing efforts and identify, intervene, and/or report bullying. Students across Colorado returned to school after the Columbine High School shooting wearing tiny patches that bore the single word "respect." The patch was designed to promote harmony among the school cliques exposed at Columbine.

4. *Teachers and Other Staff as Resources*   Teachers can include in their curriculum and instruction diversity awareness and multicultural initiatives aimed at promoting tolerance. Teachers can use inclusive language whenever possible to talk about famous gay, lesbian, and bisexual historical figures in social studies, English, and science (Lipkin, 2004). Classroom discussions can include information about issues involving gay, lesbian, and bisexual students, to the extent that institutional and community standards will support. Critically important, teachers can challenge disparaging verbal or written remarks about sexual orientation that are made in their presence.

Other educators can provide support in the form of information, acceptance, staff development, counseling, and so on. For example, the media specialist can influence the choice of library books so that gay, lesbian, and bisexual students can begin to see themselves in the curriculum. Nurses can educate teachers as to the prevalence of suicide and development issues for this at-risk group.

The guidance assistant can establish a packet of documents for teachers and other educators in order to raise awareness of the gay, lesbian, and bisexual minority. Most practitioners interviewed about their sources of knowledge regarding gay, lesbian, and bisexual youth have commented about the limited content in their preparation program and curriculum (Lipkin, 2004). The school counselor managing resources can ask the guidance assistant to provide information that will close the gap in information and understanding.

5. *Technology Resources*   Through technology, teachers and other educators can be provided with access to legal information on creating a safe respectful school climate. One example of such information can be found at http://web.lexis-nexis.com/universe/document?. Also, technology can help us track discipline referrals that involve hate crimes and tell us where the incidents are taking place and who the perpetrators are.

In addition to the coordination of CASTT, school counselors also can provide specific strategies to support individual students as well as offer activities and services that educate the wider community in order to promote a safe and respectful environment. You can develop strategies to help students ease into the discussion of sexuality. For example, have students respond to verbal or written questions in which sexuality is but one of a number of questions and given the same weight as other questions (Stone & Hanson, 2002). Encourage gay, lesbian, and bisexual students to involve their parents, and offer to be available for a joint conference. Persuade students to express the fears they hold about telling their parents. Help students anticipate their parents' reaction, and assist the student in developing coping strategies (Stone & Hanson, 2002). Display the pink triangle "safe place" stickers supplied by Gay Lesbian Straight Educators Network (GLSEN) or other support symbols to send a message to heterosexual as well as gay, lesbian, or bisexual students that the school counselor is an ally or friend. Continue to enhance collaboration between families and school. Involving parents routinely helps facilitate communication in tougher times. Practice unconditional positive regard. Gay, lesbian, and bisexual students are very vulnerable because they are fraught with guilt and know they are facing almost universal alienation and hostility. Regardless of school board policy, community standards, and their personal values, counselors must make a student feel valued while making an appropriate referral. Ignoring or invalidating a student who is struggling with a sexual identity issue is a devastating response. Acquire professional development training through workshops and/or literature on counseling strategies and legal and ethical issues involving sexual harassment for gay, lesbian, and bisexual students. Provide an on-site workshop for faculty and staff.

Supporting the right of all students, including gay, lesbian, and bisexual students, to have a safe and respectful school climate would be a daunting task if not for the multitude of resources that a school counselor can draw upon. This one example still takes tremendous coordination, resources, and time, but if we seek and find one or two talented individuals to help us, we minimize our involvement and maximize our effectiveness. (Myrick, 2003b).

TechTools

CASTT a Wider Net by using technology in your coordination role.

- School counselors often develop patterns in their recommendation letters, repeating key phrases and expressions when describing different students' academic prowess, character, athletic performance, service, and leadership. By compiling the standard phrases that you use and then creating files by type, you can go to your file, chose the paragraph that most closely matches each student, and tailor the paragraph to accurately reflect the individual student.

- Develop electronic forms, handbooks, addresses, and other information for easy use. Teachers and others can personalize and send information much more efficiently if templates are provided for them. All they need to do is personalize them so that the information is specific to their class or student(s).

- Technology plays a critical role in having accurate, timely data from student information management systems. A school counselor who uses this data increases his or her ability to be a social justice advocate; to monitor patterns of course enrollment, student access, and success in higher level academics; to deliver career and academic advising; and to manage resources to extend the reach of the school counseling program.

- Make technology your partner in career and academic advising, helping you close the information gap in areas such as helping students understand that financing a higher education is possible, assisting students in researching career clusters, helping students with interest inventories, and enabling students to virtually experience colleges.

School Counselor Casebook: *Voices From the Field*

The Scenario Reviewed

For the second consecutive year your school has been placed on the Critically Low Performing Schools list, which means that if test scores do not improve over the next two years, the state will take over the school. You believe that as a member of the leadership team, instructional success and student achievement are as much your job as they are that of the principal, teachers, and other critical stakeholders. Your principal does not assign you extraneous duties, and you have a comprehensive developmental school counseling program that is very solid and meaningful and already supports the achievement of students; yet, like everyone else in the school, you feel pressure from the possible state takeover. You want to extend your reach to support more students' academic success, but your day is already packed with very important tasks that you do not want to relinquish.

A Practitioner's Approach

Here's how a practicing school counselor responded to this school scenario:

As a counselor I would examine my resources first to see what options I have at my disposal. For example, I would look at my time and at already scheduled activities on my calendar: How much time can I personally allocate to improving our school's performance on this year's test scores? What interventions am I already doing? What interventions would I like to implement, and how much time will I need to implement them?

Next I would look at the faculty resources available: Are there other stakeholders who can assist with some of the interventions I have in mind? For example, would our school social worker, school psychologist, and other student service personnel be available to assist? Would I be able to utilize parent volunteers, students from the high school, and other community-based persons to assist? And then I would look at my financial resources: What type of funding will be needed to implement the interventions, and are those types of funds available to me through my local school budget? If not, what other types of system funds could be accessed, i.e., Drug-Free Schools, PTA mini-grants, etc.?

After examining my resources, the next step would be to meet with the school leadership team to present my ideas to them. If they are interested, then I can move forward with an action plan, but if they do not want to see a particular program implemented, I would need to explore other options. Without administrative support and the support of the school leadership team, little can be accomplished. The most significant aspect of reviewing my ideas with the school leadership team is to make sure that my suggestions fit with the school's overall strategic plan for school improvement. Our strategic plan drives our school focus and must be utilized as the overall force behind implementation of our school counseling plan.

Once the resources have been reviewed and the support from administration and the leadership team has been gained, it is time to move ahead with implementation of strategies and ideas. I would utilize an action plan format to formulate the structure and timeline of any intervention I plan to implement. This would allow me to spell out what my goals and objectives are and what strategies I want to use to reach those objectives. It will also keep me on track in terms of who is responsible for what, what my timelines are, what benchmarks I can use to gauge my success by, which national standards we are meeting, and what the final evaluation component will be.

These are some more specific suggestions for strategies I might utilize:

I would identify which students are performing below the proficient expected levels on the state or national test by examining test scores. I could also use student grades to help identify underperforming students. Once students are identified, I could assess what services these students are already receiving in terms or remediation, tutoring, and other forms of academic assistance. If there are students who are not receiving these types of services, I can find out how to get them involved in a tutorial program, afterschool help sessions with teachers, etc. If it appears that students need assistance with study skills and school success skills I can set up small group counseling sessions with these students. If I have not had the opportunity to implement classroom guidance sessions on these topics, I could also set these up with teachers.

Another useful strategy to assist students in becoming responsible for improving their own areas of weakness is to utilize individual advisement sessions with each student to review their last year's test scores and areas of weaknesses and strengths. Helping the student come up with a plan for improvement is the focus of the advisement session. For this strategy it is important to enlist other persons in the school system, including central office personnel, who are willing to come out and assist students on assigned dates. Each adviser is given a group of students to work with on a specific date and is scheduled with students every 15 minutes during that day.

Reaching out to parents of identified students in several areas, such as interpretation of test scores, how to help your child be test-wise, and other related topics is another way to work on improving your school's test scores. Parents need to know how important the test dates are for their child, and what they can do to help their child do their very best on test dates.

Finally, I would review the resources I acquired from past conferences and counselor's meetings and talk with other counselors to see what ideas they are using in their schools. I find other counselors to be the very best resource of all because they can come up with ideas that they are familiar with from their schools and then I can adapt those ideas to fit my own school. Resources exist—but it is truly a matter of identifying and coordinating them if we are going to improve the situation in our school. Who better than the school counselor to take a leadership role in making this happen!

Susan McCarthy is currently working as a middle school counselor at Sandy Springs Middle School, Fulton County Schools, Georgia, and has extensive school counseling experience at the elementary and secondary levels. Susan has also served as the state guidance consultant for the Georgia Department of Education and as a supervisor of counseling for a large suburban/urban school system in Atlanta. Susan is the editor of the Georgia School Counselors Association Journal *(GSCA), president of the Georgia Association of Counselor Educators and Supervisors, and is an ASCA national standards trainer. Reprinted with permission by Susan S. McCarthy, Ed.S.*

Chapter Summary

Coordination of Services, Collaboration, and Management of Resources

Skillful coordination, collaboration, and brokering of resources will determine the success or failure of your school counseling program. Coordination, collaboration, and management of resources are the mechanics or "how to" that guide your school counseling program. Coordination of services means prioritizing and efficiently organizing and delivering the components of your school counseling program, including individual and group counseling, classroom guidance lessons, consultation services, career and academic advising, and systemic support. Collaboration is entering into a partnership or liaison with other individuals, groups, or members of other institutions who share a common mission of student success and who work with you and other members of the educational community for the purpose of enhancing the personal-social, career, and academic outcomes of every student in the school. School counselors who broker resources can extend their reach to more students by bringing in resources such as parents, students, teachers, technology, administrators, community members, and business partners.

Coordinator of Services

The coordinator's role is to decide the goals of the school counseling program and to identify the mechanisms and resources needed to carry out those goals. The coordination role has become one of the most important roles of a school counselor because we must increasingly rely on the expertise and services of others in order to deliver optimum programs. School counselors' roles need to change from just direct service delivery to becoming staff developers, consultants, collaborators, team builders, resource brokers, and supporters of instruction.

Collaboration and Partnering

Collaboration is an important tool to help us meet the needs of all the students in our charge. By teaming with others, we have a better chance of getting our arms around all of our students to close the gaps in their information, to support their social development, and to widen their opportunities to fully participate in the U.S. economy. School counselors take ownership of individual counseling, consultation, leadership, and advocacy, which require specialized skills. There are many activities that school counselors want to see successfully completed to benefit students but that do not need to be under their exclusive purview. Standards, socioeconomic stresses, and limited resources demand that educators—especially school counselors who have been demanding student-to-counselor ratios—collaborate with each other to deliver optimum services to students. Collaboration with and among administrators, teachers, businesses, and community agencies, with careful guidance and nurturing, will improve school counseling programs and promote student success.

CASTT a Wider Net: The Benefits of Collaboration

School counselors can cast a wider net when they commit to collaboration. CASTT is an acronym that stands for Community, Administrators, Students, Teachers, and Technology. These are the people who will benefit the most from a collaborative school counseling program and who will also be our partners in this collaborative program, increasing our effectiveness and widening our reach. Technology is an efficient and effective way of disseminating information and analyzing results. The benefits of collaboration allow counselors to establish a high-profile, powerful school counseling program that will help support students to realize their dreams. Collaboration is capacity building so that the future work can be redistributed and the school counseling program will cast a wider net in a more efficient manner with minimum duplication of services. Involve others, because the payoff is increased commitment to the school counseling program and a widening of stakeholders.

Barriers, Limitations, and Collegiality of Collaboration

Limitations exist, which make partnerships in schools a challenge. External members are harder to manage than partners who are right there in the school. Lack of interpersonal skills prevents educators from establishing and maintaining collaborative efforts. Collegiality models shared decision making, multifaceted/multidisciplinary efforts, and reacts with enthusiasm to new ideas. School counselors usually have an advantage in collaboration because they generally have a facilitative leadership style, good communication skills, an understanding of the nature and function of schools, and the "sink or swim" attitude needed to make collaboration work! It helps immeasurably when there is a climate for collaboration in which the leadership of the school district and the school site encourages collaborative efforts with mechanisms such as site-based teams and shared decision-making teams.

Management of Resources

School counselor service delivery has widened from a direct service deliverer to a coordinator of resources, from an individual focus to a systemic focus, from a small percentage of the population to a program focusing on all students. The dilemma is how to achieve efficient use of time and resources to be able to address increasingly heavy caseloads for counselors. A delivery model is needed based on having the school counselor at the hub of managing different stakeholders and resources to help the efforts of the school counseling program. This model requires that the school counselor must be comfortable being a leader and motivator to get others to be part of the school counseling program.

Key Terms

CASTT p. 186
Collegiality p. 194

Coordination of services p. 180
Coordinator p. 180

Learning Extensions

1. Discuss the benefits and limitations of collaboration. Can you be collaborative without being collegial? Why or why not? What are the benefits of collegiality?

2. Briefly discuss how you plan to use each of these eleven potential resources in your school counseling program: (a) administrators, (b) regular education teachers, (c) Exceptional Student Education Teachers, (d) other educators, (e) parents, (f) students, (g) guidance assistants, (h) agency members, (i) community members, (j) colleges, universities, and other postsecondary institutions, and (k) technology. Identify other resources to bring in for partnering with your school counseling program besides the eleven named in the chapter.

3. Besides the above eleven resources, identify and explain the role of two other resources to bring in to partner with your school counseling program.

4. Think about the makeup of a pre-referral team for your future school. Who would you want to see on the team? How will you go about organizing the team? What other educator could take ownership of the team besides you? Develop a plan for your future school.

Chapter 8

Implementing the National Standards and the ASCA Model

Chapter Objectives

By the time you have completed this chapter, you should be able to:

- Understand the relationship of school counseling to the national standards movement.
- Identify the nine National Standards for School Counseling Programs (ASCA, 1997)
- Explain the relationship of the national standards to the ASCA National Model and the comprehensive model.
- Understand how to implement a national standards-based comprehensive, developmental, and results-based program.
- Give examples of how implementing the national standards can help to support student growth, development, achievement, and success in school.

School Counselor Casebook: *Getting Started*

The Scenario

For the past two weeks, several students in your caseload have complained to you about certain other students, who have been provoking them to fight. Although students often complain about "being picked on," something about this situation just doesn't seem right. The students will not tell you who is involved, but insist that you "tell" the teachers to do something about it. As you think this through, several courses of action are available to you. You decide to discuss this with the other school counselors in your building, the teachers who are involved with these students, and your building principal. In your planning, you consider how the ASCA model and the national standards will help you address this situation.

Thinking About Solutions

As you read this chapter, think about what actions you might take in this situation. How would you get the faculty involved? What activities might address the complaints about "bullying"? How would you know that these efforts were successful? When you come to the end of the chapter, you will have the opportunity to see how your ideas compare with a practicing school counselor's approach.

The National Standards Movement: An Agenda for Equity

The changing status of children and families, the needs of the work force, the dynamics of the economy, and our interrelationship with the global community have, for the past 20 years, challenged the educational community. The demands on schools for higher student achievement and the reallocation of educational resources were noted as necessary to prepare the next generation of Americans with the computational, literacy, technical, and learning skills needed to be productive participants in tomorrow's economy (Annie Casey Foundation, 1996). Reform measures for results and accountability became the basis for political platforms (Owings and Kaplan, 2000). Archibald (2000) suggested that the pressure for improvements in public education came primarily from politicians and representatives of business and industry. As a result, **national standards** were mandated as the solution for educational reform.

In every state, in every school building, and in every community, school improvement initiatives have taken hold. The annual Phi Delta Kappan poll, *Of the Public Attitudes Toward Public Schools* (Rose & Gallup, 2004), showed that 75% of the respondents supported reforming the existing public school system as the means to improve public education. Likewise, many teachers also believe that the push to raise academic standards is headed in the right direction (Olson, 2001).

GOALS 2000 (U.S. Department of Education, 1994) was the impetus to challenge the American educational system to use standards as the foundation for curriculum development. Educational leadership across the nation struggled to define what was meant by standards (Darling-Hammond, 1992; Eisner, 1993; Howe, 1991; Wiggins, 1991). The intent was that standards for what students should know and be able to do would transform American education (Alexander, 1993). Since the wave of standards-based educational reform, which began with *A Nation at Risk* (1983), every state across the nation has adopted some form of standards-based education, but not without controversy and concern for equity and equal educational opportunity for every student.

As the academic disciplines grappled with the pressures of educational reform, commissioned reports of national significance, such as *Keeping the Options Open* (1986) and *High Hopes, Long Odds* (1994), praised school counselors for the work they do and condemned them for what they didn't do. The Commission on Precollege Guidance and Counseling (1986) proposed a comprehensive set of recommendations that identified the ways in which guidance and counseling can contribute to increasing student potential and the number of students pursuing postsecondary opportunities. Disturbing issues addressed in these documents included the accusation that school counselors were gatekeepers perpetuating the accepted rules and systemic barriers that caused inequities between achievers and nonachievers based on race and socioeconomic status (Hart & Jacobi, 1992).

Although school counselors continued to work doggedly to deliver a constellation of responsive services to at-risk students in need of counselor intervention, the majority of American educators were focused on improving student achievement. Little in research was offered to connect counseling to student achievement; therefore, the studies that did mention us gained little national attention (Whiston, 2002). School counseling research examined the school counselor role, analyzed time and tasks, and explored the impact and significance of intervention and prevention activities (Borders & Drury, 1992; Johnson, 2000). Without clearly connecting the practice of school counseling to student impact, the school counselor remained conspicuously absent in the conversations that centered on reform efforts to promote higher levels of student success.

School Counseling: Finding a Place in School Improvement

Concerned that school counselors were being viewed as peripheral to the school reform agenda, ASCA took a leadership role in recasting school counseling as an integral component of the educational system (ASCA, 1994). In this era of increased educational accountability, it became vital to show how school counselors contribute to preparing students to meet the increasingly complex demands of society and the work force.

Concurrently, organizations that had an interest in the work of school counselors, such as the Education Trust (1997), defined a new vision for school counseling that emphasized leadership, advocacy, use of data, and a commitment to support high levels of student achievement. School counselors were encouraged to shift their focus from the delivery of a menu of student services to providing a structured and programmatic approach for counselors to address the needs of all students (Gysbers & Henderson, 2000).

To move this agenda forward, three important ideological transformations were necessary:

1. Counselors would shift the focus from the role of the school counselor position to the impact of the school counseling program on student achievement. Counselors would share the concerns and goals of other education professionals.

2. School counselors would look at their work from an "all students" perspective. No longer would it be enough for *some* students to profit from counselor services; every student would benefit from the school counseling programs.

3. School counselors, as potentially powerful allies in school reform, would develop programs to support student developmental growth and academic achievement, improving results by impacting the system (Clark & Stone, 2000; Dahir, 2004). School counselors would be seen as partners in school improvement, concerned with every student's ability to access a quality education.

Table 8.1

From Position	To Program	To System
Impacting Some Students	Impacting Every Student	Impacting the System to Impact Every Student
Advocacy for students on an as-needed basis.	Advocacy to ensure that every student benefits from a program that emphasizes academic, career, and personal-social developmental growth and learning.	Advocacy to ensure that school district policies and practices fairly and equitably provide educational opportunity to every student.

As depicted in Table 8.1, school counselors, embracing the law of parsimony (Myrick, 2000) have shifted their focus from a *some students agenda* to an *every student agenda* that assures the acquisition of skills and knowledge and equity in educational opportunity.

ASCA's Contribution to School Reform: The National Standards for School Counseling Programs

In response to GOALS 2000 (1994), the ASCA Governing Board committed to the development of the national standards, following the lead of the academic disciplines, which were in the process of creating their own national standards. ASCA believed that standards would motivate the school counseling community to identify and implement goals for students that were deemed important by the profession, clarify the relationship of school counseling to the educational system, and address the contributions of school counseling to student success.

Standards would provide counselors, administrators, and the general public with an understanding of what school counseling programs should contain and deliver (Perry, 1991). National guidelines assisted in establishing the overall purpose of school counseling programs and offered strategies to assess the achievement of that purpose (Schmidt, 1999). This concept of standards was not new to the school counseling profession. *Standards for Guidance and Counseling Programs* (ASCA, 1979) outlined the administrative structure, resources, and facilities needed, and presented evaluation guidelines. The document did not suggest program content or methods of delivery, but promoted consistency in practice as counseling programs were adapted to the individual school's mission.

ASCA determined that the school counseling standards, like the academic subject standards, would define what K–12 students should know and be able to do as a result of participating in a school counseling program (Campbell & Dahir, 1997).

The National Standards for School Counseling Programs (ASCA, 1997) tied the work of school counseling programs to the mission of schools, and encouraged school counselors to assume a leadership role in school reform (Bowers, Hatch, & Schwallie-Giddis, 2001). ASCA believed that national standards would:

1. Promote equitable access to school counseling programs and services for all students.

2. Establish similar goals and expectations for all students.

3. Identify and prioritize the key content components for school counseling programs.

4. Position school counseling as an integral component of the academic mission of school.

5. Identify the knowledge and skills that all students should acquire as a result of the pre-K through 12 school counseling program.

6. Ensure that school counseling programs are comprehensive in design and delivered in a systematic fashion for all students (Campbell & Dahir, 1997).

A major research study was undertaken in 1995 to analyze relevant school counseling and educational reform literature and to review existing school counseling program models developed at the state level. Two thousand ASCA members were surveyed to assess the level of support for standards development and to offer opinions about their content (Dahir, Campbell, Johnson, Scholes, & Valiga, 1997). The survey findings (Dahir et al., 1997) revealed that school counselors strongly supported national standards and believed that standards could help school counselors define program goals and a professional mission, and would raise expectations of practice.

Key Areas of Student Development

The study confirmed the continued importance of the three widely accepted and interrelated areas of student development: academic development, career development, and personal-social development. In addition, nine standards emerged from the research (Campbell & Dahir, 1997).

Academic Development

The three standards for **academic development** guide school counselors as they implement school counseling program strategies and activities to support and maximize student learning. The academic development standards are:

Standard A.   Students will acquire the attitudes, knowledge, and skills that contribute to effective learning in school and across the life span.

Standard B.   Students will complete school with the academic preparation essential to choose from a wide variety of substantial postsecondary options, including college.

Standard C.   Students will understand the relationship of academics to the world of work, and to life at home and in the community.

Career Development

The standards for **career development** guide school counselors as they implement school counseling program strategies and activities to help students acquire attitudes, knowledge, and skills to successfully transition from grade to grade, from school to postsecondary education, and ultimately to the world of work. The three career development standards are:

Standard A.   Students will acquire the skills to investigate the world of work in relation to knowledge of self and to make informed career decisions.

Standard B.   Students will employ strategies to achieve future career success and satisfaction.

Standard C.   Students will understand the relationship between personal qualities, education and training, and the world of work.

Personal-Social Development

The standards for **personal-social development** guide school counselors as they implement school counseling program strategies and activities to provide personal and social growth experiences to facilitate students' progress through school and the transition to adulthood. Personal-social development contributes to academic and career success, acquisition of effective interpersonal skills, and development as contributing members of society. The three personal-social development standards are:

Standard A: Students will acquire the attitudes, knowledge, and interpersonal skills to help them understand and respect self and others.

Standard B: Students will make decisions, set goals, and take appropriate action to achieve goals.

Standard C: Students will understand safety and survival skills.

Source: Sharing the Vision: The National Standards for School Counseling Programs (Campbell & Dahir, 1997, pp. 17–19)

Student Competencies

Expectations of student accomplishments or outcomes as a result of participating in a standards-based school counseling program are written in terms of **student competencies.** Student competencies support the goals of the national standards, guide the development of strategies and activities, and are the basis for assessing student growth and development. Competencies represent the specific knowledge, attitudes, and skills that students can acquire to support their academic, career, and personal-social success. The 122 student competencies are arranged in the three domain areas and provide pathways to each of the nine standards. Evaluating each student's acquisition of knowledge, attitudes, and skills is accomplished by monitoring the competencies, establishing benchmarks, and examining the impact of standards-based school counseling on school improvement goals.

Many state, district-level, and building-site comprehensive school counseling programs include specific competencies or outcomes that are aligned with the mission statement as well as with the academic or curriculum standards. Needs assessments, advisory committee input, teacher observations, and relevant school data are sources of information for locally developed student competencies. Competencies that guide the development of the program content for student growth and achievement in the academic, career, and personal-social domains are an integral part of individual planning, guidance curriculum, responsive services, and system support (Gysbers & Henderson, 2000). Competencies may be organized developmentally by school level and, through a comprehensive sequence of strategies and activities, reflect local school system issues, priorities, and concerns. As students struggle in assuming responsibility for their educational plans, career goals, and personal behavior (Wittmer, 2000), the standards and competencies help each student to take responsibility for her or his academic development, career preparation, and personal-social skills in order to successfully transition from grade level to grade level and to the next phase of life after high school.

Box 8.1 presents an activity that connects the goals of the national standards to school improvement. This scenario is a familiar one, especially for school counselors who work with high-school students.

This is an example of how to use the national standards in an experience that is meaningful and purposeful for students and supports their success in school. Success is not only about individual student skills; it is also demonstrated by drawing a direct line to the goals of school improvement and moving school data in a positive direction. Through teaming and collaboration strategies with a classroom teacher two purposes are served: (a) to encourage student affective growth with an emphasis on self-knowledge, motivation, taking responsibility, goal setting, and self-monitoring; and (b) to contribute to the improvement of English, language arts, and communication skills in both verbal and written forms.

Box 8.1

Putting Standards Into Practice

Title: School Success and My Future

Domain: Academic Development

Standards:

B. Students will complete school with the academic preparation essential to choose from a wide variety of substantial postsecondary options, including college.

C. Students will understand the relationship of academics to the world of work, and to life at home and in the community.

Competencies:	Students will: • Establish challenging academic goals. • Identify postsecondary options consistent with interests, achievement, aptitude, and abilities. • Understand that school success is the preparation to make the transition from student to community member. • Understand how school success and academic achievement enhance future career aspirations.
Level:	High School
Targeted Population:	Every 9th, 10th, and 11th grader in the high school.
Purpose:	The purpose of this activity is to help high-school students develop a plan of study and update it each year to reflect their educational (academic and career) goals.
Delivery Method:	Classroom Guidance; Individual Student Planning
Activity Summary:	1. Present a classroom guidance session to review course selection planning materials, graduation requirements, career pathways information, and other relevant materials. 2. The school counselor schedules follow-up appointments to meet in small groups with all students to discuss course selection that supports educational and career goals; to review current academic progress; and to share any potential obstacles to or concerns about achieving these goals.

3. The parent or caregiver of every student is invited to participate in a follow-up individual or small group meeting.

4. In collaboration with the classroom teachers, students monitor their progress on their educational plans and share their thoughts on each quarter's progress through reflective writing.

5. Students needing additional support or intervention self-refer or are referred by the teacher to the school counselor for individual sessions.

Materials Needed: Annual educational program planning worksheets, which include academic and career goals; student transcripts; achievement, aptitude and/or college entrance test scores; interest surveys, career portfolios, and course selection materials.

Results-Based Data: The results of this activity will show:
- 100% of the 9th-, 10th-, and 11th-grade students will actively participate in the design of an educational plan that supports their academic aspirations and career goals.
- 100% of parents and caregivers will be invited to participate in the educational planning process.
- Targeted efforts will result in an increase of 25% in parent participation from last year.

Connection to School Improvement:
- Student course changes and drops are reduced by 25%.

Data:
- Student participation and buy-in to this process reduces course failure by 25%.
- 75% of the students show academic improvement at the end of the school year as a result of self-monitoring their progress and connecting academic success to future career goals

Delivering a Standards-Based Program

As you can see from the sample activity, the shift to a standards-based school counseling program is most impactful when it is aligned with the educational initiatives under way in your school system or building. To help practitioners analyze school counseling practices and services, assess the gaps and assess how to move from the "what is" to the "what is to be." ASCA (Dahir, Sheldon, & Valiga, 1998) provided the field with a continuous five-step implementation process: discuss, plan, design, implement, and evaluate.

Discuss   The initial discussion about standards in your school system includes an awareness of what your program currently accomplishes. Examining school-based data will help you to identify student needs and connect school counseling to the mission of your school.

Plan   The planning process takes into consideration the knowledge and skills that students need to acquire as they progress through a pre-K through grade 12 school counseling program. Collaborative planning will help you to achieve your vision for student success and support students as they make successful transitions from grade level to grade level and to opportunities after high school.

Design   Strategies and activities are designed intentionally and purposefully, based upon the current situation of student needs and school improvement concerns. The selected student competencies should support the identified needs of your students and the goals of your school's improvement plan. Consider aligning the program design with the curriculum and academic standards for your school system and state.

Implement   Initiate what you intend to accomplish. Consider a phase-in plan for the short term, and establish benchmarks for long-term goals to help you monitor every student's progress. Implementation or program delivery involves individual and group counseling, school counseling curriculum, and system support activities that engage the faculty, staff, and community.

Evaluate   The information gained from the evaluation process tells you what students have learned and how your standards-based program has made a difference. Evaluation determines which accomplishments should be celebrated, what obstacles have been encountered, what mistakes have been made, and what challenges remain. It also helps you assess the conditions that support or challenge the success of your students and the success of your school counseling program.

National standards–based school counseling programs help students develop attitudes, knowledge, and skills in academic, career, and personal-social development that are needed in today's and tomorrow's world.

The ASCA National Model: Moving the Profession Forward

With the continued progression of school improvement and standards-based education, the American School Counselor Association (ASCA) developed the ASCA National Model (ASCA, 2003). **The ASCA model** integrates the three widely accepted and respected approaches to program development; that is, comprehensive, developmental, and results-based models (Myrick, 2003a). The ASCA model has contemporized school counseling foundation and philosophy, management and delivery systems, and accountability and aligned the program with the expectations of 21st-century schools (Myrick, 2003a). Using the national standards as the foundation for program content, the ASCA model offers a standards-based approach to school counseling that is aligned with the mission of schools, proactively responds to school improvement, and is intentional in its support of every student's development. The ASCA model forwards the Transforming School Counseling Initiative (Education Trust, 1997) by:

- Pointing counselors in the direction of improving academic achievement and eliminating the achievement gap. School counselors connect academic, career, and personal-social development to improving achievement for all students.
- Connecting school counseling to each school district's mission and the goals of school improvement. School counselors are encouraged to become leaders and systemic change agents to help ensure that no student is left behind.
- Providing school counselors with the tools to develop school counseling programs that include student competencies and outcomes based on the national standards (Dahir & Campbell, 1997); are aligned with state and district curriculum standards; and are based on measurable student learning outcomes.
- Encouraging school counselors to use data to assess student outcomes. School counselors use school-based data to understand the current situation in their school building and district and work collaboratively toward the goals of school improvement.

The outside frame of Figure 8.1 represents the transformed school counselor skills (Education Trust, 1997) of leadership, advocacy, collaboration, and systemic change that every school counselor needs to help every student succeed. The inside of the graphic depicts the four interrelated quadrants that are the essential components of successful and effective comprehensive school counseling programs (ASCA, 2003).

This is a brief explanation of the four quadrants of the ASCA model:

1. The *Foundation* of the program describes the *what* of the program, discussing what every student should know and be able to do (ASCA, 2003, p. 22). The foundation of the program, based on the national standards, reminds school

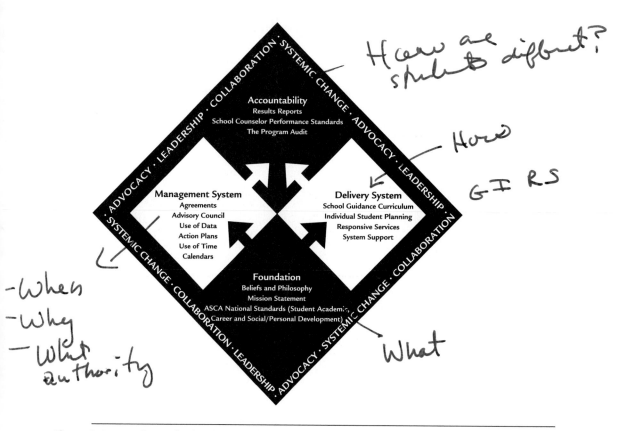

[Handwritten annotations: "How are students different?", "How GIRS", "What", "-When", "-Why", "-What authority"]

Figure 8.1 Transformed School Counselor Skills and the ASCA Model.
The ASCA National Model ® and the accompanying graphic are registered trademarks of the American School Counselor Association (ASCA). Reprinted with permission.

counselors of the importance of aligning with the school mission, having a vision for student success, and developing a proactive belief system that ensures that every student will benefit from the school counseling program.

2. *Delivery System* addresses *how* the program will be implemented and defines the implementation process and the components of the comprehensive program; that is, guidance curriculum, individual planning with students, responsive services, and system support. The model describes each of the components and offers examples and tools for implementation.

3. *Management System* addresses the when, the why, and on what authority the program is delivered (ASCA, 2003, p. 22). This section also presents the organizational processes and tools needed to deliver a comprehensive school counseling program. Sample agreements of responsibility, data application, action plans, and time and task analysis tools are presented.

4. *Accountability* answers the question "How are students different as a result of the school counseling program?" The ASCA model encourages school counselors to demonstrate accountability by presenting the effectiveness of their work in measurable terms such as impact over time, performance evaluation, and undertaking a program audit. Accountability also requires counselors to become familiar with the **use of data** and connect to the goals of school improvement in their respective buildings. Understanding data helps school counselors address issues of equity and inequity especially with regards to student achievement. Comprehensive school counseling programs support the goals of school improvement and positively impact student success.

The ASCA national model offers an inclusive approach for school counselors to design, coordinate, implement, manage, and evaluate their programs. The model encourages the school counselor's role in implementing and promoting the underlying philosophies of leadership, advocacy, and systemic change and challenges school counselors to respond to the question "How are students different as a result of what we do?" No matter how comfortable the status quo or how difficult or uncomfortable change may be, every school counselor must work diligently to support every student's quest for success. The ASCA national model directs school counselors toward a unified, focused, professional school counseling program with one vision and one voice (ASCA, 2003).

The Interrelationship of Comprehensive, Developmental, and Results-Based School Counseling Programs

Although interpretations may vary, there is consensus that comprehensive, developmental, and results-based school counseling programs are systematic in nature, sequential, clearly defined, and accountable (ASCA, 2003; Cobia & Henderson, 2003; Galassi & Akos, 2004; Gysbers & Henderson, 2000; Johnson & Johnson, 1991, 2001; Stone & Dahir, 2004).

Similar in presentation to other programs in education, components include student outcomes or competencies, activities to achieve the desired outcomes, professional personnel, materials, resources, and a delivery system. These three approaches to program development show the connection of school counseling to the total educational process and also the need to involve all school personnel (Stanciak, 1995). These program approaches share common goals, are proactive and preventive in focus (Borders & Drury, 1992), and assist students in the acquisition of lifelong learning skills by:

- providing developmental, as well as prevention and intervention programs;
- measuring student and program growth; and,

- taking into consideration the rapidly changing nature of society as well as pressures on education from business and industry, and how these impact every student's need to acquire academic, career, and personal-social growth and development.

Recent studies (Brigman & Campbell, 2003; Dimmitt, 2003; Galassi & Akos, 2004; Lapan, Gysbers, & Petroski, 2001; Sink & Stroh, 2003) have demonstrated the positive effects of comprehensive, developmental, and results-based school counseling on the academic achievement of elementary and secondary school students. The work of school counselors actively supports the goals of No Child Left Behind and contribute to the school improvement agenda nationwide.

Research suggests that high-quality counseling services can have long-term effects on a child's well-being and can prevent a student from turning to violence and drug or alcohol abuse. High-quality school counseling services can improve a student's academic achievement. Studies on the effects of school counseling have shown positive effects on students' grades, reducing classroom disruptions, and enhancing teachers' abilities to manage classroom behavior effectively. High-quality school counseling services also can help address students' mental health needs.

— *U.S. Dept. of Education, 2002b, p. 117*

Comprehensive, developmental, and results-based school counseling programs employ strategies to support student achievement and success, provide career awareness, open doors to opportunities, encourage self-awareness, foster interpersonal skills, and help all students acquire skills for life (Dahir, 2004).

Understanding Comprehensive School Counseling

The concept of the **comprehensive school counseling** program was developed by Gysbers and Moore (1981), and refined over the past 20 years by Gysbers and Henderson (2000). To operationalize the overall goals of the school counseling program, the comprehensive model has an organizational structure that consists of four components (Gysbers & Henderson, 2000) that have been adopted by the ASCA model (2003).

a. School counseling/guidance curriculum (e.g., structured groups, classroom guidance)

b. Individual planning with students (e.g., advising; assessment; placement; academic, career, and personal-social goal setting; and follow-up)

c. Responsive services (e.g., individual and group counseling, consultation, and referral)

d. System support (e.g., program management, coordination of services, community outreach, and public relations).

School Counseling/Guidance Curriculum

Counselors provide information, knowledge, and skills to students through developmental and sequential lessons. In most circumstances, the **school counseling/ guidance curriculum** is designed to serve the largest number of students possible through large group meetings and classroom presentations. The curriculum gives attention to particular issues or areas of concern in the school building or district, such as conflict resolution. School counselors often collaborate with teachers, student support services personnel, and community specialists to deliver the school counseling/guidance curriculum.

Individual Student Planning

When students have opportunities to plan, monitor, and evaluate their progress they often take ownership of their academic and affective learning and development. School counselors facilitate this process and encourage and motivate students to become engaged in their education and accept responsibility for success. Students and counselors collaborate on setting goals and developing academic and career plans. School counselors interpret, explain, and apply assessment data for students and help them apply this information to the planning process in a meaningful way. Individual student planning is most successful when a parent/guardian is involved. By personalizing the educational experience each student develops a pathway to realize her/his dreams.

Responsive Services

Responsive services include interventions needed for at-risk students, group counseling, consultation, referral to community agencies, crisis intervention and management, and prevention activities. The impetus for response and intervention is often dominated by crises in, school administration and faculty concerns; parental trepidations; and community needs. Often, through individual and group counseling, responsive services proactively address student issues such as peer pressure, conflict resolution, family relationships, personal identity issues, substance abuse, motivation, and achievement concerns.

System Support

The purpose of **system support** is to provide ongoing support to the school environment and to organize, deliver, manage, and evaluate the effectiveness of the school counseling program. Oftentimes system support consists of indirect services rather than services that are delivered directly to students. Direct services provided by the counselor typically include individual counseling, small group counseling, and classroom guidance; indirect services can include resource management, consultation, collaboration and teaming, advocacy, and the coordination of services. Indirect services are essential to impact systemic change and support the "new vision" of school counseling (Ripley, Erford, & Dahir, 2002).

Coordination of services involves managing resources and planning and connecting activities and services to goals of the counseling program in the school. For example, hosting an advisory committee helps to inform the program's direction and provides a sounding board for discussion about what is working, what needs to change, and how the comprehensive school counseling program can better support student success. Participating in the school improvement team, coordinating student service volunteers, or facilitating the school peer mediation program are some additional examples of the positive ways that system support connects school counseling to the mission of the school. System support also provides school counselors with multiple opportunities to act as leaders and as advocates by facilitating discussions around school improvement, examining data that may be impacting the success of some groups of students, and assisting with professional development and in-service activities for the faculty.

The Developmental Program

The developmental progression of student affective growth from pre-K through grade 12 can be nurtured through school counseling. This approach incorporates human growth and development theory (Piaget, 1952; Erickson, 1963; Kohlberg, 1984) by considering the progressive needs of students consistent with the stages of growth and learning. Myrick reminded us that **developmental school counseling** is for every student, and has an organized and planned curriculum that is sequential and flexible. The program is an integrated part of the total educational process, involves all school personnel, helps students learn more effectively and efficiently, and includes specialized counseling services and interventions (Myrick, 1997).

The Results-Based Program

A third approach, results-based guidance, is also competency-based. Developed by Johnson and Johnson in the 1980s, results-based programs emphasize total pupil services integration, with the student as the primary client and recipient. Students acquire competencies to achieve school success, which is demonstrated by positive transitions from school to postsecondary education and/or to employment. At the heart and center of results-based counseling is accountability. School-based issues, counselor-principal agreements, use of data, and using results guide all counselor action and activity (Johnson & Johnson, 1991; 2002).

Working From a Programmatic Perspective

Using a comprehensive school counseling mindset helps counselors to move theory into practice, responds to the needs and goals of the entire school community, and uses data to inform decisions. School counselors coordinate the objectives, strategies, and activities of a comprehensive school counseling program to meet the academic, career, and personal-social needs of all students (ASCA, 2003).

tie all together.

Once the school counseling program has an organization and structure just like any other curriculum, it is no longer ancillary but an integral component directly linked to student achievement and school success. When guidance and counseling is conceptualized, organized, and implemented as a program, it places school counselors in the center of education and makes it possible for them to be active and involved (Gysbers, 2001, p. 103).

The purpose of the ASCA National Model (2003) is to promote educational excellence through school counseling programs; encourage counselors to provide prevention and intervention programs and experiences; create a model of collaboration that integrates the expertise of school counselors, other pupil services personnel, businesses, and the community into the total program; and ensure that the program is current with the needs and expectations of the education agenda and societal issues (ASCA, 2003).

Program content is based on the national standards, grouped by domains (academic, career, and personal-social); has an organizational framework; uses varying strategies to deliver the content of the program to all students (ASCA, 2003; Gysbers & Henderson, 2000; National Consortium for State Guidance Leadership, 2000); and supports the imminent need for school counseling programs to be aligned with and tied to the mission of schools (Gysbers, 2001).

When building administrators, faculty, parents, and community members have substantial input into the development of the school counseling program, there is a willingness to assist in its design and delivery. Implementing a comprehensive, developmental, results-based program requires

- establishing a school counseling advisory committee of faculty, administrators, and representatives from all key stakeholder groups;
- determining priorities to meet the identified student needs;
- developing student competencies based on the national standards, school data, and school improvement needs;
- analyzing current services and activities and linking these to the national standards and student competencies;
- identifying gaps in the school counseling program and developing strategies;
- securing the commitment of all teachers, administrators and counselors to assist in program delivery;
- building the program based on the four ASCA model quadrants of foundation, delivery, management, and accountability.

The ASCA model (2003) encourages school counselors to

- establish the school counseling program as an integral component of the academic mission of school;
- provide for equitable access to school counseling services for all students;
- identify through the national standards and competencies the knowledge and skills that all students should acquire as a result of the K–12 school counseling program;
- ensure that school counseling programs are comprehensive in design, delivered in a systematic fashion for all students, and accountable for results.

Counselors Making a Difference

Meet Dr. Dorothy Youngs and the Counselors of the Piscataway School District

After years of reorganization, Piscataway School District administrators, teachers, and students felt that they were moving in the right direction. An Elementary School Counseling Demonstration Grant was the impetus for Dr. Dorothy Youngs to build a comprehensive national standards–based school counseling program. The school counselors examined district concerns and decided to redirect services into a programmatic framework. The counselors committed to address critical needs, such as student absenteeism, graduation rate, and state test results. As part of the program development process, the counselors initiated collaborative discussions with teachers and administration and soon learned that many of their colleagues believed that the school counselors' primary responsibility was to schedule students.

The comprehensive national standards–based model in Piscataway demonstrated to the administration and teachers that school counseling can be infused into curriculum across all the content areas and helps all students achieve academically, establish career goals, and develop the personal-social skills for success in school and with peers.

The Piscataway Comprehensive School Counseling Program soon became part of a model school counseling initiative sponsored by the New Jersey Department of Education. As part of a state and national network of school districts working with a similar focus, the counselors discovered a multitude of resources available, from networking and listservers to numerous local, state, and national supports including conferences and professional development opportunities.

The vision and the leadership of Dr. Dorothy Youngs and the commitment and dedication of the elementary, middle, and high-school counselors resulted in the Piscataway School District receiving one of two 2002 Exemplary National Standards Program awards from the American School Counselor Association.

Reprinted with permission by Piscataway Public Schools.

A programmatic approach to school counseling places school counselors in a valuable position to impact the instructional program and contribute to every student's achievement through collaboration and teaming with teachers, student support personnel, and parents.

Professional recognition of programs such as Piscataway's is extremely important. However, the investment of time and effort into the implementation of the comprehensive program also is beginning to show the type of impact that is more readily understood by the public. Recent research on fully implemented comprehensive programs conducted in Missouri (Lapan, 2001; MacDonald & Sink, 1999) has revealed that students achieve higher grades and believe that they are well prepared for their future choices.

The Transformed School Counselor's Knowledge and Skills

Comprehensive school counseling programs facilitate the " new vision" of the school counselor (House & Hayes, 2002; House, Martin, & Ward, 2002). An effective school counselor possesses the attitudes, knowledge, and skills to provide the direct and indirect components of the school counseling program. Successfully delivering the ASCA model (2003) utilizes counselor skills and competencies based on the Transforming School Counseling Initiative (Education Trust, 1997).

Transformed school counselors build on the traditional practice of services and extend their skills to deliver comprehensive school counseling programs that are standards-based and data driven (Table 8.2). These skills, in the transformed context, are briefly reviewed here.

Counseling.   Counseling in schools is the process of assisting a student in understanding, assessing, and making a change in behavior for the purpose of advancing self-awareness and understanding, increasing self-efficacy, and improving or enhancing relationships with others. As a result of the counseling process, students learn to make decisions to further improve their ability to achieve academic, career, and personal-social success in school.

Consultation.   The school counselor exchanges and shares information and knowledge with parents and caregivers, teachers, and the community to assist each student in his or her academic, career, and personal-social development. Consultation helps parents and teachers process problems and concerns, acquire more knowledge and skill, and become more objective and proactive.

Coordination of Services.   Counselors serve as a liaison between teachers, parents, support personnel, and community resources to facilitate successful student development. School counselors secure the appropriate and necessary services and supports that are essential to every student's ability to achieve.

Table 8.2

The Practice of the Traditional School Counselor (Service-driven model)	The Practice of the Transformed School Counselor (Data-driven and standards-based model)
• Counseling	• Counseling
• Consultation	• Consultation
• Coordination of Services	• Coordination of Services
	• Leadership
	• Advocacy
	• Collaboration and Teaming
	• Managing Resources
	• Use of Data
	• Use of Technology

Leadership. A comprehensive program is a proactive response to school improvement. School counselors, empowered in the restructuring process within their school systems, establish a foundation for affective education and competency-based learning. The school counselor serves as a leader as well as an effective team member working with teachers, administrators, and other school personnel to make sure that each student has an equitable opportunity to succeed.

Advocacy. The school counselor advocates for the elimination of significant performance gaps among students from different economic classes, genders, races, or ethnic groups.

Collaboration and Teaming. School counselors, as education professionals, join teachers and school administrators as partners to improve student success and achievement through a collaborative approach to developing strategies to deliver a comprehensive program.

Managing of Resources. Counselors identify, access, and coordinate the resources within the school and community that are necessary to support school success. The school counselor helps families, parents, and caregivers identify their children's needs and provides the information and assistance to access resources.

Use of Data. Data-driven results are the key to linking school counseling programs to improved levels of student achievement. Measurable success resulting from this effort can be documented by an increased number of students completing school with the academic preparation, career awareness, and personal-social growth essential to choose from a wide range of substantial postsecondary options, including college (Education Trust, 1997).

Use of Technology.   Technology tools help school counselors access and analyze data that depict the current situation of student achievement. Technology also helps school counselors monitor improvements in school climate and other student-related school factors that result from implementing a comprehensive school counseling program.

Counselors Making a Difference

Meet Dr. Glynda Cryer and the School Counseling Leadership Team in Memphis City Schools

Memphis City Schools' counselors exemplify the persistence and dedication that are necessary to change the process and content of the school counseling program. During the past 20 years, school counseling in Memphis has evolved to change with the times. The foundation of developmental counseling was started in Memphis more than 20 years ago.

In the early 1990s, Memphis became one of six College Board Equity 2000 sites integrating the principles of equity and access across the curriculum content areas. School counselors, collaborating and teaming with colleagues and communities, were committed to the systemic change that was needed to help students accomplish what they were now expected to do to achieve success.

The price of change did not come easy. Some counselors went through the traditional stages of storming and forming. Ongoing professional development was needed to keep these initiatives going. Counselors were trained to deal with the issues put forth in *Gatekeeper to Advocate* (Hart & Jacobi, 1992), and to examine the principles of leadership, advocacy, collaboration and teaming, and use of data as described in the Education Trust's Transforming School Counseling Initiative (1997).

Dr. Glynda Cryer, K–12 counseling services coordinator, made certain that the word was out that Memphis City Schools' counselors were committed to improving student achievement. Memphis City counselors had implemented the national standards and had begun to implement the comprehensive program model in order to make the shift from process and services to outcomes for students. With a clear direction in place, a comprehensive program, using individual, small group, and classroom guidance, became the way of work. In just three years, Dr. Cryer moved the district forward with implementation of the new Tennessee School Counseling Standards; development of a new comprehensive model for K–12; and the use of MEASURE, an accountability process, to align school counseling with school improvement.

The process of change, focused and deliberate, has paid off. Memphis City Schools was one of the two ASCA Exemplary Standards-Based School Counseling Program award winners for 2003.

Reprinted with permission by Jeane Chapman.

Meeting the Challenges of Renewal and Reform

ASCA (2003) has advocated that school counselors establish their identity and clearly articulate and define the role that school counseling programs play in promoting student achievement and educational success. New vision (Education Trust, 1997) school counselors work intentionally with the expressed purpose of reducing the effect of the environmental and institutional barriers that impede student academic success (Education Trust, 1997). School counselors are challenged to demonstrate accountability, document effectiveness, and promote school counseling's contributions to the educational agenda (Stone & Dahir, 2004) and are in a unique position to exert a powerful influence (Clark & Stone, 2000). Comprehensive, national standards–based school counseling programs offer a mechanism to contribute to the educational experience of every student. The contributions of school counseling can support every student's progress through school to help each emerge more capable and more prepared than ever before to meet the challenging and changing demands of the new millennium.

The 21st century presents an array of challenges and opportunities for school counselors to renew their practice and respond to the climate of school reform. Voices from the profession have called for a shift in the role of the professional school counselor from that of service provider to one of promoting optimal achievement for all students (Clark & Stone, 2000; Martin, 1998).

Advocacy, leadership, collaboration and teaming, and use of data are essential components of the repertoire of skills that a contemporary school counselor employs in today's schools (Education Trust, 1997). The school counseling profession has taken hold of the present and the future. No longer will the work of school counselors be defined by the perception of others. Comprehensive, developmental, results-based, national standards–based school counseling programs have established our presence and will define our future.

TechTools

Use the power of technology to learn more about the national standards for school counseling programs.

- Create a spreadsheet to align your current school counseling activities and strategies with the national standards.
- Develop a database to map the integration of the national standards across the content areas and curriculum. School counselors and faculty can search

for strategies, activities, and lessons that meet particular national standards in a schoolwide or districtwide database.

- Design a database so that you can monitor the delivery of student competencies and the process used (individual student planning, responsive services, guidance curriculum, and system support) for all of the students in your caseload.
- On your school counseling website, showcase the national standards that you are delivering to your students. Parents will be pleased to see that the priorities that you have for your program meet national expectations.
- Create a checklist for your students of the competencies that they will acquire this year as part of your school counseling program. They can keep the checklists in their school counseling portfolios.
- Develop an electronic portfolio for your students so that they can monitor their progress each year toward achieving the student competencies and national standards. Students can use electronic portfolios for their entire K–12 school careers.
- Subscribe to an ASCA or your state association's school counselor listservers to help you identify the best practices for program implementation.
- Go to http://nces.ed.gov/nceskids/ and use the graphing section to show student growth and achievement in academic, career, and personal-social development standards. Use the graphs and charts as part of your parent and staff newsletters. If you are looking for more of a challenge, try using Excel or Lotus for more "sophisticated" presentations.

Internet Resources

ASCA: http://www.schoolcounselor.org

K–12 Guidance Counseling Offices: http://www.looksmart.com/ (Enter "school counseling")

State School Counseling Plans:
http://coe.fgcu.edu/faculty/sabella/cerc/guidance.htm

Comprehensive Programs: http://www.indep.k12.mo.us/WC/wmccane.html

School District Websites

At the following websites, the blueprints will take you to the competencies and the domain areas, and will link to lessons:

North Carolina Public Schools
   http://www.dpi.state.nc.us/curriculum/guidance/
Orange County (Florida) Public Schools
   http://www.ocps.k12.fl.us/$zr1$5182d6c7b40676c6aa698c55704ca9c4$72
   4add715f17/framework/subject.php?subject=18

Covina Valley (California) http://www.lacoe.edu/dsss/
Montgomery County (Maryland) http://www.mcps.k12.md.us/department/dsd
Springfield, Massachusetts
   http://www.umass.edu/schoolcounseling/SpringfieldCurriculum10-03.pdf

School Counselor Casebook: Voices From the Field

The Scenario Reviewed

For the past two weeks, several students in your caseload have complained to you about certain other students, who have been provoking them to fight. Although students often complain about "being picked on," something about this situation just doesn't seem right. The students will not tell you who is involved, but insist that you "tell" the teachers to do something about it. As you think this through, several courses of action are available to you. You decide to discuss this with the other school counselors in your building, the teachers who are involved with these students, and your building principal. In your planning, you consider how the ASCA model and the national standards will help you address this situation.

A Practitioner's Approach

Here's how two Los Angeles county supervisors/consultants who work with practicing school counselors on a daily basis responded to the school counselor casebook challenge:

A prevailing school culture might discount or ignore our students who complained of being "picked on." Some adults might say it's just part of "growing up." Not so fast. If this situation came up in our school, we would implement the five-phase process of the national standards. In the discussion phase, we would talk to the students about why they believe they are being provoked to fight. If "something about this situation just doesn't seem right," then we would look further. The students want the teachers to do something about it. They actually said that. The classroom or teacher-supervised areas are good places to start. I would ask the students, "Which teachers would be the best ones to do something about the situation?"

In the planning phase, we would review the school policy and strategies for addressing bullying with these teachers. What insights do they have about these students or of the safety climate on campus?

We would then design an intervention using the information gained by identification and research. We would need to decide if certain students or teachers needed specific interventions or if the whole class, grade level, or system would benefit from a systemic approach.

We would target our implementation strategies to certain students or teachers, which might include a review of work done in Personal-Social Standards A and/or C. Our systemic strategies might include developing training for teachers and staff; reevaluating the schoolwide policy and intervention procedures; or increasing supervision and monitoring of hot spots on campus.

In the evaluation phase, we would implement both informal and formal student assessment and schoolwide appraisal (i.e., continue dialogue with our students and teachers, monitor "reportable" school safety incidents, or initiate/review school climate surveys).

Bob Tyra is a school counseling consultant with the student support services division of the Los Angeles County Office of Education. Bob has worked as a school counselor and assistant principal. He is an ASCA national standards trainer and has written numerous professional articles.

Michael Pines, PhD, is a mental health consultant with the student support services division of the Los Angeles County Office of Education. He also chairs the multidisciplinary Los Angeles County Child and Adolescent Suicide Review Team. Author of many professional articles, he is the senior editor of California Laws for Psychotherapists *(2003). Reprinted with permission by Robert Tyra and Michael Pines, Ph.D.*

Chapter Summary

The National Standards Movement: An Agenda for Equity

Educational leadership across the nation sought to determine and define what was meant by standards. Issues surrounding standards have been the focal point of national education conferences and publications. The debate continues to this day as to whether standards-based education will ultimately result in a better educated and prepared citizenry capable of competing in the global economy.

School Counseling: Finding a Place in School Improvement

Without clearly connecting the practice of school counseling to student impact, the school counselor would remain conspicuously absent in the conversations that centered on reform efforts to promote higher levels of student success. School counseling leadership sought ways to apply the language of educational reform and school improvement to school counseling programs.

ASCA's Contribution to School Reform: The National Standards for School Counseling Programs

Concerned about the absence of school counseling in GOALS 2000 and the increasing importance of standards and assessment, the ASCA Governing Board committed to the development of the National Standards for School Counseling Programs in 1994. The intent of this effort was to motivate the school counseling community to identify and implement goals for students that were deemed important by the profession, clarify the relationship of school counseling to the educational system, and address the contributions of school counseling to student success in school.

Student Competencies

Competencies are the pathway to documenting and demonstrating student growth, development, and progress toward the achievement of the nine standards. Student competencies represent the knowledge, attitudes, and skills that students need for academic, career, and personal-social success. The competencies are incorporated into a comprehensive, developmental school counseling program, which emphasizes early intervention and prevention as well as responsive counseling services.

Delivering a Standards-Based Program

The national standards represent what a school counseling program should contain and provide to every student. The nine national standards are based on the three widely accepted and interrelated areas of student development as described in the counseling literature and research: academic, career, and personal-social development.

The ASCA National Model: Moving the Profession Forward

ASCA developed the ASCA National Model (ASCA, 2003), which uses an integrated approach to the three widely accepted and respected program models—comprehensive, developmental, and results-based. The ASCA model has contemporized the foundation and the philosophy, management systems, and accountability sections to align with the expectations of 21st-century school counseling

The Interrelationship of Comprehensive, Developmental, and Results-Based School Counseling Programs

Comprehensive, developmental, and results-based school counseling are frameworks for the development, implementation, and evaluation of systematic school counseling programs. The characteristics are similar to other programs in education, such as student outcomes or competencies; activities to achieve the desired outcomes; professional personnel; materials; resources; and a delivery system. These approaches have clear goals and include an organized and sequential curriculum.

Working From a Programmatic Perspective

Programs in schools are about student growth, learning, and results. Students, not the role of the teacher, are the focal point. Therefore, it was imperative that school counselors change the focus from position to program; that is, from the role of the school counselor to the impact of the school counseling program on student achievement and school success. When all stakeholders contribute to the development of the comprehensive program, there is a willingness to support the program and assist in its implementation and evaluation.

What School Counselors Need to Know and Be Able to Do

School counselors utilize a variety of strategies, activities, delivery methods, and resources to facilitate student growth and development. In order to accomplish this, the school counselor must possess a solid knowledge of what he or she needs to know and be able to do to serve as a student advocate, provide direct and indirect services, and ascribe to the belief that all children can learn and achieve. Counselors need to be proficient in counseling, coordination of services, consultation, collaboration and teaming, case management, leadership, advocacy, management of resources, assessment and use of data, and program design and evaluation.

Meeting the Challenges of Renewal and Reform

Implementing comprehensive school counseling programs based on the national standards challenges school counselors to demonstrate the positive impact of the school counseling program on student achievement. Communities can see that school counseling programs do produce the results they are demanding and that school counselors desire the same levels of success and positive results as do parents, teachers, and administrators.

Comprehensive school counseling programs, linked directly to the mission of the school, are designed to promote and enhance the learning process, with an emphasis on ensuring that the school counseling program is an integral part of the total school program.

Key Terms

Academic development p. 211
ASCA model p. 217

Career development p. 212

Learning Extensions

1. Reflect on the scenario presented in the beginning of this chapter. What competencies would be most helpful for students in your school to acquire to intervene with "bullying" and prevent future occurrences? How can the national standards help to "bully-proof" your school?

2. The PTA has invited you to explain the school counseling program at an open meeting. The PTA president has explained that the members seem to be supportive of the counseling program but really don't understand it. Prepare an outline of the key issues that you would explain in your half-hour overview.

3. You are in the process of "rethinking" how counseling services are delivered in your school. You and your colleagues know that many students are rarely seen by the school counselors. You decide to meet with your principal to discuss how using the national standards would help to improve the quality and effectiveness of school counseling services in your school. What key issues should be brought up at this meeting? How will you get your principal to support a shift from a service-driven model to a program-based model?

4. You have decided to implement a comprehensive national standards–based program over the next two years in your building. How will you determine which standards to begin with? How will you develop competencies that reflect the needs of your students and school?

5. Prepare five presentation software (such as PowerPoint) slides about comprehensive school counseling as an introductory presentation to the faculty in your school.

6. You are meeting with the social studies teachers in your building about collaborating on classroom guidance activities. Select one standard and develop a collaborative activity that supports one of the social studies standards or curriculum goals. How will you measure the success of the activity?

Chapter 9

Accountability and Data-Driven Decision Making

Accountability: Success, Not Survival
ASCA National Model for Accountability
Accountability Defined
Time-on-Task and Results-Based Data

Building a Data-Driven School Counseling Program
Critical Data Elements or Report Card Data
Disaggregated Data

MEASURE: A Different Way of Focusing Our Work
The Six Steps of MEASURE
Systemic Changes and Other Interim Data

By the time you have completed this chapter, you should be able to:

- Describe the components of a data-driven, accountable school counseling program.
- Understand the power of data in delivering an effective school counseling program.
- Define critical data elements and measurable outcomes for student success.

- Analyze, synthesize, and disaggregate data to examine student outcomes and to identify barriers, successes, areas of weakness, etc.
- Establish accountability measures for a data-driven school counseling program.
- Assess measurable outcomes for counseling programs, services, activities, interventions, and experiences.
- Use school-based data to support decision making, to design effective school counseling interventions, and to support all students to be successful learners.
- Identify critical data elements.
- Know how and where to acquire data.
- Identify steps to move critical data elements and to demonstrate your contribution to student success.
- Identify challenges and opportunities.

School Counselor Casebook: Getting Started

The Scenario

When polled at the beginning of the school year, 91% of the students in your school responded that they were planning to enter college. However, only 27% of the students were delivering an academic performance that would widen their options to include college. What do you see as your role, if any, in helping students see the connection between academic performance and enrollment in college?

Thinking About Solutions

As you read this chapter, think about what you would do if you were a school counselor in this situation. What would you see as your role, if any, in helping students see the connection between academic performance and enrollment in college? When you come to the end of the chapter, you will have the opportunity to see how your ideas compare with a practicing school counselor's approach.

Accountability: Success, Not Survival

A school board member is discussing the budget allocations for the next school year:

> "Test scores are down, attendance is not improving, postsecondary enrollment rates
> are stagnant, and the end-of-year failure rate for students in grades 4, 8, and 9 is over

35%. Our children are slipping through the cracks in standards-based reform. The school counselors of this district work very hard. The annual report shows that you delivered 2,300 classroom guidance lessons, conducted 180 groups, and made innumerable individual contacts with student and parents. We applaud your efforts but we need you to go one step further. Add to your tally of services an explanation of how your efforts made a difference in our district's report card data. We face a dire budget next year and we have to justify the continuation of funding for each educator. We know that your school counseling programs are making a difference in our students' academic achievement. Help us add to your time-on-task numbers, data that demonstrates the impact your school counseling program is having on students' academic achievement."

This all-too-real challenge from the district school board is an example of what your future profession is being called on to do, which is to show how the school counseling program influences the **critical data elements** that are sometimes called the school's report card data. Everyone in a school setting is accountable for student success, and that includes school counselors as well as students, parents, and the community at large (Herr, 2001; Isaacs, 2003; Kiselica & Robinson, 2001; Lapan, 2001; Stone & Hanson, 2002). School board members, administrators, and others who are charged with making tough decisions about spending are asking all members of the educational community for an accounting of their contributions to student achievement (Whiston, 2002). The allocation of school resources is expected to produce a return on the investment, and no educator is above accountability (Stone & Dahir, 2004).

Accountability governs the 21st-century school. School counselors are more frequently illustrating the influence and impact of their programs through the use of data. Though they have the best of intentions, school counselors have not successfully documented that students have been more successful in schools as a result of counselors' actions and interventions (Whiston & Sexton, 1998). Sharing accountability for student success with stakeholders is a driving force for transforming and reframing the work of school counselors across the nation (ASCA, 2003; Herr, 2001; Gysbers & Henderson, 2001; Lapan, 2001; Myrick, 2003b; Stone & Dahir, 2004).

In the spirit of preparing you to be ready to connect your program to school improvement and student success, this chapter offers concrete images of the "how to" of accountability. Rather than waiting for others to determine how your school counseling program will demonstrate accountability for student success, you can enter the field with a strong understanding of how to determine accountability yourself. A data-driven approach to building your program will help garner support and secure your position as a valued player in school improvement (Hughes & James, 2001; Kachgal, Romano, & Peterson, 2001; Kiselica & Robinson, 2001; Lapan, 2001; Louis, Jones, & Barajas, 2001; Myrick, 2003a; Stone & Dahir, 2004; Thorn & Mulvenon, 2002). Your school counseling program will be aligned with the educational enterprise, will be data-driven, proactive, and preventive in focus, and will assist students in acquiring and applying lifelong learning skills.

ASCA National Model and Accountability

The development of the national standards for school counseling programs was an important first step in engaging school counselors and stakeholders in a national conversation about program effectiveness and accountability.

The **American School Counseling Association (ASCA) National Model** (ASCA, 2003) was written to guide the design and implementation of school counseling program models nationwide, bringing to the school counseling program the imperative to align with the mission of schools and to demonstrate this alignment through accountability (Myrick, 2003). The standards and ASCA model helped the profession develop a common language to describe their work and contributions to accountability (Myrick, 2003). "The language of accountability permeates the document" (Myrick, 2003a, p. 175).The ASCA National Model for School Counseling Programs (ASCA, 2003) reinforces the importance of delivering a comprehensive, developmental, and results-based program that carefully considers local demographic needs and the political climate of the community.

The accountability quadrant of the national model speaks to the importance of having an accountability system and an organizational framework that answers the question "How are students different as a result of the school counseling program?"(Johnson & Johnson, 2001). In the ASCA model, as in school counseling initiatives of the past decade, the shift has moved from answering the question "What does the school counselor do?" to the question "How are students different because of what the school counselor does?" By collecting and using data, school counselors link the effectiveness of the program to student success. The national model challenges school counselors to accept accountability as a means to demonstrate the program's impact in measurable terms. When the school counseling program goals are aligned with the mission of the school, it is inevitable that student achievement will improve as a result of the efforts of school counselors (ASCA, 2003). Accountability, as presented in the ASCA model, links the work of school counselors to student success.

Accountability Defined

> Accountability is a set of ideas, knowledge and consequential activities based on the principles of shared responsibility that involves all of the critical players in the school setting collectively removing barriers impeding learning and demonstrating their results with hard data.
>
> — *Rhode Island Department of Education, 1997*

How does school counseling fit into this idea of accountability being a shared responsibility for student learning? School counselors up until recently escaped the accountability imperative because their work mainly focused on addressing individual issues and concerns related to social and personal development for the segments of the school population that were perceived as the most talented or the most at risk. The school counseling profession responded that counseling is a personal relationship, and that it is impossible to measure a counselor's effectiveness or evaluate a series of services (Schmidt, 2000). Poverty, special needs, giftedness, exceptionality, and highly selective college counseling were some of the issues that required significant counselor involvement and fueled the cliché that 20% of the students commanded 80% of the school counselors' time. Before accountability, school counselors were viewed as working in a "support" role removed from what happens in the instructional arena of schools, and their work appeared only marginally related to teaching and learning. For these and other reasons, school counselors were not held to the same accountability standards as were teachers, administrators, and other educators. Yet, for more than 20 years, the professional literature was replete with calls for increased measures of counselor accountability (Gysbers, 2001; Gysbers & Henderson, 2001; Isaacs, 2003; Myrick, 2003a).

Time-on-Task and Results-Based Data

Methods traditionally used for assessing needs and evaluating school counseling programs are being supplemented or replaced by accountability methods required of administrators and faculty (Herr, 2001; Isaacs, 2003; Stone & Dahir, 2004; Whiston, 2002). Needs assessments, surveying, and the collection of time-on-task and results-based data are still used with good results by the profession; however, collecting student impact data is becoming the required accountability method for all educators. For example, the concept of identifying areas of need by surveying stakeholders is a positive step, but far from sufficient to increase success for every student. Looking at data to see who is failing multiple subjects, repeating for the second time, absent frequently, or in the office for frequent fighting is an essential step in identifying areas of need for focused attention.

Compiling **time-on-task** data, such as how many classroom guidance lessons were conducted, how many students were seen individually, and/or how many small groups took place, effectively contributes to an understanding of how school counselors spend their time (Gysbers, 2001; Gysbers & Henderson, 2001; Myrick, 2003a). However, as the school board member said in the scenario presented at the beginning of the chapter, ". . . we need you to go one step further. Add to your tally of services an explanation of how your efforts made a difference in our district's report card data." The school board members want to know how the counselor's work is helping to impact on student success data, such as attendance rates, discipline referrals, grades, and the going rate for postsecondary education. Time-on-task tallying is incomplete when used as the only method of accountability (Herr, 2001; Gysbers & Henderson, 2001; Kachgal, Romano, & Peterson, 2001; Kiselica & Robinson, 2001; Lapan, 2001; Whiston, 2002).

Another approach sometimes used to document success is called **results-based accountability.** For example, a school counselor may report time-on-task information, such as the fact that 20% of every day is spent in career and academic advising, including helping students understand financial aid information for postsecondary education. The counselor may take it a step further and report results-based data with the information that 60% of the student population can identify financial resources for postsecondary education. Taking it a step further, the school counselor could report the number of seniors who actually filled out the Free Application for Federal Student Aid (FAFSA) and show how this number compared to the year before and in this way the counselor has moved into a **data-driven school counseling** program reporting movement of critical data elements. Stakeholders, especially school board members, administrators, and teachers, understand the significant difference between reporting results based on information and reporting the academic outcomes for students, such as an increase in going rates for postsecondary education (Green & Keys, 2001; Lapan, 2001; Louis, Jones, & Barajas, 2001; Myrick, 2003; Stone, 2003; Thorn & Mulvenon, 2002; Whiston, 2002). The result of the school counselor's efforts to inform more students about the FAFSA would be to determine if more students continued their education after high school. Each year the data-driven school program would set a higher goal; next year, the goal might be to move from 48% to 53% for the number of students seeking higher education.

Another example of results-based accountability would be to assess the impact of your conflict resolution efforts by collecting impact data. This "one step further" would describe how your students are more successful in school because they are participating in your conflict resolution program. Relevant impact or critical data would be that the number of discipline referrals for fights and conflict went down by 9%. Time-on-task methods (for example, reporting 42 classroom guidance lessons) and results-based methods (reporting that 91% of students identified a conflict resolution technique), while helpful, do not resonate as powerfully with legislators, school board members, principals, and other stakeholders as does impact data that says, "the school counselor implemented a conflict resolution program and as a result contributed toward reducing the discipline referrals by 9% and raising our attendance rate from 78% to 83% during a four-month period."

The school counseling profession is building on the great work that has been done in the past with time-on-task and results-based data and moving in the direction of impact data. This progression is demonstrated in another example: divorce groups that are in place to help remove emotional barriers to concentration and learning. Stakeholders' questions are quickly becoming "Were the students in the divorce group suffering academically? If so, how did the divorce group positively impact these students' academic achievement? Were you able to reduce their absenteeism, raise their test scores, or improve their grades?"

It is an accepted premise that supporting a student's personal and emotional needs during the experience of parental divorce can help the student stay focused and succeed academically. However, beyond counting the number of divorce groups you conduct, can you demonstrate accountability? How would you show that the divorce group increased the students' academic success? If you could show that participants' grade point averages went up over the previous marking period or that collectively the group had 12 fewer absences, stakeholders would better understand the impact the three divorce groups were having on student success.

If you were to conduct a series of conflict resolution classroom guidance lessons, what would be your accountability measure? If you answer that you would look to see if the classes that had the series of six classroom guidance lessons had a reduced number of discipline referrals, then you are reporting accountability data that has meaning and merit for stakeholders. You have nothing to fear in seeking a data-driven school counseling program. Even if the data do not move in a positive direction, you are speaking the language of the critical stakeholders, garnering support for your program, helping students be more successful, and changing your program based on learning about what does and does not work.

Building a Data-Driven School Counseling Program

"In God we trust, all others bring data."
— *Brad Duggan, president and CEO of the National Center for Education Accountability (2002)*

What does it mean to build a school counseling program around critical data elements that are important to legislators, school board members, superintendents, administrators, teachers, and parents? There are multiple ways in which a school counselor, as part of the leadership team, can use data to support students, remove barriers, and develop a school counseling program around critical data elements. Data paint a vivid picture of a school and its students. Data draw a depiction of achievement patterns; successes and failures in teaching; equity issues; and overall effectiveness of the school to support successful learners. Data can help us understand the national picture and the district picture, but more importantly data helps us understand the individual school (Gysbers & Henderson, 2001; Isaacs, 2003; Myrick, 2003a; Stone & Dahir, 2004).

School-site data can help the school counselor determine goals for the school counseling program. A school counseling program built around data means use of numbers rather than use of assumptions or perceptions. Data, such as enrollments in college prep courses, graduation rate, retention rates, special education placements, attendance, grades, and standardized test scores, reveal a telling story of achievement patterns, equity issues, career and college connections, and overall effectiveness of the schools (Dahir & Stone, 2003; Martin, 2004).

If school counselors build their programs around the identified needs of the school they will hit the mark, because these needs are decided by the internal and external critical stakeholders of the school. For example, if stakeholders identify the poor promotion rate for third and fifth graders as a problem area, then the school counselor, as part of a collaborative team, can help develop strategies to move the promotion rate data in a positive direction.

Let's meet counselors who have established data-driven school counseling programs.

Counselors Making a Difference

Meet Linda Miller and the Louisville School Counselors

Delivering Data-Driven Programs

The school counselors of Louisville, Kentucky, increased the promotion rate for hundreds of ninth graders in 21 out of 24 comprehensive high schools! In discussing data-driven work, Director of School Program and Services Linda Miller says, "No longer will we say, 'A counselor can make the difference.' A counselor *is* the difference." The ninth-grade counselors looked at the data for the ninth grade and collectively decided that they needed to do something about the out-of-control ninth-grade retention rate. These counselors collaborated and developed strategies, which each counselor tailored to his or her school. The counselors collected baseline data from freshman retention rates, developed action plans that they submitted to the district supervisor of guidance, implemented strategies for a school year, and then looked at the impact of their work by examining the retention rate at the end of the year. Astounding the impact! Twenty-one out of 24 schools reduced their retention rates.

The strategies these counselors used to get results were those that they like to employ and that are within their area of expertise. The difference for these Louisville counselors was the focused effort, the collective collaboration, and the cooperation toward a common goal. Strategies included conducting classroom guidance lessons on "freshman survival skills" and postsecondary requirements; involving students and their parents through contracts, letters, and phone calls; providing brochures on college preparation and advanced placement credits; aligning the curriculum and setting standards to improve retention rates; conducting tri-weekly assessments of where at-risk students stand; developing an advisor/advisee program; holding small group counseling sessions for students; developing a year-long transition class for at-risk incoming ninth graders; meeting with each freshman for individual academic advising to discuss graduation plans and postsecondary education; and helping to make systemic changes, such as double time blocks for at-risk ninth graders in reading and math.

The percentages are very impressive, but this is not about numbers. The real celebration is about the difference in the lives of the students represented by these percentages. Hundreds of students are better off because their school counselor decided on their behalf that they deserved greater opportunities. This is the joy of data-driven work. When these figures are disseminated widely, the school counselor's impact is known throughout the internal and external community. The table presents the first 10 in the alpha list of 24 schools.

The Measure of Success

Decrease in 9th-Grade Retention Rates from 2000–2001 to 2002–2003	2000–2001 Baseline	2002–2003 Outcome Data
ATHERTON HIGH	29.75%	21.40%
BALLARD HIGH	13.47%	7.28%
BRECKINRIDGE	61.02%	39.13%
BROWN HIGH	1.92%	4.35%
BUECHEL METROPOLITAN HIGH	60.00%	56.82%
BUTLER TRADITIONAL/TECH. HIGH	8.25%	8.26%
CENTRAL HIGH	32.26%	6.05%
DOSS HIGH	21.85%	14.98%
EASTERN HIGH	18.16%	19.70%
FAIRDALE HIGH	24.54%	18.55%

The Louisville school counselors achieved these systemic changes:

- Institutionalized collaboration among schools to improve the promotion rate for ninth grade
- Changed practice so that every counselor and administrator will disaggregate data on a regular basis to see which students need more attention.

Reprinted with permission by Linda S. Miller.

Critical Data Elements or Report Card Data

Every school district in America has data that the school board, administration, faculty and staff, and parents would consider critical to analyze in order to assess the effectiveness of their efforts in meeting educational benchmarks. Examples of these critical data elements are attendance, demographics, graduation, going rate for postsecondary education, and standardized testing results (see Box 9.1). Closely examining critical data elements that identify the needs of your students and the schoolwide issues that cloud success is the first step to inform and guide the development and construction of an accountable school counseling program. With data, school counselors are able to paint a picture of the current situation of the students in the school, and can begin to document the students' successes and failures.

Many school counselors have databases available that contain biographical information as well as scheduling, attendance, discipline, and test history. This information is useful in itself when working with students in regard to any of the

Counselors Making a Difference

Meet Jim MacGregor

Hammering Away at the Achievement Gap

Jim MacGregor looked around his school and saw inequity. He decided on his students' behalf that he would advocate for greater opportunities for them and then persistently, for six years, hammered away at the system until he significantly impacted the achievement gap. Jim persevered until all students in his high school were supported with access to algebra and with safety nets such as double mathematics periods and tutoring. Jim MacGregor, steward of equity and access, is a hero. This quiet, unassuming, self-effacing counselor has impacted thousands of lives by giving students the opportunity to access and be successful in higher level academics. The data that follows demonstrates that Jim does not know the meaning of the words "it can't be done."

Jim did not do anything that you and I, as school counselors, would not want to do. Jim raised student aspirations by implementing a career awareness program for every student in the school to help them see the interrelationship between postsecondary education and their future economic opportunities. Jim involved parents in academics by helping them see that their children's future would be severely handicapped if the children did not participate in the rigorous courses that would prepare them for postsecondary options. These parents became supporters for changing the academic expectations for the whole student body. Jim advocated for a systemic change in course enrollment patterns to support more students' access to higher level academics. Using data and anecdotal information about student success in higher level academics, Jim was able, over time, to successfully change attitudes and beliefs about widening opportunities for higher level academics. Jim impacted the instructional program by using disaggregated test results so that teachers had better information about student weaknesses. He led large and small group sessions on motivation and problem solving; used software for four-year plans to track every student from ninth grade so that course selections were in writing and matched a student's aspirations; and established a mentoring program. For a complete list of Jim's strategies see the six-step accountability approach called MEASURE in Stone & Dahir (2004).

(continued)

Jim's MEASURE of Success

1. Increased Graduation Rates

Students Graduating with a College Core (i.e., completing 40 specified semester credits)	1994	2000
Caucasian	62.5%	78%
African American	26.7%	66%

2. Students Passing the Course

	1991–92	1995–96	2000–01
ALG 1 & 2	71%	94%	99%
GEO	66.1%	83%	96%
ALG 3 & 4	55.4%	63%	65%
Pre-CAL	31.5%	39%	46%
CAL 1 & 2	11%	20%	20%

Jim MacGregor achieved these systemic changes:

- The approach to transitioning between middle and high school became a state model for Indiana.
- The school district added counselors and funded counselors to work in the summer, based on their success rate in helping students complete higher level mathematics.
- Double mathematics periods were implemented.
- Teachers, all other educators, and community members changed their attitudes and beliefs about opening higher level academics to all students.
- The district superintendent and other central office decision makers developed an awareness and appreciation for what could happen when there is a counselor-led data-driven focus on ratcheting up academics for all students.

Reprinted with permission by James MacGregor.

Counselors Making a Difference

Meet LeAnn Pollard, Lee Kinard, Edith Vanderhoek, and Pat Schneider

Impacting Their School's Accountability Report Card

LeAnn's new principal, Mr. Cobb, came into the school improvement team (SIT) meeting to discuss which personnel had to be cut to balance a serious budget shortfall. Mr. Cobb entered the room and without a word went to the board and wrote

(continued)

"school counselor." He turned to the team and said, "Every position is up for consideration to be cut, but there is one position that is a nonnegotiable. Don't touch the school counselor." How did LeAnn Pollard, urban elementary school counselor, accomplish this vote of confidence when the year before, her position was cut only to receive a reprieve at the last minute?

It was June 2002 when LeAnn and the rest of the school received the bad news that their school had scored an "F" on Florida's accountability report card, meaning a possible state takeover if the Florida Comprehensive Assessment Test (FCAT) scores did not improve. As part of the leadership team, LeAnn went to work with all the other educators with a focused effort to see how they could support their students in reading and mathematics learning gains. Simultaneously, in other Florida schools, Lee Kinard, rural elementary school counselor, and Edith Vanderhoek, urban middle school counselor, also were engaged with their leadership teams to be part of the effort to improve their school's FCAT scores. These three counselors put into place strategies that made sense for their schools. These strategies included initiating a tutoring program; carefully pairing mentors with struggling students; implementing family outreach when children were frequently absent; incorporating into their character education lessons the higher order thinking skills found on the FCAT test; participating in the school improvement teams; advocating for systemic change, such as changing the special education and reading recovery schedules to optimize effectiveness for students; implementing behavior management and reward programs that focused on completing work; and conducting small groups on study skills. In LeAnn's school, 79% of her third grades made learning gains in math and 58% made learning gains in reading. LeAnn's work was so appreciated that her job became a nonnegotiable.

Results for Lee's students

	2001–2002 FCAT baseline data scoring 3>	2002–2003 FCAT outcome data scoring 3>
4th Math	57%	67%
4th Reading	63%	77%

Results for Edith's students

	2001–2002 baseline data scoring 3>	2002–2003 outcome data scoring 3>
8th Math	94%	96%
8th Reading	83%	88%

*The Florida Comprehensive Assessment Test (FCAT) reports scores in five achievement levels (1 [low] to 5 [high]).

High-school counselor Pat Schneider hopes to have similar results. Pat explains how she is trying to help the critically low students pass the state test (FCAT) that is required for graduation. In supporting the instructional program by shoring up students who are struggling, Pat is positioning herself as a critical player in the mission of her school. "Our school used technology to target the students with low FCAT scores, i.e., the 10th-grade students who scored in the lower quartile in the 9th grade. The counselors are working with these students on the 'bubble' [students who performed at level 2 out of 5 levels, with level 1 being the lowest]. These 10th graders will be taking the FCAT in March and must pass both sections for graduation. We are offering small groups on study skills, touching base with these students regularly to check their progress, and generally mentoring them and getting them tutors and other support so that they can pass this critically important do-or-die test." Through technology Pat was able to identify the students who needed extra attention, mentoring, and support and the counselors brought their strategies to help the identified students.

Reprinted with permission by LeAnn Pollard, Laura Lee Kinard, and Edith T. Vanderhoe.

---

information contained in the database, such as attendance, test scores, current grades, and past academic performance. By using data on the entire school population, no students are overlooked (Martin, 2004). This provides equity in analysis and guarantees that no group of students will be left out of critical calculations for a data-driven school counseling program (Stone & Turba, 1999).

Disaggregated Data

Disaggregated data, which is data separated out by ethnicity, gender, socioeconomic status, or teacher assignment, is very important in the study of student performance and in examining equity issues. This disaggregation of data makes it possible to determine how policy and practices affect issues of equity as counselors work toward closing the gap in student opportunities and achievement.

Often the discussion will center around what data elements you don't have rather than examining the data you are able to obtain. "Work for but don't wait for good data" (Martin, 2004).

When looking to create change, it is important to know which areas need the most attention. For some, the evidence may reveal itself; for others, key questions must be asked and data must be utilized to obtain the answers. Presented here are easy steps for analyzing data that will help identify areas of interest and therefore will assist in creating change. Once the data are brought together, the story they tell can be used to inform, provoke, and persuade those individuals who may not be open to change (Martin, 2004).

Box 9.1

Examples of Critical Data Elements

Direct Measures of Achievement

Test results   Examples are state exams, such as the Florida Comprehensive Assessment Test, and standardized achievement tests, such as the Preliminary Scholastic Achievement Test (PSAT), the Scholastic Achievement Test (SAT), Iowa Tests, ACT, ASVAB, etc.

Number of credits taken per year

Retention rates   (also, dropout rates)

Postsecondary enrollment   For example, four-year-college, community college, apprenticeship, career and technical, military training

Grade Point Average

Rank in Class

Indirect Measures of Achievement

The following areas do not "measure" achievement but impact achievement:

Course enrollment patterns that demonstrate commitment to high achievement

Enrollment in honors, AP, IB, or college-level courses

Enrollment in general, remedial courses

Exceptional Student Education screening and placement

Gifted screening and enrollment

Alternative school enrollment

Other Informative Critical Data Elements

There are other elements that can inform the work of school counselors, such as these:

Demographics of the internal and external school community

Entry and withdrawal information

Ethnicity

Gender

Number and type of discipline referrals, to include suspension rate

Attendance rate

Single family situations

School geographic areas

Free or reduced lunch students and other available socioeconomic measures

Before you begin, remember that simple kinds of data analysis can go a long way; providing complex statistics is not the best way to present data to others. Start with simple statistics, such as averages and percentages. Then disaggregate or "slice" that piece of data into different units. For example, if you are putting a bully-proofing program in place and you want to report the results of the program on discipline referrals, you could report that the number of schoolwide discipline referrals dropped from 278 to 156. To learn more about the decrease in discipline referrals, you could report the results by grade level (see Figure 9.1). This is called disaggregated data; you took your total discipline referrals and began to cut your data into smaller pieces so that you could learn more. The disaggregated data show you which grade levels are responding most favorably to the bully-proofing program and which grade levels may need increased attention.

Next, look for data as it relates to time. This process will add yet another dimension to the data by adding longitudinal elements. For example, when looking at the pattern in discipline referrals over a five-year period, as shown in Figure 9.2, it is unmistakable that the bully-proofing program had a positive impact on discipline referral rates.

Finally, as shown in Figure 9.3, cross tabulate the data by comparing two sets of disaggregated data. Compare not only the scores of students across different ethnicities, but also compare them with other variables, such as the classes in which they are enrolled.

Cross tabulation can be obtained by following these easy steps. Ask questions that will lead you to the data you are looking for: (a) What are you trying to measure? (for example, postsecondary completion rate); (b) What is the first characteristic to be used to divide this data into groups? (for example, it could be divided by race); and (c) What is the second characteristic to be used to divide this data into groups? (for example, it could be divided by high-school curriculum). The answer to question b produces the results shown in Figure 9.4.

When the answer to question c is added, Figure 9.5 is the result.

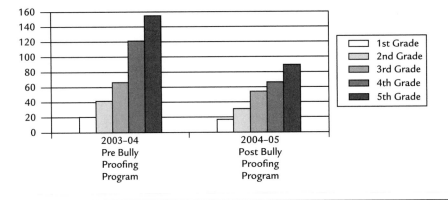

Figure 9.1 The Impact of a Bully-Proofing Program on Discipline Referrals Disaggregated by Grade Level.

Remember, you do not have to know and use the technology to disaggregate data. As long as you understand the power of data and know the right questions to ask, you can get others to help you with the technology or to provide the disaggregated data for you. Lack of familiarity with the technology should not make school counselors fear using data. Make noise about needing good data when you hit roadblocks to retrieving data. Knowing the power of data, which data elements you need, and who to ask for help to retrieve the information in a form you and the

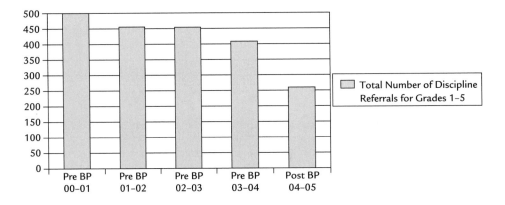

Figure 9.2 Total Number of Discipline Referrals each year and the impact of the 2004-2005 Bully-Proofing (BP) Program.

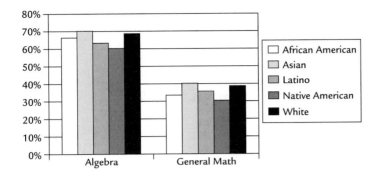

Figure 9.3 Graph of Cross-Tabulated Data.

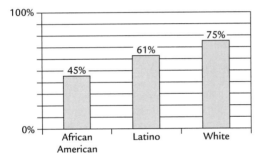

Figure 9.4 Postsecondary Completion Rates by Ethnicity.

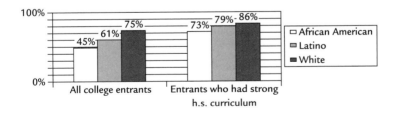

Figure 9.5

other members of the leadership team can use is an exceptional start toward creating an accountable school counseling program.

MEASURE: A Different Way of Focusing Our Work

MEASURE is a six-step accountability process that helps school counselors demonstrate how their programs impact critical data, which are those components of a school report card that are the backbone of the accountability movement (Stone & Dahir, 2004). Implementing a MEASURE is an easy way to connect to the school leadership team and demonstrate that you are helping to drive data in a positive direction (Stone & Dahir, 2004). MEASURE stands for Mission, Elements, Analyze, Stakeholders-Unite, Reanalyze, Educate. MEASURE will help organize your efforts and show your results. MEASURE is a way of using information to target critical data elements, such as retention rates, test scores, and going rate for postsecondary education, and to develop specific strategies to connect school counseling to the accountability agenda of today's schools (Dahir & Stone, 2003). Simply put, MEASURE helps you grab baseline data, which is data that tells you where your students are currently functioning in areas such as attendance, test scores, promotion rates. MEASURE helps you develop strategies to move this baseline data, and then look at the results to see if your strategies made a difference. If you don't begin with a picture of current functioning, baseline data, then you don't know if your efforts helped students. Starting with baseline data helps you educate everyone as to how you contributed to moving data.

The Six Steps of MEASURE

Let's learn how to use the six steps by using a very common goal for school districts: to improve the going rate for postsecondary education.

Step 1: Mission

Connect the design, implementation, and management of the school counseling program to the mission of the school and to the objectives of the annual school improvement plan. The mission statement of every school in America has the common theme of supporting student achievement. If we place the school's mission at the heart of our school counseling program, we will have taken the first step to begin our accountability work. By stating that your school counseling program is to be held accountable for furthering the school's mission of academic achievement for all students, you have clearly articulated that you are concerned about the same accountability fire to which every other educator's feet are held.

Example

The mission of our school is to promote the conditions necessary so that each student experiences academic success. Each student will have the course work required to choose from a wide array of options after high school.

Step 2: Elements

As a member of the school's leadership team, you need to identify and examine the critical elements of the available data that are important to your school's mission. What indicator of school success are you trying to positively impact? Grades? Test scores? Attendance? Promotion rates? Rate for postsecondary going? School counselors play a pivotal role in this process as they work collectively with all stakeholders to focus on areas of concern for student success. Critical data elements usually can be found on the school's district or building report card. School systems routinely collect and store academic and **demographic data** in a retrievable form.

Example

A key critical element in accomplishing our school mission is the rate for postsecondary going. Currently 50% of our students access postsecondary education (college and other educational opportunities after graduation).

Step 3: Analyze

Analyze the critical data elements to see what it reveals, to identify the problem areas, to establish your baseline, and to set your goal. School counselors can initially determine which elements to tackle first and which elements the school counseling program can move in a positive direction to specific targets.

Example

Baseline: Currently, 50% of our students access postsecondary education.
Goal: A one-year increase of 5% in the rate of postsecondary going.

Analysis will determine the institutional or environmental barriers that may be impeding student achievement and adversely influencing the data elements. A quick look at data alone does not tell the whole story. It is important to disaggregate the critical data elements on which you are focusing, and to look at them in terms of gender, race/ethnicity, socioeconomic status, and perhaps by teacher to shed light on areas of success or on areas in need of attention. The analysis will reveal how far away the data are from your school improvement goal.

What other information do you need to know? The counselor in the example might want to know which student groups are among the 50% accessing postsecondary education. Which students compose the 50% not accessing this option? Disaggregate the data to answer these and other questions. You can disaggregate data in a number of ways: gender, ethnicity, socioeconomic status (SES), home location, teacher or counselor assignments, course-taking patterns, feeder schools, and so on. This information can be gathered through the student information management system, school report card, or by similar means.

Let's suppose that in the example situation, the data reveal (among other important things) that of the 50% of the students seeking postsecondary education, the majority, or 34%, came from one particular feeder middle school where all students are assigned to algebra classes in eighth grade and are supported with mentors and tutors to be successful. The feeder middle school practice to place every student in algebra is a positive practice that could be replicated by the other feeder schools.

Step 4: Stakeholders-Unite

First, identify stakeholders to become part of a team to be involved in addressing the movement of the critical data elements. All concerned members of the internal and external school community should be included. Determine how to secure their commitment and who will bring them together. If possible, use an existing school action committee. Accountability for school counselors is about collaborating with other stakeholders and avoiding tackling issues in isolation. Table 9.1 lists examples of stakeholders.

Next, unite with stakeholders and develop and implement strategies to move critical data elements in a positive direction. The team will

1. define targeted results;

2. decide what information is needed and how to gather it;

3. determine the strategies to move the data;

Table 9.1 Internal and External Community Stakeholders

Internal Community	External Community
Principal	Agency Member
Teacher	Business Representative
School Board Member	Faith Representative

4. identify skills and resources needed and assign responsibilities to appropriate stakeholders;

5. develop a timeline and a way to assess interim progress and final results.

With your stakeholders, begin to develop and implement an action plan that contains strategies, a timeline, and responsibilities in order to move the rate of postsecondary going to 55%. Table 9.2 gives a high-school example of stakeholders and strategies that could be used to increase rate of postsecondary going. Similar tables can be created for middle and elementary schools based on the target established in Step 3.

Step 5: Reanalyze

Even if the targeted results were met, there still is reflection and refining to do. Did the results of everyone's efforts show that the **interventions and strategies** successfully moved the critical data elements in a positive direction? If so, reassess your efforts to develop your next steps toward continuous school improvement, including any changes in the school counseling program.

What if the targeted results were *not* met? The next step would be to reanalyze and refocus the efforts to determine why the interventions were unsuccessful in moving the data in a positive direction. Identify the components of the effort that worked. Reanalyzing means replicating what is working and developing new or different strategies for what did not work. Based on your analysis, determine what changes need to be made to the school counseling program to keep the focus on student success. We become vulnerable if we hold fast to programs and strategies that do not help our students become more successful learners and productive citizens. There is too much work and too little time to accomplish all that needs to happen for our students. If a particular strategy is not making a difference, then we have to rethink our investment of time and energy.

It is always necessary to reanalyze and refocus to determine whether you met your targeted results. If the targeted results were met, set new targets, add new strategies, and replicate what was successful. If the rate of postsecondary going increased by only 2% and thus fell short of the targeted results, it will be necessary to refocus efforts to determine which strategies were successful and which need to be replaced or revised. All stakeholders, including the school counselor, can determine which of the efforts worked well, and which strategies need to be modified, adjusted, or perhaps changed altogether. The next steps will be to revise the action plan for the following year and to continue to move the critical data elements in a positive direction.

Example

Reanalyze   (Restate the baseline data. Where is the data now? Did the strategies have a positive impact on the data?) Result of reanalysis: The goal was not only reached, but exceeded! Our 50% rate of postsecondary going grew by 6% to 56%.

Table 9.2 Stakeholders and Strategies for Increasing the Rate of Postsecondary Going

Beginning date: September of this school year

Ending date: June of this school year

Action Plan Goal: Increase rate of postsecondary going

Stakeholders	*Strategies*
School Counselors	• Implement a career awareness program for every student in the school to help each see the interrelatedness between postsecondary education and his or her future economic opportunities. • Advocate for a systemic change in course enrollment patterns to support more students to access higher level academics. • Use data and anecdotal information about student success in higher level academics to try to change attitudes and beliefs about widening opportunities for higher level academics. • Provide additional group and individual counseling to high-risk students on motivation and problem solving.
Teachers	• Social studies teachers have students research their career goals and project how their career paths fit with economic trends and the business climate. • English teachers have students write essays for scholarships. • Mathematics teachers integrate financial aid calculations into lessons.
Administrators	• Provide professional development for the faculty on raising aspirations. • Orchestrate collaboration with feeder schools to see how to replicate the practices that are proving successful in raising aspirations.
School Social Workers	• Work with parents and caregivers on teaching students the importance of attendance for school success.
Clerical Staff	• Monitor student progress in submitting applications for postsecondary admissions. • Organize group meetings between the counselors and the students who are not submitting information to postsecondary institutions in a timely manner.
School Clubs	• Invite community leaders to talk about career opportunities and the education and skills needed to be successful in the work environment. • Help close the information gap by sponsoring awareness activities regarding postsecondary opportunities.
Parents	• Assist in establishing a tutoring program. • Create a phone chain to call parents to remind them of important school events.

Table 9.2 continued

Stakeholders	Strategies
Volunteers	• Work with individual students on the power of financial aid to impact their future.
Business Partners	• Assist in establishing a mentoring program.
	• Provide site visits to their businesses.
	• Help organize and participate in career fairs.
Community Agencies	• Assist in establishing a mentoring program.
	• Run evening and Saturday programs with school personnel for parents and students on raising aspirations, homework help, technology awareness, etc.
Colleges and Universities	• Host "College for a Day" programs for elementary and middle school students.
	• Offer diagnostic academic placement testing to 10th and 11th graders.
	• Provide targeted interventions for underrepresented populations.

Reflect   *(Reflect on why the stakeholders were successful or unsuccessful in executing the action plan.) Result of reflection: All of the strategies executed by the stakeholders contributed to our success.*

Revise   *(Which strategies should be replaced? Added? Based on what you have learned, how will you improve the action plan in the future?) Result of revision: No change in strategies noted at this time. Next year we are going to focus on the discrepancies in the rate of postsecondary going among Caucasians, African Americans, and Hispanics.*

Step 6: Educate

Disseminate to internal and external stakeholders the changes in the targeted data elements that show the positive impact that the school counseling program is having on student success. Publicizing the results of an effective school counseling program is a vital step in the accountability process and key to garnering support for your program. This can be a time to celebrate success and recognize and applaud your partnerships.

Example

Look at our high-school profile now! Now 56% of our students are accessing postsecondary opportunities, slightly better than our goal of 55%. What did we learn from this process?

- *Critical data element analyses helped us focus our efforts.*
- *Districtwide systemic change issues must begin in elementary school.*

- *Stakeholders across all levels were willing to share responsibility for moving critical data elements.*
- *Changes in data clearly demonstrated the intentional focus of the school counseling program on improving the postsecondary going rate.*
- *Collaborative efforts made the changes happen.*
- *The school counselors' commitment as key players in school improvement was well established and acknowledged.*
- *Strategies delivered K through 12 positively moved this data forward.*
- *Measurable results showed how the school counseling program worked to increase the rate of postsecondary going through a systemwide focused effort.*

Through this education, stakeholders will have a deeper understanding about the contributions of a school counseling program focused on student achievement. School counselors will be seen as partners in school improvement who have demonstrated a willingness to be accountable for changing critical data elements. Because of these efforts, school counselors are viewed as essential to the mission of the school.

Systemic Changes and Other Interim Data

As you work together with the other stakeholders toward meeting your goals, you will have interim success stories that are both anecdotal and hard data. You will implement systemic changes. Capture these successes and note them on your report card.

When you tackle delivering a data-driven school counseling program, you become a systemic change agent impacting policies and procedures that will widen opportunities and empower more students to be successful learners. If the system were working optimally then a MEASURE would not be necessary; we can't drive data without changing systems. So, when you are gathering stakeholders and developing strategies, make certain you implement a MEASURE that intentionally tackles systemic barriers. Give yourself credit for impacting systems. Impacting systems means (a) replicating successful programs and interventions, (b) identifying barriers that adversely stratify students' opportunities to be successful learners, and (c) developing strategies to

- change policies, practices, and procedures;
- strengthen curriculum offerings;
- maximize the instructional program;
- enhance the school and classroom culture and climate;
- provide student academic support systems (safety nets);
- influence course enrollment patterns to widen access to rigorous academics;
- involve parents and other critical stakeholders (internal and external to the school);
- raise aspirations in students, parents, teachers, and the community;
- change attitudes and beliefs about students and their abilities to learn.

Box 9.2 provides an example of how to educate others. The report card, called a SPARC, is the result of the Piscataway elementary and middle school counselors' 2002–2003 MEASURE.

Box 9.2

School Counseling Program Accountability Report Card (SPARC)

Our MEASURE of Success: School Counseling Program Accountability Report Card (SPARC)

District:	Piscataway Elementary and Middle Schools
Enrollment:	K–8 4,688
Principals:	Susan Chalfin, Wayne Rose, Barry Glickman, Dr. Willa Pryor, Alice Rothberg, Shirley Eyler, Dr. Suzanne Westberg, Mr. Mario Tursi, Mr. Richard Gardner
Assistant Director for Counseling:	Dr. Dorothy J. Youngs
Counselors:	Jill Brown, Gillian Roth, Susan Manley, J. Courtney Boyd-Moscowitz, Irene Guarino, Carmen Campoverde, Sherri Griffith, Jaime Schnirman, Rebecca Walker, Ildiko Henni-Jones, Robyn Rosenthal, Deirdre McClafferty, MaryAnn Lombardi, Margo Shapiro, Marge Delaney, C. Alex Gray, Dan Rothberg, Wendy Johansen

Director of Counselors' Comments

Collaboration was key to our success this year with elementary and middle school counselors working together to build on skills and knowledge that students acquired in the elementary schools. The school district's suspension rate was strongly impacted as a result of this effort. Training was provided for staff in conflict resolution skills to manage student behavior. We pulled together toward the common goal of creating a climate of caring and respect in our schools.

School Improvement Issues

Suspension rates were at unacceptable levels.

Critical Data Element(s):   Reduce the number of K–8 suspensions

(continued)

Box 9.2 continued

Systemic Changes

1. The elementary and middle school counselors began the process of annually establishing goals and collaborating to achieve them.

2. A safe and respectful school climate became a focus of each school with multiple stakeholders seeking attainment.

3. Choosing a goal and having the entire faculty focus on that goal became the district practice, with a safe and respectful school climate becoming the first such goal.

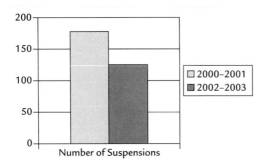

Number of Suspensions

Results

Number of Student K–8 Suspensions

2000–2001	2002–2003
176	124

Faces Behind the Data

Shortly after Irene Guarino taught her second graders anti-bullying strategies, a second grader ran up to her. "Mrs. Guarino," she excitedly said, "here's the story. So far I told them to stop. I stood up to the whole group. I told them how I felt. I gave them an "I" message. And now I'm telling a grownup."

Counselor Marge Delaney always goes out of her way to compliment her students when she "catches" them doing something good! One student looked quizzically at her and responded, "but I just listen to you."

Stakeholders

Counselors: Involved students in the Peace Pledge program; developed anti-bullying classroom guidance lessons; trained peer mediators; implemented a schoolwide program; collaborated with counselors across schools to continue the skills taught in K–5; taught conflict resolution skills; used disaggregated data to identify problem areas

Administrator: Encouraged mediation first; enforced consequences; used conflict resolution strategies with students

Teachers: Reinforced conflict mediation skills; created bully-free class environments; referred students for mediation as an alternative to discipline

Parents: Participated in workshops that focused on resolving conflict peacefully; reinforced the code of conduct at home

Students: Created an anti-bullying school; served as peer mediators; took the "peace pledge," learned when to seek help from an adult and how to confront bullying

Higher Education: Provided mentors and tutors for children who displayed at-risk behavior

Business Partners: Spoke to students about the importance of working together.

Remember, the Steps Will Rarely Be Nice and Neat

The six steps will not always follow the sequence as outlined. You may enter this accountability process at different points or you may follow a different sequence. For example, you may want to look at the issue raised by the school board by first bringing the stakeholders together, as in Step 5.

Sharing accountability can be messy and difficult, and the results sometimes disappointing. It is very frustrating when, in collaboration with other stakeholders, your goal still remains elusive. Whole-school efforts in collaboration and teaming are critical toward moving data elements. Do we give up after one year? Systemic change takes time. Remember, change is a process, not an event (Fullan, 1993, 2002).

Change Is Hard

In implementing a data-driven school counseling program, you are often asking people to work in a different way than they have become used to working. This is especially true if you are part of a school counseling department with counselors prepared in the traditional approach. Teachers and administrators may not view the school counselor as someone who can help impact the academic success of students because it has not been their experience that school counselors have worked in this way. Change is hard, and the very stakeholders you want to bring to the table to help you make a difference for students may be the stakeholders who do not agree

We can't measure what we do.

I don't have the time.   The problem is too complex.   Too risky!

It's not reality.   No matter what we do, things will never change.

It's pie in the sky.

It's impossible!   That's not my job.

We tried that before.   It's too expensive.   What's wrong with the way things are?

It can't be done.   It takes too long.   We've always done it this way.

This is fiscally impossible.   It is a political hot potato.   We don't have the staff.

The principal will not support it.   This too shall pass.

I am too close to retirement to change now.   There are too many variables.

Figure 9.6 The Naysayers.

with your approach. You will experience naysayers and roadblockers. You will hear a litany of reasons why you should not work differently. As shown in Figure 9.6, the "Yes Buts" can be endless.

These three counselors have proven that data can really help counselors garner support for their programs and more important, support more students. Are our sights too high, our goals too lofty, the work impossible for us to implement? Not at all! The wonderful amazing work you will be doing to change students' lives will be enhanced by adding the next step, accountability, which will demonstrate your value to the mission of your school. Don't let the data naysayers deter you. Failure to establish recognizable school counselor results for student achievement is tantamount to being counted out (Martin, 2004). In the world of schools today, where increased academic performance for all students is the mandated goal, school counselors must take this critical step—they must become routine users of data to inform and sharpen their focus. Data, those cold hard numbers, actually move us closer to children because now, with assurance, we affirm that the school counselor has made an impact on students' learning (Stone & Dahir, 2004).

TechTools

Technology can help you retrieve data in order to get a clear picture of student achievement. Data will help you identify the areas of concern and the patterns of achievement that inform you as to where your school counseling program is most needed. Accountability and a data-driven school counseling program depend on student information.

- Work for good data through your school or district student information management system. Ask questions of the managers of student information for the district. Continue to ask questions and gently push until you get reports in a form that is usable to you.
- Monitor student progress by querying databases to see which students are not progressing, need special attention, or are being successful.
- Make informed decisions about individual students and large groups of students by accessing data about students, such as scheduling, attendance, discipline, test history, test scores, current grades, and past academic performance. For example, if you find that certain students are chronically absent, you have critical information for looking into why these students are absent so often and for seeking ways to encourage them to come back to school.

School Counselor Casebook: *Voices From the Field*

The Scenario Reviewed

When polled at the beginning of the school year, 91% of the students in your school responded that they were planning to enter college. However, only 27% of the students were delivering an academic performance that would widen their options to include college. What do you see as your role, if any, in helping students see the connection between academic performance and enrollment in college?

A Practitioner's Approach

Here's how a practicing school counselor responded to the school scenario:

The counseling staff would immediately try to get to the cause of the gap between aspirations and reality. Here are strategies to use to close this gap:

We would begin by carefully looking at the course enrollment patterns and grade distributions for the students at each grade level. We might discover that the majority of the students had grades that would be marginally acceptable to college admissions counselors. Many of the seniors were taking elective courses just to fill their day, with little connection to what they would need in order to have a successful freshman year at college.

As a result of the findings, my colleagues and I would develop an action plan that would focus on motivating and encouraging students to raise their aspirations. We would work with our faculty to discuss motivation and aspiration with our students. This problem is one that every faculty member needs to get involved with if we are going to be successful.

The action plan we would propose would have both short-term and long-term so-lutions to the problem and would utilize the group guidance periods that we have already established in our school.

Short-term solutions: First, we would schedule group guidance meetings with all students in their classrooms (homeroom time). The purpose of the meetings would be to illustrate the direct link between high-school performance and college admis-sion. For 9th and 10th graders, we would emphasize the importance of the strength of high-school curriculum. Since it's a little late for juniors and seniors to change their courses, we would emphasize the need to work on getting a high GPA. We would spend more time with the older students talking about options for college and how decisions are made, encouraging them to meet with a member of the guid-ance department or with a teacher they trust to talk about their future plans. Second, we would request the opportunity to speak to parents at "back to school night" about the importance of strong academic performance and college admis-sion as well as giving hints about how they might help their children achieve. We have had great success in the past using a National Association for College Admission Counseling (NACAC) exemplary program called PACT (Parents and Counselors Together). Using very simple overhead transparencies, the program out-lines the importance of education in obtaining career opportunities and gives some basic information about admission, financial aid, and the importance of high-school curriculum. Although it is geared toward middle school parents, it can be very useful for 9th- and even 10th-grade parents. It is available in Spanish as well. This would help us to be prepared to deliver information to parents and caregivers.

Long-term solutions: We would meet with the principal to discuss the mission of the school and the need for promoting the goal of college entrance for all students who want it. We would propose creating a more formal and extensive group guid-ance program for each grade level, which would focus on the relationship between achievement and reaching future career goals. We would want to include faculty in the program, because they are the people who see the students most frequently, and also because they can act as "mentors" for the students. The program would also include bringing current college students to talk to our students and might even include visits to local colleges to give the students a firsthand look at majors offered. Ultimately, we would like to be able to go into the middle schools that feed into our high school to talk to administrators, parents, teachers, and seventh- and eighth-grade students about the importance of being prepared to enter college prep classes in ninth grade.

School counselors must use data to contribute to student success and show that they too are accountable for results. Having information and understanding the facts is very powerful. We know that 91% of the students are planning to enter col-lege, but only 27% are doing what they need to realize the goal. The population is di-verse in all aspects, including financial ability to pay for college. What the students and their parents need to understand is how to match the high school course curriculum to their goals. Through a strong career and academic advising program, students will learn to strengthen their transcripts, GPA, and desire to learn. These are important factors in acquiring the goals to which they aspire.

Joan Mudge has been a college counselor in an independent school for 28 years, and she currently also holds the position of dean of the faculty at that school. She is a past vice president for professional development of NACAC (National Association for College Admission Counseling), past chair of the Middle States Regional College Board, and has been actively involved in the leadership and professional development activities of the Potomac and Chesapeake Association for College Admission Counseling. Reprinted with permission by Joan W. Mudge.

Chapter Summary

Accountable Data-Driven School Counseling Programs

In this age of accountability, it is essential that school counselors contribute to the school success agenda and clearly tie successful outcomes for students to the counselors' presence in the school. Documenting the results of our efforts is key to assessing program effectiveness. Time-on-task and process data has sufficed in the past for accountability, but student impact data is the logical next step. The accountable school counseling program utilizes student data to create vision and targeted change. Accountability measures involve systematically collecting, analyzing, and using data to inform and guide the development and construction of a school counseling program. Accepting the challenge of accountability propels us to demonstrate by words and actions that we accept the responsibility of removing barriers to learning and achievement and promoting success for those students from whom little is expected.

ASCA National Model and Accountability

The ASCA National Model and the Transforming School Counseling Initiative were critical in starting the conversations about measurable results. The ASCA National Model speaks to the importance of having an accountability system and an organizational framework that documents and demonstrates how students have changed as a result of the school counseling program.

Time-on-Task and Results-Based Data

Counting services delivered and looking at posttests for learning gains are important aspects of program evaluation, but they are soft data. When you couple this soft data with evidence of the school counseling program's impact on critical data elements, the program will be aligned with the accountability agenda of the school and school district.

Building a Data-Driven School Counseling Program

A school counseling program built around data means using numbers rather than relying just on assumptions or perceptions to determine where to focus the efforts of the school counseling program. The school counselor examines critical data elements to identify students' gaps and needs; then, in collaboration with other stakeholders, the counselor develops and applies appropriate strategies. Enrollments in college prep courses, graduation rate, retention rates, special education placements, attendance, grades, and standardized test scores are just a few of the critical data elements that may receive attention in a data-driven school counseling program. Use of data to provide a telling story of achievement patterns, equity issues, career and college connections, and overall effectiveness of the school is a central tool in the school counseling program.

Disaggregated Data

Disaggregating data means looking beyond averages and percentages to separate out the data by categories, such as ethnicity, gender, socioeconomic status, and teacher assignment, to reveal where the needs are greatest or the successes to replicate the strongest.

MEASURE: A Different Way of Focusing Our Work

MEASURE, an acronym for Mission, Elements, Analyze, Stakeholders-Unite, Reanalyze, and Educate, is a six-step accountability process that helps school counselors develop a data-driven school counseling program. MEASURE shows school counselors how to begin the process with baseline data, develop strategies with other stakeholders to move the data in a positive direction, and then report the results in hard data.

Key Terms

American School Counseling
    Association (ASCA) National Model
    p. 238
Critical data elements p. 237
Data-driven school counseling p. 240
Demographic data p. 253

Disaggregated data p. 247
Interventions and strategies p. 255
MEASURE p. 252
Results-based accountability p. 240
Time-on-task p. 239

Learning Extensions

1. Read the case scenario that follows. Develop a MEASURE for the case by filling out the first four steps as if you had really met with stakeholders and everyone developed strategies.

   Scenario: It is an unwritten policy of the teachers and administration of your school that all students who are in danger of being retained for the second time be screened and tested for possible placement into special education classes. Special Education (SE) students can have testing accommodations if they have identified disabilities and are offered different promotion and graduation policies. You believe that in your particular school there is an overreliance on SE as an intervention without aggressive searches for other effective means to support students before they get to their second retention. There is a disproportionate number of minorities placed into SE programs. What will be the role of your school counseling program in curbing the trend for SE placement as an intervention?

2. Visit a school counselor and retrieve a real piece of data that is troublesome for the school counselor (follow confidentiality rules). Sit down with the counselor and explain MEASURE, and help the counselor think through how he or she could implement a MEASURE. Finish the first four steps of the MEASURE.

3. The school improvement plan for the year calls for an improvement in the orderliness and safety of the school's learning environment. It is believed that the disruptions in the environment and the bullying behavior are contributing to the decline in test scores and grade point averages. What are some strategies you can use to enhance the school learning community? Discuss how you will gather baseline data and then how you will demonstrate that your strategies have been a success.

Chapter 10

Addressing Diversity in Schools

Promoting a Social Justice Agenda

Examining Personal Beliefs and Behaviors

Diversity and Multiculturalism
    Social Class Distinctions
    Gender Equity
    Sexual Minority Youth
    Learning Differences

Creating a Culturally Compatible Climate
    Challenging Beliefs and Changing Behaviors

Chapter Objectives

By the time you have completed this chapter, you should be able to:

- Explore your personal beliefs, attitudes, and knowledge about working with diverse student populations.
- Ensure that each student has access to a comprehensive school counseling program that advocates for all students in diverse cultural groups including affirmation of all ages, ethnic/racial identities, social classes, disability statuses, languages, immigration statuses, sexual orientations, genders, gender identities/expression, family types, religious/spiritual identities, and appearances (ASCA, 2004).
- Explore the impact of poverty and social class on student achievement.
- Identify the impact of family culture upon student performance.

- Use data to close the gap among diverse student populations.
- Identify resources and methods of support for English language learners and students engaged in bilingual support.
- Acquire knowledge of strategies and skills for promoting student success through culturally sensitive advising and counseling.
- Develop consultation strategies to raise the consciousness level of faculty, administration, and staff to better serve students from an increasingly diverse population.

School Counselor Casebook: Getting Started

The Scenario

At the end of the first quarter, a classroom teacher asks you to come to observe four students whom he believes are not working up to their ability. The students are not getting along with others in the class and not completing assignments in a timely manner. The bottom line is that the teacher does not believe that the students are keeping up with the expectations for the fourth-grade class and not sure if they are appropriately placed in a regular education classroom. You agreed to observe the students and review the findings with him. You are also aware that these four students represent various racial and ethnic backgrounds.

Thinking About Solutions

As you read this chapter, imagine yourself in the role of leader and advocate for these students. What factors will you look for that might be contributing to the students' lack of success? What diversity influences may be contributing to the teacher's concern about these four students? How will you address your findings with the classroom teacher? When you come to the end of the chapter, you will have the opportunity to see how your ideas compare with a practicing school counselor's approach.

Promoting a Social Justice Agenda

"Too many children who enter school with equal yearning soon falter under the harsh light of adult assumptions and American cultural history. Our lowered sights precede their own."

— Roberts, 1997, p. 23

Today's schools mirror the changing demographics of the neighborhoods and communities that reflect the **diversity** of America. Public schools are the place where children can learn to get along with others, and they continue to be the primary institutions that create cohesion among diverse groups (Center on Education Policy, 1998). Not all public schools bring together children from various racial and ethnic backgrounds, or children whose families are rich with those who are poor. Some public schools today are racially and economically isolated, but this does not diminish the importance of teaching children to be accepting of differences, to understand and appreciate each other's culture, and to respect other people's point of view (Center on Education Policy, 1998). School counselors have a responsibility to observe, monitor, and modify adult and student behaviors in order to foster a learning community in which every student, regardless of color, wealth, or ability, can flourish.

In the mid-19th-century wave of immigration, public schools were responsible for building a common culture and teaching democratic principles and ideals (McDevitt & Ormond, 2002). As large waves of new immigrants landed on our shores, they were encouraged to quickly assimilate. The cultural standard for immigrant children was to quickly master English, accept the normative culture, and become "mainstreamed" into American society; newly arrived children were labeled "culturally deprived" or "culturally disadvantaged" (Sadker & Sadker, 2005). The debates between **assimilation** and acculturation resulted in an acceptance of the beliefs that "native culture" was inappropriate or perhaps inferior (Woolfolk, 2004). Students who recently immigrated to the United States developed internal self-doubts regarding their ethnic and cultural identity. Conflict among students was a direct result of the resulting confusion that students experienced (Goldstein & Kodluboy, 1998). During the 1960s and 1970s some ethnic groups desired to sustain their unique pride, culture, and heritage and were less inclined to fully assimilate into the American mainstream(McDevitt & Ormond, 2002). The focus of attention was no longer only on color and race; **ethnicity** and cultural tradition assumed a new prominence. **Multiculturalism** and the **integration** of cultural awareness in the schools became a goal of educators (Woolfolk, 2004).

Today, in the tens of thousands of schools across our country, educators in classrooms and in school counseling offices respond to the complex influences of diversity. In large urban areas such as Los Angeles or New York City, upwards of 80 different languages are found in ESL classrooms, each representing a group of children whose heritage and ethnicity are far from the norm of what is considered traditional American culture (Shore, 2001). By the year 2050, it is predicted that there will be no majority race or ethnicity in the United States; every American will be a member of a minority group (Banks, 2001; Halford, 1999; Payne & Biddle, 1999). Of the 45 million students enrolled in public schools and in private elementary and secondary schools during the 1990s, almost 30% represented groups designated as racial minorities (National Center for Educational Statistics, 2002).

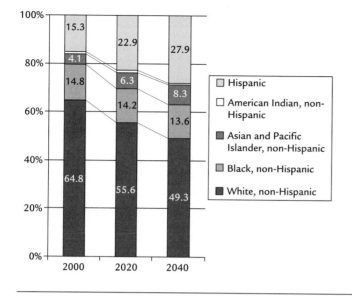

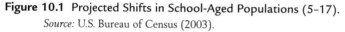

Figure 10.1 Projected Shifts in School-Aged Populations (5–17).
Source: U.S. Bureau of Census (2003).

School counselors are ethically obligated (ASCA, 2004) to deliver a comprehensive school counseling program to every student from culturally diverse backgrounds and need the requisite awareness, knowledge, and skills to do so.

Differences are not limited to race, ethnicity, or language; school counselors also must address identity, generation, cultural customs, geographical origin, community, and family traditions (Capuzzi & Gross, 2003). Blending ethnicities, culture, and heritage can place educators in a cultural "minefield" where they must navigate a caring and respectful path that addresses the needs of many groups (Franklin, 2001; Holcomb-McCoy, 2004). A child's worldview of harmony or discord will be influenced in great measure by his or her educational experience (Center on Education Policy, 1998). With a renewed interest in creating safe and respectful school environments (NCLB, 2001) public schools have promoted an affirmation of human rights by focusing on social harmony, **tolerance,** and respect. By seeking ways of bringing together children from all races and ethnicities, **prejudices** and biases are reduced or eliminated (Teaching Tolerance, 2003). According to the National Center for Education Statistics (2003):

- Twenty percent of the children in school are immigrants or have parents who are immigrants. Most new arrivals to our nation come from Central and Latin America.
- In 2002, 35% of children under the age of 18 were from minority groups. By the year 2020, this proportion is expected to increase to 45%.

- The United States is becoming more religiously diverse, with Islam becoming the fastest growing religion in the nation.
- One in five children under the age of 18 was born poor, and one in six is poor now.
- One in five children has a foreign-born mother.
- Nearly 50% of all African-American children are poor.
- By the year 2020, approximately 46% of all students in the United States will be students of color, many of whom will be the children of new immigrants.

The data tell the story. As the lines continue to blur between what had been perceived as majority and minority populations, school counselors, as social justice advocates, should encourage students and faculty to be knowledgeable, open-minded, and respectful of all cultures and all aspects of diversity. School counselors explore, understand, and work with the multiplicity of variables that compose diversity and have a responsibility to value culture, race, ethnicity, gender, **socioeconomic status (SES)** and social class, and sexual orientation, and to promote awareness and **acceptance** among all student groups. These variables have a profound influence in students' lives and will continue to do so as they approach adulthood.

School counselors are in an influential position to challenge the status quo, and assist those who have been victims or are potential victims of social and educational problems (Kiselica & Robinson, 2001). Embracing a social justice agenda requires school counselors to "possess the awareness, knowledge, and skill to intervene not only at the individual level, but at the system-wide level" (Lee, 1998, p. 9). Working from a social justice mindset requires school counselors to give special care to those who historically have not received adequate educational opportunities or services, including students of color, students from low socioeconomic backgrounds, students with disabilities, and students with non-dominant-language backgrounds (ASCA, 2004).

Examining Personal Beliefs and Behaviors

School counselors also recognize and acknowledge personal biases and prejudices that can influence counseling, guiding, advising, and encouraging students. As counselors heighten their awareness as to how one's personal membership with regard to race, ethnicity, and culture can influence attitudes and beliefs, they have an obligation to participate in activities that allow them to explore their own identity (Constantine & Gainor, 2001). Personal sensitivity to diversity also helps school counselors to determine how culture influences a student's perception of the problem and the choice of intervention. School counselors have an ethical obligation to be mindful of the influences of bias and prejudice (ASCA, 2004) and are responsible to act as "path finders," not "gatekeepers" (Hart & Jacobi, 1992), for students from all walks of life and backgrounds.

Box 10.1

Reflections

Self-reflection is an important component of professional identity (Council for Accreditation of Counseling and Related Educational Programs, 2001). Here are some questions that will guide you in reflecting upon your own cultural identity and beliefs. (Later in this chapter you will find additional reflection questions. When you do, stop and reflect on them before continuing on.)

1. What were the prevailing issues (social, historical, cultural, etc.) of your "developmental years" that helped to shape your thinking, your belief system, and your attitudes?

2. How did these issues influence or affect you, your family, and your relationships with your family?

3. How did the sum of all of these components create the person that you have become today?

4. How does your worldview impact how you work with or will work with students?

An individual's development is the totality of experiences and is greatly influenced by variables such as the era in which one was born as well as the color of one's skin. Examining one's personal identity is a first step before one can explore the cultural norms and the diversity that represent others. Generational location strongly shapes how you see and live your life. Generations are influenced by the times and traditions that prevailed in any given period. The 1970s were about "breaking rules," the '80s about "clouding conventions," and the '90s about "getting by" in an era in which traditional rules no longer applied; these generational perspectives shape decisions, choices, and values (Howe & Strauss, 2000).

Diversity and Multiculturalism

When educators and community members refer to diversity in conversations in faculty rooms and classrooms, race and ethnicity often are what first come to mind. These terms are not interchangeable. Woolfolk (2001) defines race as "a group of people who share common biological traits (such as skin color, hair texture, etc.) that are seen as self defining by the people of the group" while ethnicity is presented as "a cultural heritage shared by a group of people" (p. 165).

Box 10.2

Self-Assessment for Counseling Diverse Students

Consider where you are on the continuum of acquiring knowledge and honing skills. Answer each question; then develop a plan for professional and personal growth.

1. Am I familiar with strategies that promote equity in a multicultural society (e.g., utilizing culturally/gender relevant counseling practices, empathizing with and understanding the students' worldview)?

   Yes ____   Need to know more ____   No ____

   Action planned: _____

   _____

2. Am I familiar with verbal and nonverbal language patterns of different ethnic/racial groups?

   Yes ____   Need to know more ____   No ____

   Action planned: _____

   _____

3. Do I have high expectations for all students and assist students to acquire resources and opportunities necessary for success?

   Yes ____   Need to know more ____   No ____

   Action planned: _____

   _____

4. In working with a diverse student population, do I consider the interaction of gender differences, class differences, language differences, and cultural differences?

   Yes ____   Need to know more ____   No ____

   Action planned: _____

   _____

5. Do I provide career counseling on the basis of the students' abilities, interests, and skills rather than according to traditional roles based on gender, race, disability, or ethnicity?

   Yes ____   Need to know more ____   No ____

   Action planned: _____

   _____

6. Do I encourage students to take courses nontraditional to their gender, race, disability, or ethnicity if a student shows an interest in one of those areas (for example, mathematics, science, computer technology for girls; early childhood education for boys)?

Yes ____   Need to know more ____   No ____

Action planned: _____

_____

7. Do I assess my own values, attitudes, and beliefs and have the ability to refrain from imposing them upon the student?

Yes ____   Need to know more ____   No ____

Action planned: _____

_____

8. Do I participate in professional development programs or special skill sessions for counselors dealing with culturally diverse students?

Yes ____   Need to know more ____   No ____

Action planned: _____

_____

9. Do I meet with students outside of the office to show an interest in their needs beyond the classroom?

Yes ____   Need to know more ____   No ____

Action planned: _____

_____

10. Do I use a multidimensional approach to identify the level and scope of a student's ability before recommending course selection, placement, and future schooling and career opportunities?

Yes ____   Need to know more ____   No ____

Action planned: _____

_____

In a broad context, diversity refers to the range of cultures and subcultures that represent attitudes, beliefs, values, rituals, symbols, norms and conventions, customs, behaviors, and ideologies (McDevitt & Ormond, 2002). School counselors recognize that diversity impacts and influences the dynamics of learning, personal-social development, and school climate. The term diversity-sensitive counseling has been coined to reflect this wider range of variables (Baker, 2000). School counselors who seek further specific skill development acquire and develop intervention techniques that are appropriate to particular individuals or groups (Holcomb-McCoy, 2003).

The school experience can be supportive or disabling to our student populations. Regardless of the level of the work setting, school counselors must make a commitment to create a climate of caring and respect. Whether it is a racial slur or a comment about a student's ability to learn, school personnel are all too familiar with the tales told about some aspect of insensitivity in the school setting that has had a profound impact on student performance.

After race and ethnicity, culture is oftentimes the next thing that comes to mind when considering diversity. Culture is the sum total of ways of living, including core beliefs, societal values, esthetics, patterns of thinking and communication, and behavioral norms which a group of people have developed to assure their position in a particular environment (Cooper, 1998). Culture is the response of a group of human beings to the valid and particular needs of its members and includes knowledge, values, traditions, and attitudes that guide the behavior of a group of people (Pedersen, 1991). Banks (2001) reminds us that "membership in a particular group does not determine behavior but makes certain types of behavior more probable" (pp.13–14). We can gain insight about an individual's behavior, but we cannot assume to predict behavior. Most of us hold membership or have an identity with more than one group.

Traditionally, race and ethnicity are the terms that educators tend to consider when discussing the concept of multiculturalism. However, school counselors can take on a broader worldview that requires a look at multiculturalism as a "serious scholarship that includes all American peoples" (Halford, 1999, p. 9). Halford also says, "When we look around us, we realize that not all of us came from Europe. Many immigrated from Africa and Latin America, and others were already here in North America" School counselors must be most cognizant of norms that stem from the majority culture when working with students and their families (Holcomb-McCoy, 2004).

Multiculturalism is an awakening to our global interdependence. When working with children and youth, school counselors rely upon an ability to understand and appreciate differences, and focus on the potential rather than on the prejudice. School counselors could approach all counseling as multicultural because each individual presents his or her unique blending of culture, heritage, and ability at the counselor's door. Pedersen (1991) suggested that multicultural counseling is a situation in which two or more persons, with different ways of perceiving their social environment, are brought together in a helping relationship; thus cultural norms and expectations may vary between the counselor and the client (student).

Chisholm and Trumbull (2001) proposed a model that addresses a framework of individualism and collectivism, which helps counselors better understand some of the large differences between the dominant Euro-American culture and new immigrants. For example, Hispanic students usually want to share what they have, even at the expense of giving away a pen or pencil that leaves them without one to use in class, and they tend to want to work together to problem-solve or help each other out with an assignment or directions (Chisholm & Trumbull, 2001). Asian students often present dress and religious affiliations that may stand out in a school setting (Axelson, 1999). Counselors and teachers who understand that these cultural differences impact classroom behavior will clearly delineate the difference between students' working together and working alone. "Singling out an individual's achievement can be seen as a negative in collectivistic groups because of its implicit slighting of other's abilities" (Chisholm & Trumbull, 2001, pp. 3–4). This depth of understanding comes from taking the time to get to know the children, their families, and their culture through continuous communication. With the prediction from the U.S. Bureau of the Census (2002) that as many as 1 in 10 children will be foreign born by the year 2040, the value of understanding cultural differences becomes even more important to ensure student success in schools.

Cultural differences in our schools are often addressed by multicultural education, which teaches the value of cultural diversity (Sadker & Sadker, 2005). This is one response to the increasingly racial, ethnic, and cultural diversity of our schools. Schools, as centers of learning, are in the best position to foster multicultural awareness in children and youth to encourage them to accept and appreciate cultural differences. Students and faculty need opportunities to acquire the experience, skills, awareness, and understanding to transcend the perceived barriers of differences (Johnson, 1995). Banks (1994) promotes multicultural education from a holistic perspective and emphasizes that it is much more than classroom instruction. One also faces challenges associated with enculturation in which the student identifies with the attitudes, behaviors, and values of the predominant culture (Lee, 2001a). Many young people seek to adapt to the dress, style, and lifestyle of the "American youth culture" and master the task of balancing an ethnic identity with one that will provide access to the mainstream culture. Students frequently find themselves caught in between the two cultures (Lee, 2001).

What responsibility does the school counselor have in fostering a climate that is respectful of cultural diversity? School counselors can help focus attention on the overall impact of creating an empowering school climate that fosters an atmosphere of participation and acceptance. After identifying practices that may be inhibiting equity and access, it is necessary to seek ways to motivate staff and student interaction that transcends ethnic, cultural, and racial lines (Banks, 1994). These efforts extend far beyond moment-in-time interventions such as "Human Rights Days" and multicultural events. To systemically and positively impact attitudes and beliefs about racial, ethnic and cultural mores, programs must be:

- multifaceted (varied in activity and services);
- inclusionary (engaging all school personnel, all students, and involving the community);
- developmental (proactive, not reactive in nature);
- continuous (ongoing);
- have the support of the school district (Johnson, 1995).

Social Class Distinctions

There was a time when social class identification was synonymous with wealth, power, stature, and prestige. Children are acutely aware of upper-class, middle-class, and lower-class economic and social characteristics (Sadker & Sadker, 2005). Power and prestige are not always synonymous with wealth. Politicians and professors may have influence, but often do not have the economic baseline to access upper-class social circles. Social class is influenced by perception. Values have begun to transcend what had been previously perceived as racial and ethnic barriers to demographic change, whether these reference child-rearing practices or manicured lawns. Neighbors find that they have more in common with those of similar wealth, who share similar values, and are more accepting of racial, ethnic, and cultural differences (Woolfolk, 2004).

Educational aspirations are reflective of communities and school systems, and the gap continues to widen among the "haves" and the "have nots" (Haycock, 2004). Low-income youth, those from middle-income families, and children from affluent communities should have the same access to educational opportunity (House & Martin, 1998). This may not always be the case. Although there are exceptions, poor students who attend poverty-stricken school systems usually have less opportunity. This is more apparent as we examine the college attendance rates shown in Table 10.1.

The data on the low socioeconomic status of students of color and their families is cause for alarm. The 2003 census data reveal that 13.8% of all families of all

Table 10.1 Four-Year College Attendance Rates by Income

Achievement Level in Quartiles

	Low Income	High Income
First (low)	8%	25%
Second	16%	42%
Third	31%	70%
Fourth (high)	58%	86%

Source: Adapted from NELS: 88, Second (1992) and Third Follow up (1994), in USDOE, NCES, NCES Condition of Education 1997, p. 64.

races had incomes below the poverty level. The percentage of families in this category increased dramatically for minority families. McLoyd (1998) reminds us that African-American and Hispanic children are more likely to experience persistent poverty, and continue to live in areas of concentrated poverty. The rise in the numbers of children of color has also increased the proportion of those living below the poverty line. Children who live in high-poverty communities have different life exposures, which include minimal access to public services and quality health care, poorly equipped schools, street violence, homelessness, drug racketeering, etc. (McLoyd, 1998). Children of poverty often live in single-parent homes, and most often, the single parent is a woman. When the head of household is female with no husband present, the poverty level almost triples (U.S. Bureau of the Census, 2003).

Studies show that high SES students stay in school longer and have higher levels of achievement (Conger, Conger, & Elder, 1997; Garrett, Ng'andu, & Ferron, 1994; McLoyd, 1998). Students who are caught in a cycle of poverty are also caught in a cycle of low expectations. These cycles are self-perpetuating unless there is direct intervention on the part of educators to focus their efforts on both the obvious and the underlying symptoms. McLoyd (1998) also speaks to several other contributing factors, such as low expectations, learned helplessness, peer influences, and resistance. Each of these factors offers school counselors additional insight into the world of poverty. For example, students with limited financial resources may not wear the "trendy" clothes that other young adolescents and teens consider as essential to their wardrobes, and they may have little or no experience with cultural icons such as museums, theaters, and public libraries.

Self-Confidence

Students of poverty may also believe that it is extremely difficult or next to impossible to be successful (Conger, Conger, & Elder, 1997; McLoyd, 1998). As you may recall from Chapter 1, income is directly related to educational attainment. Low SES children, particularly students of color, may firmly believe that they do not have access to participate in mainstream America (McLoyd, 1998). For some students, making it in school socially, being academically successful, and getting involved in sports, activities, and clubs, is translated by their peers to mean that they sold out or are acting "white," acting "black," or acting "middle class" (McLoyd, 1998). This perspective impacts students' ability to maintain stature in their peer group and they must reject the behaviors that would make them successful (Bennet, 1999). Students may be insecure about jumping into classroom discussions or choose not to participate in field trips because of a lack of self-confidence and low self-esteem (Conger, Conger, & Elder, 1997). Yet many adolescents are high achievers, despite their economic situation or pressure from peers (O'Connor, 1997). Regardless of each student's economic status, school counselors are in an ideal position to identify the issues that stratify opportunity and to work collaboratively with faculty and staff to close the achievement gap.

Tracking

The national debate around tracking continues to place attention on gatekeeping versus gate opening. Many educators believe that it is simpler for students with similar skills, aptitude, and intellectual ability to learn together in a homogeneous class (Sadker & Sadker, 2005). When educators follow this belief, they sort students into groups based on their abilities, which sets the students on an educational path that can predetermine their futures. *Tracking* is the term given to this process.

Although there are many complex arguments that focus on tracking and detracking, for purposes of this text, two basic philosophies are presented. The first one promotes homogeneously grouping students of similar ability together for purposes of remediation and acceleration. The second emphatically asserts that tracking stands in the way of equal educational opportunity (Loveless, 1999). What is the appropriate, ethical way to proceed? Reflect on the role that school counselors have played in the past in this commonplace practice of tracking or ability grouping by class.

School counselors have been part of the system that sorts and selects students according to perceived ability and/or achievement (Hart & Jacobi, 1992). School counselors have supported tracking systems by failing to inform students appropriately about the outcome and consequences of course assignment and placement (Hart & Jacobi, 1992). Tracking students has been the modus operandi in American education for many years. Children learn at an early age that they are sorted, selected, ranked, re-grouped, and classified according to ability as they compete each day for teacher approval, stickers, rewards, grades, bumper stickers, and access to honors and upper-level courses. Tracking also adds a socialization dimension to education. Expectations of teachers and parents differ and are dependent upon student placement. Oftentimes differentiated instructional materials are selected for use in class, and adjustments are made in the rate of learner response and in the teacher's delivery of the curriculum. Students, even the very youngest, are aware of where they are placed and what level of achievement is expected of them.

A study by Stone (1998) revealed that placement into ninth-grade algebra was largely dependent on a student's socioeconomic status and school assignment. The ninth-grade mathematics placements for 6,000 students in an urban school district were examined. Low SES students in the upper quartile on eighth-grade mathematics were not uniformly placed into algebra, despite their ability. Instead, they were placed into the general mathematics courses. Placement also was directly related to the attendance boundaries that defined which middle school a student attended. These also reflected the socioeconomic environment of the local community. Schools in the affluent areas of the city placed upper quartile mathematics students into algebra at much higher rates, while the low SES schools largely ignored algebra as an option for their students.

Critics of tracking suggest that it can be eliminated and that students who arrive to school with very diverse backgrounds can learn from each other and together

(Sadker & Sadker, 2005). Detracked schools can become learning communities, but teachers need time and support so that all can succeed—students and teachers.

School counselors have a moral and ethical responsibility to examine practices and policies that impact any student's right to a quality education. Predetermining a student's future is an action that speaks louder than words. School counselors can either support or challenge the philosophies and procedures that stratify opportunities for students.

Gender Equity

There has been a tradition of thinking that suggests

- girls do better in some subjects than boys do;
- some careers are for men and some careers are better suited for women;
- science and math are difficult for girls;
- girls and boys use computers for different purposes;
- men and women receive unequal pay for equal work in certain job titles (Sadker & Sadker, 1994).

The challenges of becoming a diversity-sensitive school counselor require an examination of the impact of gender differences on student success in school. For many, this may not be as obvious as race, ethnicity, and cultural differences when we work with students. Gender differences can influence what is expected as the "norm" and can contribute to some of the fundamental differences in personality development for boys and girls in the traditions of some cultures (Lee, 1998). Erickson's identity and intimacy stages influence male and female development differently and influence relationship building (Gilligan, 1993). However, like other forms of **discrimination,** messages of sexism may be subtle (Sadker & Sadker, 1994). Counselors and teachers may not always be aware of the messages that are communicated and how these impact student behavior and student choices.

Gender refers to the judgments that are made about femininity and masculinity, and often these are influenced by culture and context. This differs from sex, which refers specifically to biological differences (Woolfolk, 2004). Gender identities form at an early age, when girls and boys take on social and cognitive roles that are associated with a specific orientation of masculine or feminine. As their concept of their world develops, young children receive clues about distinctions between what is considered male and female. This is evidenced in that girls play with dolls and boys play with trucks; girls wear pink and boys wear blue. As children grow older they become more attuned to role models of their own gender. Their awareness of gender differences takes on a greater level of sophistication, and this has implications for their self-concept and behaviors. As students move into adolescence their ideas about gender help them determine how they measure up to gender roles. Children and adolescents form mental images of what girls are supposed to do and what boys are supposed to do. Parents contribute to stereotypical expectations by setting different boundaries for girls and boys when it comes to personal safety. Societal influences and those of family, peers, and the larger community can reinforce the need to stay within boundaries (Ruble & Martin, 1998).

Traditional gender role orientation has impact and influence not only on how we view students and raise children, but also on our personal worldview. Sometimes this appears as a bias in behavior, which is translated into verbal phrases such as "boys will be boys" when classroom or playground behavior becomes unruly. Researchers also have discovered that teachers tend to interact more with boys than with girls (Bailey, 1993; Sadker & Sadker, 2005). Oftentimes teachers, parents, and even school counselors reinforce stereotypical expectations by not insisting that both male and female high-school students continue their studies in math and in the sciences. Exceptions are made for female students more frequently than for male students, thus reinforcing expectations around achievement related to gender (Sadker & Sadker, 1994).

Gender expectations can also affect students' career decision making, course-taking patterns, desire for "good grades," involvement in afterschool activities and sports, and hobbies. Recently, educational aspirations and postsecondary education completion have become female dominated. It is projected that women will earn the majority of associate's, bachelor's, and master's degrees through the year 2011 (National Center for Education Statistics, 2004). Educators' opinions of students can drastically affect student motivation and achievement. If a student believes that a counselor or teacher does not care about his or her contributions in class because of gender, or for that matter because of any other individual characteristic, a student can unconsciously and permanently lose interest and the willingness to work harder and to pursue his or her dream. What can school counselors do? Here are some areas that are worthy of attention:

- School counselors need to be cognizant of any unintentional biases that may exist in delivering group or classroom activities. This bias could involve grouping students by gender or favoring one gender over another in the delivery or processing of the activity.
- School counselors can use current data and analyze the trends that affect the aspirations and motivation of the student population in their care.
- School counselors need to encourage all students to explore their interests and realize their dreams. We need to pay close attention to the **stereotyping** of career paths and to what are considered traditional and nontraditional occupations from both our perspective and that of others (Graham & Taylor, 2002). Career decision making is closely aligned with educational planning.
- School counselors must be "gate openers," not "gatekeepers." We can play an influential and impactful role in every student's course selection to ensure

that talent and interest are nurtured. Upper-level math, science, and technology courses must become part of every student's academic portfolio to ensure later success and access to quality postsecondary opportunities.

- School counselors must be aware of the influence of bias in language. Using words such as "chairperson" instead of "chairman" is more in tune with an equal opportunity environment. Additionally, language should be inclusive and affirming and not discriminate in its intent.

School counselors can put aside personal gender prejudices and biases to encourage student initiative and can motivate colleagues to do the same. Working with teachers to foster cooperative learning and teamwork in the classroom will help students feel that contributions of their own gender are important and noteworthy.

Sexual Minority Youth

Sexual minority youth, as they progress through elementary, middle, and secondary schools in the United States, are confronted every day with taunts, epithets, and a host of other negative, insulting, and derogatory words from their peers, all of which are intended to bring them into conformity with the dominant majority culture's view of sexuality, that is, a heterosexual or opposite-sex sexual orientation (Pope, 2004, p. 31). Peer-to-peer interactions can at times be cruel, especially during these formative years. Students who are questioning their sexual identity are often subject to stereotypical taunting or ridicule, and fear being shunned as a classmate, friend, team member, and/or club participant (McFarland & Dupuis, 2001). All students, regardless of their sexual identity or sexual orientation, are entitled to learn, grow, and develop in a bias-free environment. School counselors have a responsibility to be sensitive to gender bias, sexual discrimination, sexual harassment, and sexual orientation and promote a school climate that permits students to study and socialize without fear of repercussion or stigma. Research suggests that sexual minority youth will first disclose that they are gay, lesbian, or questioning students to a school counselor rather than other school personnel (Harris & Bliss, 1997). Professional school counselors must be prepared to work with sexual minority students when they present themselves for counseling (Pope, 2004). As advocates and leaders, school counselors can develop and implement policies that eradicate the verbal and physical harassment of all students, including sexual minority students (Pope, 2004). All students are entitled to learn in an environment that is free of bias and harassment.

Learning Differences

School counselors and many educators subscribe to the belief that all children can learn and all children can achieve. All school personnel should be sensitive to the time needed to learn, even at a level of minimum proficiency. Learning ability is distinct to the individual; each child has unique talents, skills, and limitations (McDevitt & Ormond, 2002). School counselors are in a unique position to collaborate with faculty and to identify the essential resources and support systems that each student needs to be successful (Stone & Dahir, 2004). Some students need the additional tools, time, and specialized instruction to achieve at a minimum proficiency. Learning ability or disability is another aspect of diversity.

Ability is a student's capacity or aptitude to master a skill, task, or concept; disability describes a student's incapability to accomplish or acquire the same skills, task, or concept in certain situations (Woolfolk, 2004). A learning disability can be defined as a deficit in one or more cognitive processes and/or a problem with the acquisition and use of language (McDevitt & Ormond, 2002). Students who are learning disabled may have difficulty with reading, writing, reasoning, or mathematics, and special education services may be required (Woolfolk, 2004).

For some educators, the designation of learning disabled helps to explain why and how some students struggle with language, communication arts, and math without other apparent signs of impairment. Labels can simultaneously stigmatize and provide opportunity for students (Keogh & MacMillan, 1996).

Understanding Special Education

One area of education that is deeply rooted in the application of designation or labeling is special education, a relatively new field. The passage of The Education for All Handicapped Children Act (1975), which is commonly known as Public Law 94-142, protected the rights of all children and required states to provide a "free and appropriate education" for all children between the ages of 3 and 21, regardless of the handicapping condition or disability. PL 94-142 is the basis for **special education,** as it is commonly known across the fifty states. Special education encompasses the entire range of learning, emotional, and physical disabilities, and in some states also includes students who have special abilities, gifts, or talents. Reauthorized in 1991 and again in 2005 as the Individuals with Disabilities Education Act (IDEA) the word **_handicapped_** was eliminated and **_disabled_** was used in its place. IDEA requires that every disabled child have access to the program of study that will most effectively approximate a normal child's educational program. The Individualized Education Plan (IEP) is the written record of the needs of each student and the procedures that will be used to provide services. The IEP must include

1. long- and short-term goals, which include a statement of the student's performance;

2. a description of the instructional services designed to meet the stated goals;

3. an overview of the methods that will be used to monitor progress toward the attainment of the goals.

Student placement into special education is a complex process involving many school professionals in addition to parent(s), guardian(s), or caregivers(s). The school counselor often is sought out to initiate the referral by either a teacher or parent(s). The process for referring a student for special education involves several steps and many professionals. The following steps may occur in a different sequence, dependent upon local district guidelines and state regulations:

1. After the request for an evaluation of eligibility is made, the student's situation is presented at a Child Study meeting for an initial review.

2. The Child Study Team is composed of student services professionals, including the school counselor, and school psychologist, school social worker, and school nurse, teacher(s), administrator(s), parent(s), any individual from the school setting who has specific knowledge about the child, and sometimes the student herself or himself. Documentation is presented as to previous strategies that were implemented, and a determination is made whether a full evaluation is warranted. This comprehensive evaluation often consists of a social history; an educational/achievement evaluation; a psychological assessment, which can include ability or intelligence testing; a classroom observation; behavioral information; and a teacher report. When a comprehensive evaluation is deemed necessary, the documentation must be collected and submitted to the Committee on Special Education (CSE) within 60 days.

3. The Committee on Special Education (CSE) reviews the complete docket of assessment, achievement, aptitude, ability, psychological information, social and developmental history, health records, and other information presented by the professionals involved in assessing the student's needs.

4. Based on the results of the evaluation, members of the CSE determine whether a student is eligible for services. If the parent(s)/guardian(s) disagree with the decision, they can request a hearing.

5. The CSE always must seek an educational setting that is considered the least restrictive environment. A fully mainstreamed designation means that the student is placed into the regular education program; oftentimes when this occurs, related services such as a resource room or counseling as a related service are offered. Another option is placement into a self-contained special education classroom, which mandates a lower student-teacher ratio and a specialized learning environment for students with disabilities. The CSE has 30 days to develop the Individualized Education Plan (IEP) and the IEP is signed by the parent(s). The IEP describes the level of services and specifically how services will be provided.

6. The student's academic program is reviewed and updated annually as the student's academic, social, emotional, and other needs are enumerated in annual goals and in short- and long-term objectives.

7. Every three years an evaluation is conducted, which requires a comprehensive analysis and assessment of the student's placement and services. This triennial evaluation determines to what degree services should be reduced, expanded, or eliminated.

Adapted from *Special Education in New York State for Children Ages 3–21: A Parent's Guide*, 2004).

Many schools across our nation are establishing inclusive environments, in which students with disabilities, including those with severe disabilities, are integrated into the traditional mainstream classroom setting. Here the special education teacher and the regular classroom teacher work together to serve the needs of all of the children assigned to the classroom. Although some students appear to be in need of special education or exceptional student services, school counselors have a responsibility not only to seek the least restrictive environment, but also to provide to every student the most challenging educational opportunity possible. School counselors, by virtue of their training in human relations, group dynamics, and interpersonal skills, can play a vital role in inclusive education (Quigney & Studer, 1998). School counselors will also encounter situations in which teachers, parents, and administrators believe that a self-contained special education placement is the only option for a student's success. It has been well documented that black students are often overrepresented in special education classrooms (Zehr, 2004). In contrast, the U.S. Department of Education (2004) recently has concluded that English language learner (ELL) students are underrepresented, with only 9.2% of English language learners receiving special education services as compared to 13.5% of the overall population nationwide. State and local policies and practices may require a wait time and an immersion in English classes prior to initiating a special education referral.

Working with 504 Plans

Section 504 of the Rehabilitation Act of 1973 prohibited the exclusion of any individual from any program or activity that received federal assistance and increased the range of services offered to students with special needs. Section 504 offers provisions for students who have a mental or physical disability that substantially limits a major life activity. The disability can include impairments such as vision, speech, attention deficit hyperactivity disorder, as well as short-term disabilities such as a broken leg. Program modifications under Section 504 may be different from special education services and may include extended time to complete an assignment or test; tests read out loud; separate location for testing; and use of specialized equipment (calculators, tape recorders, etc.) to help with class notes or assignments. These modifications are made to the learning environment so that the student has access to an equitable educational opportunity.

Learning Styles

Although special education and 504 plans provide supports that alleviate some of the challenges that inhibit a student's academic success, other factors can limit or extend learning. Some theorists describe the individual's ability to learn and demonstrate success in the context of intelligence. Gardiner's theory of multiple intelligences (1999), Sternberg's triarchic theory of intelligence (1985), and Goleman's theory on emotional intelligence (1995) provide insight into how children, adolescents, and adults gather and apply information to solve problems and behave intelligently. These theorists view learning as multidimensional and offer alternative explanations and rationales to the traditional measures of intelligences that are often used to "label" students. When intelligence and learning are viewed in the context of a process, there is a greater array of options available to advocate for appropriate student services and supports (Goleman, 1995). Individual learning styles and preferences also influence how a student accepts, processes, understands, and applies knowledge (Gardiner, 1999).

According to Woolfolk (2004), **learning preferences** are individual inclinations for a particular modality and/or environment. For many students the traditional "talking head" lecture format does not spark a deeper level of understanding that can lead to an appropriate application of knowledge to skill. For others, a kinesthetic approach involving an active "hands on" experience becomes the most meaningful method of learning.

It is difficult, perhaps almost impossible, for a classroom teacher to address the dominant **learning style** of every student that he or she comes into contact with on a daily basis. However, each student can benefit from understanding her or his individual learning preference and acquire the knowledge as to how to learn to adapt to different instructional situations and different styles of teaching (Dunn & Dunn, 1987).

School counselors who are knowledgeable about learning preferences and learning styles can help individuals and groups of students explore an important dimension of self-knowledge, and adapt that understanding to the teaching and learning environment (Dunn & Dunn, 1987). Effective school settings are committed to identifying all of the possible resources for those students who are slow learners, hyperactive, artistic, English language learners, from low-income families, newly immigrated, or technically inclined (Sadker & Sadker, 2005). Effective educators challenge students to focus on their strengths and overcome the obstacles that are inhibiting their ability to learn.

School counselors must be aware that special education students and/or students with 504 plans are viewed as second-class citizens in our schools (Sadker & Sadker, 2005). This perception is frequently held by some mainstreamed students, as well as by some teachers and parents. Like newly immigrated students, students from low-income families, and others who don't fit neatly into the "norm," special education students need to be treated equitably and respectfully (Quigney &

Studer, 1998). All students deserve a quality, challenging, and successful educational experience, and school counselors have an ethical responsibility to protect the rights of every student and his/her family (Stone, 2004). Advocacy and leadership are critical to ensure that students with learning differences are treated with the same respect and are given the same opportunities as all of the students who are considered part of the mainstream.

Creating a Culturally Compatible Climate

Demographics and conceptual changes are reshaping America's schools. Given all of the variables that compose diversity, school counselors and educators are challenged on a daily basis to respond to the needs of every student. Culturally compatible schools ensure that an atmosphere of respect, understanding, and caring for students is at the heart of the learning community. School counselors play an important role in fostering this environment.

ASCA reminds us that school counselors can use a variety of strategies to heighten the awareness and sensitivity of students and parents to culturally diverse persons, and thus enhance the school environment (ASCA, 1999). Counselors have the ability to consult with school personnel to identify the alienating factors in attitudes and beliefs that impede the learning ability of culturally diverse students and to ensure that student rights are respected (ASCA, 1999).

The Association for Multicultural Counseling and Development (AMCD) developed competencies (Arredondo et al., 1996; Sue, Arredondo, & Davis, 1992) around three domains: counselor awareness of own values and biases, counselor awareness of client's worldview, and culturally appropriate intervention strategies. Within each domain are competency areas: beliefs and attitudes; knowledge; and skills. There are 117 behavioral, outcome-based explanatory statements (Arredondo, Toporek, Brown, et al., 1996) which can serve school counselors well as learning goals (Arredondo & Arciniega, 2001).

Although one can acquire knowledge from a textbook, nothing can replace the awareness gained and the skills acquired from getting to know the students, their families, and the community in which they live. As you observe students' interactions, be sensitive to their beliefs, and try to understand the impact of culture and ethnicity and how that may influence their way of thinking and responding.

One of ASCA's nine national standards specifically targets respect and states, "students will acquire the attitudes, knowledge, and interpersonal skills to help them understand and respect self and others" (Campbell & Dahir, 1997). This serves as a reminder for school counselors to look beyond self-esteem and to focus attention on students' knowledge of self as well as on learning how to extend respect to relationships with others. School counselors can powerfully influence colleagues to move beyond the traditional cultural exchange and focus the conversation on all aspects of diversity. Thus all members of the school community can better understand the influence of culture on learning and lifestyles and consider class, race, ethnicity, gender, socioeconomic status, sexual orientation, and language. Cultural norms and expectations can also influence developmental benchmarks, sexual behavior, and educational choices.

In a culturally compatible climate, the concept of respect for self and others is woven throughout the fabric of our schools and becomes part of the teaching and learning environment. The institution itself is oriented toward social harmony and cooperation. School counselors can provide the initiative and leadership to ensure that developmentally appropriate activities are an integral part of the school counseling program and are directly linked to fostering a climate built on respect and caring.

School counselors can reinforce and extend awareness from the school to home and community and promote the need for effective school communication between home and school. Parents and/or caregivers need to feel welcome to ask questions, understand expectations, and learn strategies to help their children succeed. School counselors have a moral responsibility and ethical obligation to bridge the gap between school and home, because student success relies heavily on parental support and parental involvement. School counselors accept and embrace an advocacy role for newly immigrated parents, guardians, or caregivers; for those who are culturally or ethnically different from the majority in your community; and for those who are uncomfortable with situations that are intimidating because of their personal educational attainment or experience.

Challenging Beliefs and Changing Behaviors

Education has changed, and now all educators can be open and sensitive to the preconceived attitudes and biases that may exist about students. Twenty-first-century schools are social arenas in which students who represent truly diverse behavioral styles, attitudes and orientations, and value systems are brought together with one goal in mind, which is to maximize their potential as human beings (Lee, 1998).

School counselors face the challenge of working with a student population that is like no other previous generation. Unique in its diversity, this is a generation that has aspirations for financial success, high expectations for educational achievement, and has significant social pressures. It is also the first generation that has experienced emotional trauma as a result of a declaration of war by terrorists here on home soil. Youthful uniqueness and the many aspects of diversity that exist in schools is a positive force, not to be shunned or ignored. School counselors are in a unique position to

- examine policies and practices that address student placement in course work and student activities to ensure equity and access among all student populations;
- provide professional development on key diversity issues at faculty meetings;
- encourage faculty to explore issues of culture and diversity in the context of the curriculum;

- work with school leadership teams to promote cultural sensitivity;
- seek awareness, knowledge, and skill to work with the diversity of the student population that constitutes your school;
- support students who have declared their sexual orientation as gay, lesbian, or bisexual;
- sponsor family groups to help new immigrants understand and address meaningful issues, such as negotiating the school system;
- advocate for a fair student code of conduct, and equitable course-taking options and educational attainment;
- act as a visible and vocal advocate for students and families whose first language is not English.

Changing attitudes and beliefs is no easy task; school counselors will face denial and resistance from colleagues: "If I wait long enough this will go away, or they will go away." Many will say, "We don't do that; we are not prejudiced" or "We treat all students equally." Educators as a rule are good people with good intentions. Colleagues sometimes need support to examine their belief systems, and not focus on what was. Without sincere reflection on current practices, schools cannot move forward and create systemic change (Stone & Dahir, 2004). Resistance will be the modus operandi, and it is often accompanied by self-doubt, blame, anger, discord, and withdrawal. Similarly, it is important to also help students and colleagues eliminate pervasive stereotyping that can impair their ability to assess others appropriately (Axelson, 1999). School personnel can explore biases and prejudices that result in stereotyping and then search for alternative practices and seek ways to eliminate practices that do not foster equality, harmony, and respect. School counselors must take action to ensure that strategies are in place to promote diversity within the school environment and beyond.

The 50th anniversary of the *Brown v. Board of Education* Supreme Court decision (1954) reminds us that without public education, children would be likely to be segregated into school settings that reflect their own racial, ethnic, cultural, or religious backgrounds. Without the common denominator of public school, perhaps people in general would be more divided and more fearful of those different from themselves. Schools, as important learning and social communities, are significant conduits in promoting understanding, acceptance, respect, and harmony.

School counselors must seek methods of collaboration that address diversity in our schools in a meaningful way. This is not only a challenge, but a moral and ethical responsibility. Acting as advocates and leaders, school counselors ensure that the diverse needs of our students are reflected in the teaching and learning environment of the place called school. Only by changing attitudes and behaviors can positive and constructive change occur. Part of this responsibility is the reflection and introspection that is essential for school counselors to grow personally as well as professionally (Holcomb-McCoy, 2004). Accountability and responsiveness to both the obvious and the subtle needs of our diverse student populations presents a challenge that reflects the very nature of participating in a democratic society and investing in the future.

TechTools

- Explore the U.S. Bureau of Census website to follow trends and shifts in population demographics nationally. Compare your findings to your state and local demographics.
- Want to know more about your own heritage? Genealogical websites provide insight about your family's background. You can use these tools to better understand your ethnic and cultural heritage.
- Keeping up with federal and state laws to ensure compliance with the needs of special and exceptional student education is a challenge. Go to the Office of Special Education Programs (OSEP) at http://www.ed.gov/offices/OSERS/OSEP/
- Stay abreast of current initiatives and legislative changes in IDEA. Check out the part of your state department of education's website that is devoted to exceptional/special education. Also go to the Council for Exceptional Children at http://www.cec.sped.org for information and resources.
- Consider the ethical and legal implications of technology, including issues of equity and access. Take a look at the ASCA Ethical Standards at http://www.schoolcounselor.org and consider the implications.
- You have learned that socioeconomic status influences school success. Review the Children's Defense Fund website at http://www.childrensdefense.org/ to find out more about what you can do to advocate for the needs of every child.
- Use the test locator published by Buros Institute of Mental Measurement to research various instruments that are used in your local school district at http://www.unl.edu/buros/
- Polish up your presentation skills by looking at websites such as http://www.ncjrs.org/pdffiles1/ojjdp/178997.pdf. You will need to download Adobe Acrobat Reader (a free download) to read PDF files such as this one. Then use presentation software as a tool to educate, guide, and inform students, faculty, colleagues, and parents about the diverse need of student in our schools.
- The National Center for Education Statistics at http://nces.ed.gov/nceskids/ has a Student Classroom on its home page. Check out the easy-to-use "How to Make a Graph" section to present data you have about your students.

School Counselor Casebook: Voices From the Field

The Scenario Reviewed

At the end of the first quarter, a classroom teacher asks you to come to observe four students whom he believes are not working up to their ability. The students are not getting along with others in the class and not completing assignments in a timely manner. The bottom line is that the teacher does not believe that the students are keeping up with the expectations for the fourth-grade class and not sure if they are appropriately placed in a regular education classroom. You agreed to observe the students and review the findings with him. You are also aware that these four students represent various racial and ethnic backgrounds.

A Practitioner's Approach

Here's how a practicing school counselor responded to the school counselor casebook challenge:

I decided that I would begin by observing the students' peer interactions and each student's independent and group work. My goal is to attempt to identify the factors that contribute to the behavioral disruptions and also contribute to the students' poor achievement.

When I visited the classroom, I realized that there were very few students in this class from culturally diverse backgrounds. I realized that the teacher may be unfamiliar with their cultural heritage, social/economic status, parental employment and level of education, and family configurations. Although the students are only fourth graders, he may be worried about their future success in school and their ability to move successfully from grade level to grade level. I would also look for signs of respect and understanding among the children for each other's diversity. Lack of understanding may be a contributor to the behavioral disruptions.

I would ask the classroom teacher to speak to each of the students individually and share his concerns regarding each student's academic and social progress. I would ask the teacher to focus on each student's uniqueness and talents and connect these to the class material and work. The classroom teacher may also want to develop a behavioral contract that is worded in such a way as to reward each student when positive behavior is displayed.

I would look into each student's progress to date and each student's school history to determine if there are learning issues that may be contributing to the behavioral problem. Additionally, I would connect the students to support services such as the academic center or tutoring and work with the teacher to help each student become better organized and to improve studying skills. By working with the teacher to create a plan that involves counseling, academic support, and parental involvement, together we can carefully and intentionally work through all of our options and do our best to help these students meet the grade-level expectations for fourth grade.

Deborah Hardy worked as a bilingual school counselor prior to assuming the chairperson position at Irvington High School in New York. She is a past president of the New York State School Counselor Association and an adjunct professor at Mercy College in the School Counseling Graduate Program. Reprinted with permission by Deborah Hardy.

Chapter Summary

Promoting a Social Justice Agenda

Today's schools mirror the changing demographics and diversity reflected in our communities. Census data shows that minority population growth in the United States is based upon age distribution, birthrate, and immigration patterns (Bureau of the Census, 2003). Public schools are a place where children can learn to get along with others in a diverse society (Center on Education Policy, 1998). Schools must become the primary institutions to create cohesion among diverse groups. School counselors have a responsibility to value culture, race, ethnicity, gender, socioeconomic status and social class, ability and disability, and sexual orientation, and to promote awareness and acceptance among all student groups.

Respecting and Promoting Diversity

In a broad worldview, diversity refers to the range of cultures and subcultures that represent attitudes, beliefs, values, rituals, symbols, norms and conventions, customs, behaviors, and ideologies. School counselors focus on those aspects of diversity that impact and influence the dynamics of learning, personal-social development, and school climate.

Examining Personal Beliefs and Behaviors

Each individual develops as the result of the totality of life experiences and is greatly influenced by variables that include the era in which one was born as well as the color of one's skin. Generational location strongly shapes how life is viewed and valued.

Students too are influenced by similar variables, which can have a profound influence on their lives and will continue to do so as they approach adulthood.

Multiculturalism

When we think of diversity, culture is what usually first comes to mind. Culture is the sum total of ways of living including core beliefs, societal values, patterns of thinking and communication, and behavioral norms that a group of people have developed to assure their position in a particular environment (Cooper & Denner, 1998). Culture is also the response of a group of human beings to the valid and particular needs of its members and includes knowledge, values, traditions, and attitudes that guide the behavior of a group of people. Students and faculty need opportunities to acquire the experience, the skills, awareness, and understanding to transcend the perceived barriers of differences (Johnson, 1995).

Social Class Distinctions

Social class impacts culture and has begun to transcend what had been previously perceived as racial and ethnic barriers to demographic change. Although educational aspirations are reflective of communities and school systems, the gap continues to widen among the haves and the have nots. Economically disadvantaged students in our middle and more affluent communities should have the same access to educational opportunity as do their classmates, but this is not always the case. School counselors can either support or challenge the philosophy and procedures that stratify opportunities for students that will impact their future success.

Gender Equity

Examining the impact of gender differences on student success in school may not be as obvious as race, ethnicity, and cultural differences when we work with students. Gender differences can influence what is expected as the "norm" and can contribute to some of the fundamental differences in personality development for boys and girls in the traditions of some cultures (Lee, 1998). However, like other forms of discrimination, messages of sexism may be subtle (Woolfolk, 2004). Counselors and teachers may not always be aware of the messages that are communicated and how these messages impact student behavior and student choices.

Sexual Minority Youth

Students who are questioning their sexual identity are often subject to stereotypical taunting or ridicule, and fear being shunned as a classmate, friend, team member, and/or club participant; however, students are entitled to learn, grow, and develop in a bias-free environment. School counselors have a responsibility to be sensitive to gender bias, sexual discrimination, sexual harassment, and sexual orientation and to promote a school climate that permits students to study and socialize without fear of repercussion or stigma.

Learning Differences

School counselors subscribe to the belief that all children can learn; all children can achieve. However, we must be sensitive to the time needed, the special tools that provide support, the nature of cognitive processing, and the ability or disability that impacts performance. Each child's learning ability is distinct; each child has unique talents, skills, and limitations. As a generalization, our classrooms in public schools teach to the average student of average ability. We know that within the concept of "average" there are many unique components, and these must be addressed in our schools and in our classrooms.

Understanding Special Education

The passage of the Education for All Handicapped Children Act (1975), which is commonly known as Public Law 94-142, protected the rights of all children and required states to provide a "free and appropriate education" for all children between the ages of 3 and 21, regardless of the handicapping condition or disability. This law is the foundation for the special education movement. Special education encompasses the entire range of learning, emotional, and physical disabilities, and in some states also includes students who have special abilities, gifts, or talents.

Working With 504

The Americans with Disabilities Act of 1990 provided opportunities for students to receive accommodations and assistance as long as the student qualifies as a person with a disability. The term *disability* can include impairments such as vision, speech, and attention deficit hyperactivity disorder, as well as to short-term disabilities such as a broken leg.

Creating a Culturally Compatible Climate

The primary goal for creating culturally compatible schools is to ensure that an atmosphere of respect, understanding, and caring is at the heart of the learning community. Colleagues can move beyond the traditional cultural exchange and focus the conversation on all aspects of diversity and thus better understand the influence of culture on learning and lifestyles, which includes class, race, ethnicity, gender, socioeconomic status, sexual orientation, and language.

Changing Behaviors

Education has changed; we need to change attitudes about students too. Schools have become the social arena in which students who represent truly diverse behavioral styles, attitudes, orientations, and value systems are brought together with one goal in mind, which is to maximize their potential as human beings (Lee, 1998). School counselors have a moral and ethical responsibility to act as advocates and leaders, ensuring that the diverse needs of students are reflected in the teaching and learning environment of the place called school.

Key Terms

Acceptance p. 272
Assimilation p. 270
Disabled p. 284
Discrimination p. 281
Diversity p. 270
Ethnicity p. 270
Gender p. 281
Handicapped p. 284
Integration p. 270

Learning preference p. 287
Learning style p. 287
Multiculturalism p. 270
Prejudice p. 271
Socioeconomic status (SES) p. 272
Special education p. 284
Stereotyping p. 282
Tolerance p. 271

Learning Extensions

1. Get in touch with your personal beliefs and attitudes by completing the following statements:

   a. Special education students are . . .
   b. When I meet a new Hispanic student I think . . .
   c. African-American youth are . . .
   d. When I meet an Islamic family I think . . .
   e. Our Asian students . . .
   f. The gay and lesbian students in our school . . .

   Think about your responses. Share them with a classmate or peer. Did you note any patterns? How are your perceptions similar, different?

2. What do you think about when you hear about "changing demographics"? How has your community changed over the past ten years? Which ethnic groups have shown the greatest increase in population?

3. American society used to be referred to as a "melting pot." How does this differ from the model of multiculturalism that we use today?

4. Explore the impact that your name, first and last, had on your personal identity. Share this with a classmate. Consider how your name relates to your growth and development from a variety of diverse perspectives, including race, ethnicity, and culture.

5. How does your school system respond to the diverse needs of students in your community? What aspects of diversity are the most important to address?

6. What can school counselors do to foster a multicultural atmosphere in their schools?

7. What traditional biases are you aware of that impact a student decision about his or her future goals?

8. Download your school district report card information, and then select one school to analyze in your community. What does it tell you about achievement of the diverse groups of students that compose your community?

9. What resources exist in your school and community that support diversity in its fullest meaning?

10. Reflect on the scenario presented at the beginning of the chapter. What intervention strategies did you implement as an alternative to initiating the referral process for special/exceptional student education?

Chapter 11

Legal and Ethical Issues for School Counselors

Negligence in Academic Advising

Negligence in Abortion Counseling

Sexual Harassment

Continuing Your Professional Development

Chapter Objectives

By the time you have completed this chapter, you should be able to:

- Understand the difference between ethics and the law.
- Identify the steps in making ethical decisions.
- Discuss privacy, confidentiality, and privileged communication.
- Understand the Family Education Rights and Privacy Act.
- Identify the components of negligence, and apply negligence and malpractice to cases involving school counselors.
- Apply informed consent and confidentiality to group work.
- Discuss principles established by court cases that have implications for the school counselor's work.
- Advocate for students' rights and respect parental rights.

School Counselor Casebook: *Getting Started*

The Scenario

One of the three counselors in your school plans to conduct three small groups this semester. The first group will be for students whose parents are newly divorced or are going through a divorce; the second will be for students who are chronic referrals for aggressive or violent behavior; the third will be for students who are not getting their class work or homework completed. Your colleague comes to you and asks your advice on her choice of topics for these groups. She also asks you if she should get written or oral parental permission before beginning any of the groups.

Thinking About Solutions

As you read this chapter, consider how you would answer your colleague's questions. How might you caution her from an ethical perspective? When you come to the end of the chapter, you will have the opportunity to see how your responses compare with the advice of a practicing school counselor.

Professional Ethics

All school counselors are governed by the American School Counselor Association (ASCA) **code of ethics and standards of practice** called Ethical Standards for School Counselors (2004), and the American Counseling Association's (ACA) Code of Ethics and Standard Practice (2005). By becoming a member of ASCA and/or ACA, the school counselor is agreeing to abide by the code of ethics of the organization. This professional relationship strengthens the case of the counselor who faces a legal or ethical challenge to their behavior (assuming he or she was within the bounds of ethical behavior as interpreted in standard of practice). Nonmembers can reference the codes, but there is no evidence that they ever agreed to abide by them, which is problematic if the counselor has to defend himself or herself in a legal or ethical wrangle (Nancy Perry, former executive director of ASCA, personal communication, July 12, 2003).

Ethics are the customs, mores, standards, and accepted practice of a profession (Corey, Corey, Callanan, & O'Phelan, 1998; Fischer & Sorenson, 1996; Huey & Remley, 1988). Ethical codes are an attempt by the profession to standardize professional practice for the purpose of protecting students and also to protect the school counselor. Codes are guides, and as such have to be interpreted in context because there are few right or wrong answers in real situations in which a counselor may find him or herself. "Codes are not intended to be a blueprint that removes the need for judgment and ethical reasoning" (Welfel & Lipsitz, 1983, p. 6). Codes guide us to meet the needs of individual situations but are rarely appropriate for rote application, because it is the context of the dilemma that matters. It is only the school counselor, in consultation with other professionals, who can determine how to apply a code to further the best interest of the student. Codes do not hold the answers to our specific ethical problems, but coupled with help from our professional colleagues, the codes do provide guidance. Codes are the ideal to which school counseling professionals should aspire, while **laws** are the minimum standard that society will tolerate (Fischer & Sorenson, 1996). The legal representatives for the American Counseling Association (ACA) recommended that school counselors read the codes and discuss the codes with colleagues (American Counseling Association, 1994). This may sound unrealistic because time is always in short supply for school counselors, but we cannot afford to be ignorant of the codes in a profession that is responsible to minors. School counselors have a responsibility to know the codes and what constitutes ethical actions for the reasonably competent professional.

Ethics and the Law

The law is the minimum standard that society will tolerate (Fischer & Sorenson, 1996). Laws are found in federal and state statutes, case law that spun out of court cases, and district and school board policies (Fischer & Sorenson, 1996). If in a rare incidence the law and ASCA's ethical codes were to conflict, the law would override the codes. Daily, a school counselor's work involves both legal and ethical considerations. For example, in many states **confidentiality** is a legal imperative requiring that school counselors respect the confidences of their students to the extent possible. Even if not legally binding, confidentiality is an ethical imperative for all school counselors. Reporting child abuse is both a legal and ethical imperative for all counselors.

The legal system requires that you behave as the reasonably competent professional would. If faced with a lawsuit, would you pass the "standard of care" test? **Standard of care** is the benchmark the courts use to determine what would be the actions of the reasonably competent professional school counselor. The operative word is "reasonably." The courts are not asking for extraordinary care, only reasonable care. The ethics of the profession help school counselors aspire to exceptional care, but the courts do not demand this level. The message to you, the school counseling candidate, is to know your codes and abide by them, exercise skill and care in every action you take as a professional, and wrestle with dilemmas you face by applying the model of ethical decision making explained here.

A Model of Ethical Decision Making

In reviewing models of ethical decision making, it was discovered that commonalities exist, but some key considerations for school counselors were omitted. The following suggested steps for ethical action have been created by incorporating the principles set forth by a number of authors, including American Counseling Association (1993a), Corey et al. (1998), Kitchener (1986), and Stone (2001).

For school counselors, Steps 1, 4, 5, and 6 were added to the traditional ethical models, and Step 2 was clarified to give importance to rumors and hearsay in a school setting. The traditional models include these steps: examine the facts, review the relevant ethical guidelines; identify the nature and dimensions of the problem; consult or seek supervision; consider possible and probable courses of action; examine the good and bad consequences of various decisions; and implement your course of action. Because of the unique nature of counseling in schools, we must also add several steps: identify your emotional reaction; consider parental rights; consider the setting; and consider the student's chronological and developmental levels. These additions were made because it is critically important to consider that ethical considerations are context specific. Because our clients are students in a setting called schools, parental rights, students' developmental and chronological age, and our own emotional reactions to dilemmas carry additional weight and meaning. Although the model is presented sequentially, it will rarely be a sequential deliberation when you are in the throes of making an ethical decision.

1. *Identify your emotional reaction.* It is important to keep in the forefront of your mind your first reaction to the problem. What did you immediately want to do to help this child? This emotional reaction is important because it helps us protect and guard our students' confidences. We don't act on the emotional reaction without considering the other steps in making an ethical decision, but because we care about our students we also don't want to discard the emotional reaction.

2. *Examine the facts.* Take the necessary steps to gather the facts, separating out innuendos, rumors, hearsay, and hypotheses. However, in school settings we cannot rule out the hearsay or rumors, because this is often how school counselors discover the truth about situations that involve their students.

3. *Review the relevant ethical guidelines.* Ask yourself whether your code of ethics offers a possible solution to the problem. Remember to apply the codes in context of the situation as the codes can only offer general guidelines and must be applied with careful consideration of the uniqueness of the particular ethical dilemma in which you find yourself.

4. *Consider parental rights.* You must consider the rights of parents to be the guiding voice in their children's lives, especially in value-laden decisions. Clear or imminent danger is not necessarily an uplifted knife in which a child is directly in harms way. Rather, clear imminent danger for a minor in a school setting may be an 11 year old's pregnancy or a 12 year old's cutting behavior. Because of the school setting and the fact that our clients are minors, parents have a right to be informed and involved when their children are in harms way.

5. *Consider the setting.* You must consider the dilemma in the context of the school setting. Ethical dilemmas in a school, which is a setting designed for academics, take on a different meaning than do ethical issues in other contexts. Students come to school for academic instruction; when they enter into the personal emotional arena in this setting we cannot discount that this may carry obligations to involve and inform other educators and parents.

6. *Consider the student's chronological and developmental levels* How does the student's developmental level impact the dilemma and how you will approach it? This step is critical, yet it has been left out of decision-making models. It matters how old a child is, and how he or she demonstrates ability to make informed decisions.

7. *Identify the nature and dimensions of the problem.* Consider the basic moral principles of autonomy, beneficence, nonmaleficence, justice, and loyalty (Kitchener,

1986) and apply them to a particular situation. It may help to prioritize these principles and think through ways in which they can support a resolution to the dilemma. Kitchener (1986) was one of the first to apply the virtues of autonomy, beneficence, nonmaleficence, justice, and loyalty to ethical decision making. Her evaluation model was discussed in depth in Chapter 5 and will be briefly reviewed here.

Autonomy refers to promoting students' ability to choose their own direction. The school counselor makes every effort to foster maximum self-determination on the part of students. *Beneficence* refers to promoting good for others. Ideally, counseling contributes to the growth and development of the student, and whatever counselors do should be judged against this criterion. *Nonmaleficence* means avoiding doing harm, which includes refraining from actions that risk hurting students. *Justice*, or *fairness*, refers to providing equal treatment to all people. This standard implies that anyone—regardless of age, sex, race, ethnicity, disability, socioeconomic status, cultural background, religion, or lifestyle—is entitled to equal treatment. *Loyalty*, or *fidelity*, refers to staying connected with your students and being available to your students to the extent possible. School counselors often carry heavy caseloads, and for them loyalty takes on a dimension that may not be included in what an agency counselor might consider to be loyalty. Loyalty for the school counselor does not necessarily mean that we have 50-minute sessions once a week with our students. Staying loyal may include connecting with students by encouraging them to stop by before and after school, visiting them at the bus loading zone, or stopping briefly at a student's classroom. All of these activities further the virtue of loyalty or fidelity in spite of the barriers of caseloads, time constraints, and roles.

8. *Consult or seek supervision.*   Always discuss your case (without identifying the student if this is appropriate) with a fellow professional, preferably a supervisor, to help you illuminate the issues. In the throes of an ethical dilemma it is sometimes difficult to manage to be as thorough as we should be or to see all of the issues that are involved. Seeking supervision is the one step that we must always do.

9. *Consider possible and probable courses of action.*   In this process of thinking about many different possibilities for action, it is helpful to write down the options and also to discuss options with another person.

10. *Examine the good and bad consequences of various decisions.*   Ponder the implications of each course of action for the student, for others who are related to the student, and for you. List the good and bad consequences of each decision.

11. *Implement your course of action.*   Go forward with your decision after you have considered the previous steps. Risk will be present regardless of your decision, but following these steps will allow you to make the best decision possible based on the advice and information you had at the time. School counselors cannot practice risk free, but we can reduce our risk and raise our support for students by using ethical reasoning.

The Complications of Confidentiality in the Context of Schools

What mitigating factors do school counselors consider when wrestling with the difficult dilemma of confidentiality? School counselors must consider not only student rights but parental rights when approaching the issue of whether to protect or breach confidentiality. Parents are continually vested by our courts with legal rights to guide their children (*Bellotti v. Baird*, 1979; *H. L. v. Matheson*, 1982). School boards and administrators adopt policies that counselors are ethically bound to obey. Teachers, when informed regarding children's special needs and circumstances, are in the best position to impact positively on a child's life during school and often beyond the school day. The ASCA codes dictate that school counselors have a primary obligation and loyalty to students. All of these issues contribute to the complex nature of working with minors in schools (Isaacs & Stone, 1999; Stone, 2001b). The setting in which school counselors work defines the student–school counselor relationship.

Confidentiality, found in Standard A.2 and Standard B.1 and B.2 of the American School Counselor Association (ASCA) Ethical Standards for School Counselors (2004) gives us guidance in protecting the privacy of minors while respecting parents' rights to be involved in guiding their children. However, the very nature of confidentiality makes it the most complex of all the legal and ethical issues that school counselors face; therefore, each of the confidentiality codes are addressed in the case studies that are presented later in the chapter. The ASCA ethical codes that address confidentiality and parental rights appear here, and a brief discussion follows.

A.2. Confidentiality

The professional school counselor:

a. Informs students of the purposes, goals, techniques and rules of procedure under which they may receive counseling at or before the time when the counseling relationship is entered. Disclosure notice includes the limits of confidentiality such as the possible necessity for consulting with other professionals, **privileged communication,** and legal or authoritative restraints. The meaning and limits of confidentiality are defined in developmentally appropriate terms to students.

This code instructs the professional school counselor to give **informed consent** at the beginning of counseling sessions and as often as necessary throughout the counseling session so that the counselee will know the purposes, goals, techniques, and rules of procedure under which she or he may receive counseling. The meaning of confidentiality is given in developmentally appropriate terms and helps the student understand that school counselors will try to keep confidences, except in cases when the student is a danger to self or others; the student or parent requests that information be revealed; or a court orders a counselor to disclose information.

A.2. Confidentiality

The professional school counselor:

b. Keeps information confidential unless disclosure is required to prevent clear and imminent danger to the student or others or when legal requirements demand that confidential information be revealed. Counselors will consult with appropriate professionals when in doubt as to the validity of an exception.

This code protects the confidentiality of information received in the counseling relationship as specified by federal and state laws, written policies, and applicable ethical standards. Such information is only to be revealed to others with the informed consent of the counselee, consistent with the counselor's ethical obligation. In a group setting, the counselor sets a high norm of confidentiality and stresses its importance, yet clearly states that confidentiality in group counseling cannot be guaranteed.

Loyalty and a sense of obligation to students are at the heart of our profession. The school counselor must provide a safe and secure environment in which trust can be established and maintained. Without the assurance of confidentiality, many students would not seek help. Counselors must keep confidential any information related to counseling services unless disclosure is in the best interest of students, or is required by law.

B.1. Parent Rights and Responsibilities

The professional school counselor:

a. Respects the rights and responsibilities of parents/guardians for their children and endeavors to establish, as appropriate, a collaborative relationship with parents/guardians to facilitate the student's maximum development.

d. Is sensitive to diversity among families and recognizes that all parents/guardians, custodial and noncustodial, are vested with certain rights and responsibilities for the welfare of their children by virtue of their role and according to law.

B.2. Parents and Confidentiality

The professional school counselor:

a. Informs parents/guardians of the counselor's role with emphasis on the confidential nature of the counseling relationship between the counselor and student.

Parents send their children to school for curriculum instruction. When children's emotional needs are being addressed by school counselors, conflict can result between the parents' right to know what is happening in their child's life and a student's right to privacy (ACA, 1993; Fischer & Sorenson, 1996; Remley & Herlihy, 2001; Stone, 2001b). School counselors face a dual responsibility to their minor students and to their parents. The challenge of protecting their students extends beyond students to include the parents of minor students.

Students' Rights and Responsibilities

The legal status of minors is complicated. In the ACA Legal Series, Salo and Shumate (1993), in discussing the difficulties of working with minor students in schools, pointed out that the inconsistencies in juvenile and tort law affect our ability as counselors to rely on clearly stated principles of legal policy. "Minors generally cannot be bound by their contracts, but they can be held liable for intentional and negligent injuries inflicted on others. When a child approaches a counselor without parental knowledge or consent, immediate tension arises between the child's right to privacy and the parent's right—on the child's behalf—to provide informed consent for counseling. Generally, the younger the child, the more rights are vested in the parents. Once minors reach teenage years and display increasing capacity for rational decision making, both the common law and statutory law recognize this capacity by providing more legal autonomy for minors in carefully prescribed areas" (pp. 9–10). Minors are emancipated or free from parental or guardian control when they reach the age of 18, enter the military, marry, or a court of law declares them emancipated (Stone, 2003b).

Students' rights and responsibilities are defined by federal legislation, state statutes, and school board policy. For example, the Protection of Pupil Rights Amendment (PPRA) (20 U.S.C.§ 1232h) protects the rights of students by requiring written parental permission before any analysis, evaluation, or survey can be conducted that reveals the student's or parent/guardian's political affiliation, sexual behaviors or attitudes, income level, or any embarrassing mental and psychological problems. State statutes outline student responsibility to avoid unlawful activity, sexual behavior, use of drugs or alcohol on school grounds.

Parents' Rights and Responsibilities

In addition to the points discussed, parents have the right to be the guiding voice in their children's lives in value-laden decisions. the **Family Educational Rights and Privacy Act (FERPA)** (U.S. Department of Education, 1973), a federal law that governs the disclosure of information from educational records, gives parents certain rights, including the right to talk to teachers and school administrators about their children, to see their children's educational records, and to decide if their children will participate in a questionnaire, survey, or examination regarding a parent's personal beliefs, sex practices, family life, or religion. FERPA allows parents to request that information that they believe to be inaccurate or misleading be purged from their children's **educational records** (FERPA, 1973).

Confidentiality and Community Standards

How school counselors address ethical problems depends in large part on the culture and/or standards of the community. The message here is to understand the culture and the prevailing written and unwritten standards of the community, school district, and individual work site and behave sensitively toward the culture and consistently with **community standards.** For example, some communities have established support groups for gay, lesbian, and bisexual youth. In some areas of the country, school counselors make this information available to students. Even though unwritten, in some communities disseminating this information would be unacceptable. In one very conservative U.S. city, the courts decided that a gay/lesbian/bisexual club must be allowed to meet on school grounds, but the city denied all clubs the ability to meet on school grounds in order to escape the requirement.

Confidentiality and Privileged Communication

Although all school counselors have a confidentiality responsibility, their relationships with students are rarely privileged. In most states, students, unlike patients, do not have privileged communication, which is given in state statutes to the clients or patients of certain professionals, such as lawyers and psychiatrists. A few states, such as Kentucky, grant partial privilege, which protects a student's confidences except when the counselor is required by a court of law to breach those confidences. Full privileged communication such as granted to the students of Idaho, renders the counselor incapable of testifying to information related in confidence. The school counselor's ethical responsibility to keep confidential almost all communications with students is complicated because of the school setting.

Ethics and Group Work in Schools

The legal and ethical complexities of working with minors in schools require that school counselors remain vigilant as to the rights and responsibilities of students and their parents and the implications of those rights on their work. A school counselor's **multiplicity of responsibility** in a setting designed to deliver academic instruction complicates the legal and ethical world of school counseling. These complications are acutely present in the personal counseling arena of group work because other students are present to hear possible discussions of the private world of students and their families.

Confidentiality and Informed Consent

Working with minors in groups requires that school counselors must come from the posture that whatever is said in a group will be repeated. We are risking the emotional safety of students when we expect developmentally maturing students to respect confidentiality. The ASCA codes tell us that confidentiality cannot be guaranteed in a group (A.6. . . . The professional school counselor establishes clear expectations in the group setting and clearly states that confidentiality in group counseling cannot be guaranteed.). Because we cannot guarantee confidentiality in groups, even adult groups, we must avoid putting risky faith in minors in a very social setting called schools. Minors often change friends and loyalties, and with this fluid behavior there is the danger of a student gaining attention, seeking revenge, or just thoughtlessly, without malice, revealing another student's personal pain. For every group we form, regardless of whether the topic is as innocuous as School Success Skills or as value-laden as Children of Alcoholics, Children in Divorce Situations, or Victims of Date Rape, it is imperative that we remind ourselves that confidentiality will be breached. We must continually ask ourselves, "Will the potential emotional cost to students and their families be worth any gains that we may accomplish?"

Competence, voluntariness or voluntary participation, and knowledge are necessary elements if students are to give us informed consent to participate in a group. Are middle schoolers able to understand that they will be discussing a sensitive topic, and their private revelations may well be repeated in the halls and locker rooms? An adolescent may developmentally be unable to understand the ramifications of discussing painful personal information in the presence of other students.

Appropriate Topics for Group Work in Schools

Are there topics that are not appropriate for group counseling in a school setting? For example, can we adequately address tough therapeutic issues, such as eating disorders, that are resistant to change even in residential treatment programs and other specialized settings designed to tackle eating disorders? In classroom guidance lessons we can tackle the issue of body image and nutrition for the benefit of all students, but there are some topics that can't be adequately or safely addressed in schools.

Adequacy of Counselor Skills for Group Work

It is unrealistic for members of the school and larger community to expect that we should have all the skills and knowledge necessary for group work with the many serious clinical topics that many of our students face. For example, agency counselors who spend considerable time and training focusing on self-mutilating students often find trying to impact change in these students a daunting responsibility.

School counselors work to shore up and support all students to be successful learners. While students with serious emotional issues often cannot learn if their needs are not met, it is unfair of the school and wider community to expect that the school counselor can address all the serious problems and dysfunctions presented by students. Many school counselors are becoming managers of resources, reaching beyond the walls of their schools to reposition mental health support into their schools or to develop a mechanism for helping students find support outside their schools. It isn't that the school counselor is less talented or competent than their colleagues in agency or community settings; it is that the needs are bigger than can be managed by the school counselor alone. The mental health needs of our youth must become the responsibility of the larger community as we work desperately to give every student the gift of becoming a successful learner. More information about working with groups is available in the Voices From the Field section of this chapter.

Working Through Case Studies

There are court cases, state and federal legislation, ethical codes and standards, and school board policy that inform our practice. Following are hypothetical and real cases addressing case notes, educational records, parental rights, **negligence,** suicide, letters of recommendation, HIV+ students, sexually active students, group work, negligence in academic advising, abortion counseling, and sexual harassment. Working through these cases will illuminate principles of law and practice that we can apply to our day-to-day work.

Counselors' Case Notes or Sole Possession Records

You have been seeing Stephen for individual counseling for three months. You have received a request from Stephen's mother, who is incarcerated in another state, for copies of all Stephen's education records. His mother has also asked for your case notes. Are you legally required to provide her with education records? Must you provide her with your case notes?

Noncustodial parental rights are often misunderstood. FERPA (1973) makes it clear that both parents have equal access to education records. Even incarcerated parents, parents who have refused to pay child support, and abusive parents have rights to education records under FERPA unless there is a court order expressly forbidding a parent to have education records. Must case notes be sent also?

The American Counseling Association (1997) has helped clarify whether school counselors' case notes are education records. Case notes to be exempt from education records must be "sole possession records." Not all of the information collected about students and maintained by schools and school employees is subject to the access and disclosure requirements under the Family Educational Rights and Privacy Act (FERPA, 1973). One of the five categories exempt from the definition of "education records" under FERPA is "Records made by teachers, supervisors, counselors, administrators, and other school personnel that are kept in the sole possession of the maker of the record and are not accessible or revealed to any other person except a temporary substitute for the maker of the record."

The exemption of sole possession records from the definition of education records is narrow and very specific. To be considered sole possession records, written case notes must meet four requirements: (a) the information must be a private note that is created solely by the individual possessing it, (b) the information must be a personal memory aid, (c) the information must not be shared or accessible to any other person except the individual's temporary substitute, and (d) case notes will only qualify for the sole possession exemption if they record personal observations about the behavior of students or conclusions the counselor has drawn on the basis of interactions with a student or others. "Notes containing information about the substance of the interactions, particularly the content of conversations, would not be exempt" (American Counseling Association, 1997, p. 6).

Rights for Noncustodial Parents

Rouel, a fourteen-year-old student of yours, occasionally seeks your help with relationship issues with her mother. Rouel's parents are divorced and generally at war over everything, including how best to raise Rouel and her sister. Rouel describes her mother as being "very strict and closed off." Rouel, who lives with her mother, sees her father almost every weekend. A teacher expressed concern that lately Rouel's grades have been plummeting, she seems to have lost interest in her studies, and she rarely smiles or engages in conversation with others. All these behaviors are in marked contrast to how Rouel usually behaves. After meeting with Rouel you believe you need to involve her parents. Rouel begs you to call her father instead of her mother. It is Friday and Rouel explains that she is going to her father's home right after school. You believe Rouel's mother will be enraged that you contacted Rouel's father. Can you consult Rouel's father without seeking permission or notifying her mother, the custodial parent?

School counselors can find guidance in the court case *Page v. Rotterdam-Mohonasen Central School District* (1981). John Page had visitation rights for his fifth-grade son Eric, but repeated requests to the school district to provide him with educational records went unheeded. Mikado Page, Eric's mother, sent a statement to the school (at what was believed to be the school's request) explaining that she has legal custody of Eric and that she did not want John Page to have Eric's education records, participate in teacher-parent conferences, or in any way engage in the educational progress of Eric. When the matter landed in court, the court found that John Page was not trying to alter custodial rights but simply wanted to participate in his son's educational progress. The court found that school districts have a duty to act in the best educational interest of the children committed to their care, which means providing educational information to both parents of "every child fortunate to have two parents interested in his welfare" (Fischer & Sorenson, 1996; Huey & Remley, 1988; *Page*, 1981). Parents, whether or not they have legal custody, do not have to give up their rights to be psychological guardian. The court concluded that in the event of the death of one parent "it would be disastrous for the welfare of a child if an uninformed and ill-prepared parent were suddenly cast into a custodial role upon the occurrence of such a misfortune."

Negligence and Malpractice Involving Suicide

You have been told by a student that her friend Rolanda is threatening suicide. When you call Rolanda in, she vehemently denies it and scoffs at the idea that she would ever harm herself. You are convinced and you drop it without discussing it with anyone. Is there an ethical or legal dilemma?

The law of negligence, which composes a large part of the law of torts, involves injury or damage to another through a breach of duty owed to that person. Four elements must be present for negligence. First, a duty must be owed by one person to another. Until *Eisel v. Board of Education of Montgomery County* (1991), courts consistently found that school counselors did not owe a duty to their minor students to prevent suicide. The *Eisel* case changed the way school counselors must look at suicide prevention. The second element that must be present in a negligence case is that the duty that was owed was breached. The third element is that there must be sufficient legal causal connection between the breach of duty and the injury and then last, injury or damages must be present (ACA, 1994).

The Maryland Court of Appeals in *Eisel* determined that school counselors had a duty to notify the parents of a 13-year-old student of suicidal statements she made to fellow students. Nicole Eisel apparently became involved in Satanism and told several friends and fellow students of her intention to kill herself. Some of these friends informed their school counselor of Nicole's intentions, and this individual in turn informed Nicole's counselor. The two counselors questioned Nicole about the statements, and she denied making them. Neither the parents nor the school administrators were notified about these events. Shortly thereafter, in a public park away from the school, the other party to the suicide pact shot Nicole and then herself (ACA, 1994).

The court cited as critical the ***in loco parentis*** doctrine, which means the school counselors were standing in the parents' stead. *In loco parentis* brings a legal responsibility or special duty to exercise reasonable care to protect a student from harm. The court concluded that "school counselors have a duty to use reasonable means to attempt to prevent a suicide when they are on notice of a child or adolescent student's suicide intent" (*Eisel*, 1991). The court in *Eisel* broke new ground and found a **special relationship** sufficient to create a **duty of care** when an adolescent in a school setting expresses an intention to commit suicide and the counselor becomes aware of such intention. Pursuant to this duty of care and in light of the slight burden on the counselor in warning the parents, future cases that follow *Eisel* are likely to hold counselors negligent for a failure to warn parents of suicidal intentions of students (*Eisel*, 1991).

Simpson (1999) stated: "In recent years, parents have filed a slew of court actions trying to hold school employees legally liable for student suicides. The results are mixed. Courts in at least five states have rejected these kinds of cases. But courts in three others have ruled that, in certain circumstances, school employees' failure to act can make them or the school legally responsible for a student's suicide" (p. 12). Zirkel (1999) outlined a case in New Mexico decided by a federal appeals court in which a 16-year-old special education student shot himself after being suspended for threatening a teacher. The court ruled that the school principal and counselor could be held liable if, as the parents alleged, they took the student home knowing he was suicidal, alone, and had access to firearms, and yet failed to notify his parents. In a 1997 Florida case, another federal appeals court held the Polk County School Board partially responsible for the suicide of a 13-year-old. The court said school officials were negligent because they knew that the student had tried to hang himself at school but neglected to inform his parents (*Wyke v. The Polk County School Board*, 1997).

Courts in other states have refused to impose liability in these kinds of cases, primarily because of state laws granting immunity to public schools and their employees. For example, an Illinois appellate court in 1997 absolved a school counselor of legal liability where the counselor failed to tell the student's parents about his threats of suicide. All of the cases that imposed liability, however, involved employees who failed to notify parents that their children had written or talked to others about killing themselves (Simpson, 1999). The Code of Ethics for the American School Counselor Association explicitly permits disclosure when there may be "clear and imminent danger" to the student or others (ASCA, 2004).

In addition, the Seventh Circuit Court of Appeals has ruled that a school district lawfully can punish a counselor for failing to report a student's "suicidal tendencies." Whether you believe a student is serious about suicide or not, the expression of **suicidal ideation** is a cry for help. It is never advisable to ignore a suicidal threat. Adolescents who are threatening suicide are too volatile or fragile to be ignored.

Remley and Sparkman (1993) discussed what they considered school counselor's limited legal liability. "Skilled school counselors who practice in an ethical manner should not be overly concerned about the possibility of lawsuits related to student suicides being brought against them because there are few available options that will ensure the safety of nine suicidal students (short of hospitalization). Lawsuits may always be filed in our system of justice, but only counselors who lack appropriate skills or who are negligent in their care of students will be held accountable by courts for suicide attempts or deaths of their students" (p. 164).

The school counselor's legal liability ends when school authorities or parents have been notified that a student is at risk and appropriate actions have been recommended. The appeals court in the Eisel case was not giving school counselors the impossible dictate of preventing suicide. Rather, the court was saying that the consequence of the risk of not involving parents is too great and that parents must be allowed to intervene. If students are not helped after notifying parents or other responsible and significant adults, the counseling needs of the student certainly have not been met (Wellman, 1984, pp. 167–168). The next step might well be to notify child protective services.

Letters of Recommendation

Emily is applying to a very competitive university and your letter of recommendation will be a critical part of her admission. Emily's freshman year was dismal academically. She confided in you that she was being physically abused by her boyfriend during her freshman year but ended the relationship after seven months. Emily has been a stellar student since her sophomore year and is not the same person who allowed herself to remain in an abusive relationship. You are considering explaining all this in your letter of recommendation in hopes that Emily will only be judged based on what she has done since leaving this abusive relationship. Legally and/or ethically, can you include this information in a letter of recommendation?

School counselors conscientiously work to behave legally in writing letters of recommendation and find their guidance primarily in the Family Education Rights and Privacy Act (FERPA, 1973). Some of the ethical considerations involving letters of recommendation are: (a) letters and confidential, sensitive information, (b) writing letters for problem students, and (c) supporting weak students.

Confidentiality and Letters of Recommendation

In an informal survey of school counselors (Stone, 2003b), counselors reported that they would never put sensitive, confidential information in a letter of recommendation without student and parental permission. However, in Emily's case counselors report that they would not include this information with or without Emily's permission. Even when it comes to confidential information that, if known, would benefit a student, counselors would rather secure the student's permission to include an invitation in the letter to call the counselor to discuss the student's special circumstances.

Legally, school counselors can include anything in a letter that is common knowledge and observable (Fischer & Sorenson, 1996), such as, "Kennard has never let the fact that he is wheelchair-bound keep him from being an active and high-profile school leader, engaged in numerous school activities including . . ." However, best practice is to always get a student's consent to include such information. It is best practice to leave out sensitive, confidential information; if you believe that it is important to include the information to benefit the student, then secure student and parental permission to relay what they may not want known.

Writing Letters for Problem Students

Counselors report (Stone, 2003b) that if they cannot write a strong letter of recommendation, then they prefer not to write a letter at all. A response to the student such as, "I am not a good choice as you would get a stronger letter from someone who knows you better" will send the message that your letter would not be helpful.

Writing Letters for Weak Students

Counselors are skilled at advocating for their weak students who deserve a chance. Counselors know how to focus on students' assets without bending the truth, skirting the major issues, or in any way painting a false picture. As one school counselor said to an admissions representative, "Let me tell you what you can't learn about Roger from his application and transcripts. Roger has been on this long cultural journey and has developed survival and problem-solving muscles that can never be measured by standardized tests or grades. Roger has demonstrated he is an astute and determined person who has aspirations and ambitions that will make your university proud to have admitted him. For example, Roger has taken care of three siblings." Counselors often focus on life skills when a standard approach to recommendation letters will not help a student (Stone, 2003b).

HIV+ Students and Confidential Communications

An autistic preschool child entered your school. You accidentally acquire the information that this 4-year-old child is HIV+. The principal has warned you that you are not to reveal the child's HIV+ status to the teacher. This 4-year-old is not potty trained and is a biter. It is inconceivable to you that this information is being withheld from the teacher. You are seriously considering dropping some hints to the teacher, such as, "This school year you need to be especially careful to use your rubber gloves when cleaning up after your students." Is there an ethical dilemma here? Is there a legal dilemma here?

The Family Education Rights and Privacy Act (FERPA) gives parents the **privacy rights** of their minor children with regards to education records. School counselors can find guidance in FERPA (1973) if their state does not have a statute addressing the privacy rights of HIV+ children in schools. FERPA gives parents the authority to release records to third persons; therefore, it follows that parents can decide who in the school will know that their child is HIV+ or has AIDS. Most states have statutes protecting the privacy rights of HIV+ people to protect them against the fear and prejudice directed toward them. Schools need protective safeguards to be in place to keep sensitive information from being acquired accidentally.

Additional guidance can be found in *Martinez v. School Board of Hillsborough County* (1989), in which a federal district court ruled that a 7-year-old boy who had AIDS could not be excluded from his Trainably Mentally Handicapped (TMH) class. The court said the fear that the child would transmit the virus because he was not toilet trained and had blood in his saliva was unfounded. The court ruled that the overwhelming medical evidence is that AIDS in not transmitted in schools through casual contact and, therefore, the court would not exclude a child from a free appropriate public education because of "theoretical possibilities" of transmission (*Martinez*, 1989). The Individuals with Disabilities Education Act (IDEA) and Section 504 of the Rehabilitation Act guarantee this child a free education in the least restrictive environment. Supported by legislation and recommended by the Centers for Disease Control (CDC), students who are HIV+ should be afforded a free appropriate public education. The CDC recommends that school age children who are HIV+ be allowed to go to school even though their immune systems are compromised which places them at greater risk for infection. The benefits of being able to go to school counterbalances the risk to the HIV+ student. The children should be allowed to attend school and after-school day-care and be placed in a foster home in an unrestricted setting" (Centers for Disease Control, 2002).

Ethically, a school counselor is responsible to follow federal and state laws and the policies and procedures of their school district. To reveal that this student was HIV+ was illegal and unethical.

Accepting employment in a school district is an agreement to follow their laws, policies, and procedures. Ethically, as an advocate, you can work in appropriate ways to change policy and procedures that you believe work against students and other members of the school family, but as long as the law or policy stands, it must be followed.

HIV+ Sexually Active Students

A 17-year-old counselee tells you she is HIV+ and is having unprotected sex with her boyfriend, Alan. She says she will lose him if she shares her HIV+ status with him. What are your ethical responsibilities in this case? Your legal responsibilities?

Guidance for this case comes from the profession's ethical standards and, in most states, from statutes. ACA and ASCA invite, but do not demand, that counselors can notify partners of HIV+/AIDS status students (ACA Code B.1.c.). The steps in partner notification are:

1. the patient notifies the practitioner of the identity of the partner(s);

2. the practitioner recommends that the patient notify the partner(s) of his or her positive status and refrain from engaging in activities that are likely to transmit the virus, and the patient refuses to do so;

3. the practitioner informs the patient of his or her intent to notify the partner(s); and,

4. the practitioner perceives himself or herself as required to inform the partner of the patient's status as a result of a perceived civil duty or ethical guidelines.

If there is not a state statute forbidding you to disclose a person's HIV+ status to a partner, then mental health professionals are permitted to notify partners in keeping with their ethical codes, but are not required to do so. Moreover, in most state statutes there is language that says that mental health professionals may not be held civilly or criminally liable for failure to notify their students' partner(s). It is wise to consult with fellow professionals and an attorney about the interpretation of the state statutes and about the specifics of the case in which you are involved before disclosing information to a partner.

Negligence in Academic Advising

*Bruce Sain, a senior in Cedar Rapids, Iowa, had talent as an all-state basketball player. In 1996, he was awarded a five-year basketball scholarship to Northern Illinois University to start as a freshman. In the summer prior to his freshman year, Sain was notified in a letter that he did not meet the National Collegiate Athletic Association (NCAA) regulations for incoming fresh-man athletes at Division I schools. Sain fell short in the required English credits because his one-third English credit in Technical Communications was not on the list of classes that his high school submitted to the NCAA for approval. Sain's family filed suit against the Cedar Rapids School District citing the school district as negligent and the school counselor, Larry Bowen, as guilty of **negligent misrepresentation** in his role as an academic adviser (Parrott, 2001; Reid, 2001; Sain v. Cedar Rapids Community School District, 2001). How did a scholarship opportunity for Bruce Sain turn into shambles, and how did Larry Bowen find himself at the center of a lawsuit?*

Sain was dissatisfied with his second trimester English course and asked Bowen to place him in another English class. Allegedly, Bowen suggested Technical Communications and explained to Sain that it was being offered at the school for the first time, but that the Initial-Eligibility Clearinghouse would approve the high school course and that he would have no problem with his NCAA eligibility. The summer following his graduation, the NCAA Clearinghouse declared Sain ineligible because Technical Communications was not on the list of approved NCAA eligibility courses for Sain's high school (Sain, 2001; Zirkel, 2001a). With his scholarship offer voided, Bruce Sain turned to the courts to claim negligent misrepresentation against Bowen for erroneously telling Sain that he was safe to take Technical Communications (Sain, 2001). It was never implied or expressed that it was the school counselor's responsibility to submit courses for approval but rather that it was the school counselor's responsibility to give proper academic advice.

The lower court rejected Sain's suit but on appeal, the Iowa Supreme Court remanded the Sain case back to the lower court to be tried (Sain, 2001). The case was settled out of court for an undisclosed amount of money.

It is important to note that the Iowa Supreme Court did not find for guilt or innocence but left that to the lower court to decide. However, in the school counseling profession we pay attention to this case because the state supreme court found that the claim of "negligent misrepresentation" had merit and should not have been dismissed by the lower court. The majority opinion for the Iowa Supreme Court said that school counselors are liable for providing information to students about credits and courses needed to pursue post-high-school goals (Parrott, 2001; Reid, 2001; *Sain*, 2001).

The allegedly erroneous advice given by the counselor was equated to negligent misrepresentation in professions such as accounting and the law and others whose business requires that they give accurate and appropriate information (Zirkel, 2001a). The court has determined that school counselors have a similar business relationship of giving accurate advice to students when the student has a need to know. The court explains that just as accountants and lawyers stand to gain financially from giving accurate advice, so do school counselors, as that is what they are paid to do. Therefore, negligent misrepresentation can be applied to the school counselor–student relationship when erroneous advice means a student loses a lucrative scholarship. The Iowa Supreme Court says this is a classic case of negligent misrepresentation (Sain, 2001; Zirkel, 2001a).

The court acknowledged that the ruling could have a "chilling effect" on academic advising by school counselors. However, the court cautioned that the ruling should have limited effect, as negligent representation is confined to students whose reliance on information is reasonable (such as, does this course meet NCAA eligibility?) and that the school counselor must be aware of how vital the information is to the student. This explanation was intended to comfort school counselors and to keep them from overreacting to the principles outlined by the *Sain* case (Sain, 2001).

The following are recommendations for avoiding negligence in the role of academic adviser:

1. Educate yourself to the extent possible in the areas needed for competent academic advising and check your facts as often as appropriate. With care you will be able to demonstrate that you tried to keep yourself abreast of critical

information. Ask for professional development from your school district, counseling organizations, and/or literature in the area of academic advising.

2. Manage resources and equip selected professionals to be a key component in the career and academic advising roles. For example, the coaches can be in charge of advising students about NCAA regulations.

3. Widely publicize academic information for all students and parents. Newsletters, form letters, and e-mail listservers can all help you in the advising role and demonstrate that you are proactively trying to disseminate critical, timely information.

4. Require that students and parents sign off when they have been given critical, timely information. For example, when you give seniors their personal credit check for their remaining graduation requirements, have them sign off an acknowledgment that they have been told and understand what they need to do.

5. Consult. You never stand alone unless you fail to consult with others who are in a position to help you.

Negligence in Abortion Counseling

You have been working with a young woman who finds herself pregnant and unwilling to carry the pregnancy to term. You live in a state in which a student can secure an abortion without parental involvement. She is asking for your support as she wrestles with the abortion decision. She wants your help in finding an abortion clinic and in finding financial assistance to pay for the abortion. She has asked you to go with her when she has the procedure. What are your ethical and legal obligations in this situation?

The legal and ethical complications of working with minors in schools pose daily dilemmas, and never more so than in value-laden issues such as abortion counseling, which usually involves a family's religious beliefs, values about sexual conduct, privacy rights, freedom of choice, parental rights to be the guiding voice in their children's lives, and other rights. Respecting students' confidences requires school counselors to balance the rights of minors with the rights of their parents (Isaacs & Stone, 2001; Kaplan, 1996). Legal rulings and the ASCA codes for ethical behavior offer suggestions and guidance in the complexities of confidentiality. However, it is ultimately the responsibility of the school counselor to determine the appropriate response to the individual student who puts her or his trust in the security of the counseling relationship.

Under what circumstances will a counselor be held liable for giving abortion advice? In *Arnold v. Board of Education of Escambia County* (1989), Jane and John, two high-school students, filed suit along with their parents against the School District of Escambia County, Alabama, alleging that the school counselor, Kay Rose, and the assistant principal, Melvin Powell, coerced and assisted Jane in getting an abortion. Further, the accusation was that Powell and Rose hired the two students to perform menial tasks to earn money for the abortion. John, the father of the baby, and Jane claimed that their constitutional rights were violated, including involuntary servitude and free exercise of religion. The parents claimed that their privacy rights were violated when they were not informed by the school counselor and assistant principal that Jane was pregnant and when school officials allegedly urged the students not to tell their parents. The trial court dismissed the suit and the plaintiffs appealed (*Arnold*, 1989; Zirkel, 2001b).

The 11th Circuit Court of Appeals partially reversed the decision of the trial court and found Jane's privacy claim and both students' religious claim as worthy of further consideration by the courts. If Jane and John's religion prohibited abortion and Rose and Powell coerced Jane and John to proceed with Jane's abortion, then the students' constitutionally protected right of freedom of religion was violated, and therefore, the court remanded the case back to the trial court to be heard (Zirkel, 2001b).

In fact finding, the trial court established that Jane visited a physician who confirmed she was pregnant and provided her with abortion information upon her request. John and Jane told Rose that they did not want their parents to know about the pregnancy because they were not supposed to be seeing each other and also that Jane left home because she was being abused by her stepfather. Rose presented various alternatives, but the students rejected all alternatives except abortion, including consulting with their parents. Rose reported the alleged abuse by the stepfather to the child protective services, which sent a representative to meet with Jane. The representative urged Jane to consult with her mother, and offered alternatives such as foster care and adoption. When Jane rejected all alternatives, the representative assisted Jane in trying to get financial assistance and Medicaid. Jane and John said they felt pressured by Rose when she asked them how they planned to care for the baby and where they were going to take the baby. During the process of discovery, Jane admitted that these were good questions, that she alone made the decision to have an abortion, and that she was not coerced by Rose or Powell. The trial court concluded that the students were not deprived of their free will, had chosen to obtain an abortion, had chosen not to tell their parents, and that there was no coercion on the part of school officials. The principles established by the 11th Circuit Court of Appeals have implications for the school counseling profession; that is, coercion by school officials in private matters is unconstitutional (*Arnold*, 1989; Zirkel, 1991; Zirkel, 2001b).

Counselors in the course of fulfilling their job responsibilities can assist students with these value-laden issues if they are competent to give such advice and if they proceed in a professional manner. "However, just because a 15-year-old has a right to contraceptive information and devices and even an abortion if they so desire, does not mean that counselors may carelessly advise them in these matters"

(Fischer & Sorenson, 1996, p. 69). "If an immature, emotionally fragile young girl procures an abortion with the help of a counselor, under circumstances where reasonably competent counselors would have notified the parents or would have advised against the abortion, liability for psychological or physical suffering may follow. The specific facts and circumstances must always be considered" (Fischer & Sorenson, 1996, p. 60).

Can school boards adopt policy forbidding school counselors to engage in any discussions with their students about contraception, abortion, and sexual activity? School boards can (and some do) adopt policy forbidding counselors to address certain topics or instructing them to immediately call parents if such topics are brought up by their students. However, in the absence of a school board policy expressly forbidding them to discuss abortion, school counselors can discuss such options with their students. The caveat is that the school counselors must be ready to defend their behavior as that of the reasonably competent professional. School counselors must refrain from coercion and imposing one's values on a minor student in order to avoid liability for negligence.

You can avoid negligence in a situation like the one just described if you follow these recommendations:

1. Know your school board policies.

2. When working with minors on value-laden issues, it is especially important to consider the chronological and developmental level of the minor in order to determine whether intervention is needed and how much is required. To promote the autonomy and independence of minors is to decide whether they can continue on the path they have chosen without interference or whether some level of intervention or breach of confidentiality must be exercised. Primary to the counselor's ethical decision making is the seriousness of a minor's behavior in the framework of his or her developmental milestones and the minor's history of making informed decisions (Stone, 2001b).

3. Consider the impact of the setting. Parental rights are more complicated when the minor is in a school setting, because parents send minors to school for academics, not for personal counseling. Therefore, when a minor seeks counseling in a value-laden area such as abortion, which may impact on parents' religious beliefs and/or rights to be the guiding voice in their children's lives, consideration must be given to parents (Isaacs & Stone, 1999).

4. Encourage students to involve their parents in value-laden difficult dilemmas such as abortion. Use all your skillful techniques to help them make the decision to involve their parents, such as offering to be with them when they tell their parents.

5. Consider diversity issues. Each ethical dilemma must be made in context and must consider a minor's ethnicity, gender, race, and sexual identity.

6. Consult with a supervisor and/or respected colleague, examining the good and bad consequences of each course of action, striving to minimize the risk to the student while respecting the inherent rights of parents. It is ethical, lawful, and beneficial to inform and consult with supervisors and colleagues. Consult again after you implement your course of action to process the results and strengthen the probability of making more appropriate decisions in the future (Stone, 2002c).

7. Know your own values in sensitive areas such as abortion and understand the impact of those values on your ability to act in the best interest of your students. Professionals know they cannot leave their values out of their work, but they also understand when those values can interfere. Refer students to a colleague when you can no longer be effective (Stone, 2001c).

8. The professional school counselor would never provide referrals to birth control clinics or agree to take a counselee for any kind of medical procedure, especially one as controversial as abortion (Stone, 2002c).

Sexual Harassment

Fourteen-year-old Regina is subjected daily to sexually suggestive remarks by a group of boys in the hallway near her math class. Regina has started to come to math class late to avoid the taunts and jeers of the boys. Regina's math teacher, Ms. Lopez, unaware of the situation, has sent Regina to the office for tardy slips but without effect to change her behavior. Now Regina is in danger of being suspended. Ms. Lopez, sensing that something unusual is happening to her conscientious student turned truant, asks you, the school counselor, to talk with Regina. You begin to learn the truth of Regina's misery when she confides about the harassment. Regina describes her embarrassment, and her attempts at coping by "laughing it off," "avoiding them," "taunting back" (which she said only made her feel more dirty), or "dressing in really baggy clothes." She begs you not to tell anyone because "it [the harassment] will only get worse." Must you report the sexual harassment to the administration of your school? Can you keep Regina's identity confidential? Can the school administration keep Regina's identity confidential when confronting the perpetrators?

Through the case of Regina, let's explore the legal muscle that school counselors have been given to advocate for Regina and other victims of sexual harassment, including males and the most vulnerable students for abuse, gay and lesbian students. Regina fits the profile of the harassed student; self-blame, self-doubt, using avoidance techniques, and wanting to be free of the harassment but enduring it rather than risking being victimized twice when students find out that she is a "snitch," "narc," or "informant." The impact that sexual harassment has had on Regina's education and the lengths to which she will go in order to avoid the harassment both underscore the seriousness of sexual harassment. Once regarded as harmless peer interaction deemed to be flirtatious or playful, sexual harassment is now widely understood to be destructive, illegal, and adversely impacting a student's education (Stone, 2001b).

A recent Supreme Court ruling, *Davis v. Monroe County Board of Education* (1999) has given sexual harassment a prominent place on the national agenda and has established that public schools can be forced to pay monetary damages for failing to address student-on-student sexual harassment. Sexual harassment can no longer be ignored or given cursory attention by school districts, as *Davis* demands action against known sexual harassment (*Davis*, 1999).

The *Davis* case involved L. Davis, a fifth-grade girl, who repeatedly during a five-month period reported sexual abuse behaviors by G.F. to her teachers and principal, but to no avail. The abuse continued. L. was unable to concentrate on her studies (her previously high grades dropped) and her father found a suicide note. Mrs. Davis, who had also reported the abuse on more than one occasion to the educators of the school without redress, finally filed a complaint with the Monroe County, Georgia, Sheriff Department, and then G.F. pleaded guilty to sexual battery. Mrs. Davis then filed a $1,000,000 lawsuit under the **Title IX** prohibition of sex discrimination in schools (*Davis*, 1999). The Supreme Court's 5-to-4 ruling in favor of Mrs. Davis emphasized a stringent standard, stating that the harassment must be known to educators and must be "so severe, pervasive, and objectively offensive that it can be said to deprive the victim of access to the educational opportunities or benefits provided by the school" (*Davis*, 1999, n.p.).

The *Davis* case clearly encourages more protection against sexual harassment and gives school counselors legal muscle to exercise an advocacy role to assist individual victims and to help establish a respectful school climate. With 80% of students experiencing sexual harassment and fewer than 10% of that number reporting the harassment to an adult at school, it is obvious that there is a need for students to have a safe confidential place to report harassment. The Hostile Hallways study (Harris/Scholastic Research, 1993) informed us of the prevalence of the problem, and the *Davis* case and the U.S. Department of Education's **Office of Civil Rights** gave us legal muscle to encourage students to come forward, to support students who have been harassed, and to contribute toward changing hostile school climates into healthy ones.

Must you report the sexual harassment to the administration of your school? School counselors are required by law to report the sexual harassment to school officials. "A school has actual notice of sexual harassment if an agent or responsible employee of the school receives notification" (U.S. Department of Education, Office of Civil Rights, 1997, p. 12037). Once Regina confided that she was being harassed, this constituted "notice" and triggered the school counselor's legal requirement to report the harassment and the school's responsibility to take "corrective action" (ACA, 1997b, p. 9).

Can you keep Regina's identity confidential? The Office of Civil Rights (OCR) promotes protecting confidentiality, understanding that breaching students' confidences will often discourage reporting of harassment, which already is a horrific problem in many schools. If your school has a procedure or policy in place by which the victim is identified on the report, then your advocacy role can spark change in this practice. Reporting is critical—identifying the victim is not! The school counselor will need to educate Regina about the legal requirement to report the sexual harassment and, if appropriate, encourage Regina to allow her identity to be known to support addressing sexual harassment. However, the OCR does not require that educators breach confidentiality just to ensure that the perpetrators are disciplined; rather, they require that educators have to address the harassment. This can take many forms.

Can the school administration keep Regina's identity confidential when confronting the perpetrators? OCR realizes that withholding the name of the victim may interfere with the investigation and infringe on the due process rights of the accused. In the context of each situation, school counselors and school administrators will need to wrestle with the difficult decision to honor an alleged victim's request for confidentiality, yet also "remedy the harassment and take steps to prevent further harassment" (U.S. Department of Education, Office of Civil Rights, 1997, p. 12037). A student's request for confidentiality should be respected even if this hinders the investigation. The school should make every effort to address the harassment in another way such as holding a schoolwide assembly or classroom guidance lessons on sexual harassment in an effort to impact the school climate if an investigation and discipline of an individual perpetrator means identifying the victim. Regina's confidentiality needs might outweigh the need for disciplinary action against the accused. If disciplining the individual perpetrator is not possible without revealing Regina's identity, then other strategies might have to be employed, such as a schoolwide sexual harassment workshop, a student survey that tries to determine the prevalence of harassment, and classroom presentations. Techniques such as positioning a teacher in the hall during class changes, so that the teacher can observe and report the harassment, is preferable to a peer report, in which the identity of the victim can be surmised. Depending on the seriousness of the harassment and the age of the victim, the identity of the victim may have to be revealed as a last resort.

Students will not report harassment and risk being victimized twice. Students need assurances that everything possible will be done to protect their identity. The case of Regina is a small snapshot of the problem and ways to protect sexual harassment victims. School counselors can be instrumental in helping to heighten the awareness of the sexual harassment problem, assist in helping to establish a safe school climate, and can advocate for protection of a student's privacy rights in reporting harassment. School counselors can be a source of strength for the individual student who needs help in confronting and dealing with sexual harassment. The legal and ethical complications of working with minors in schools continue to pose daily dilemmas, and never more so than in sexual harassment issues. Respecting students' confidences can send a message that the school counseling office is a safe place to report sexual harassment.

Continuing Your Professional Development

This chapter is an introduction to a few of the most common and/or crucial legal and ethical areas that impact the work of school counselors. For more detailed information, it is suggested that you read texts by Fischer and Sorenson, Stone, and Remley and Herlihy (see References), attend all legal and ethical workshops presented in your area, and consider taking a university course when seeking opportunities for professional development requirements or when renewing your certificate. Workshops and courses help you develop a sensitivity to ethical decision making, which is difficult to accomplish using reference materials alone. Always remember to consult, consult, consult. You never stand alone legally and ethically if you seek guidance from your fellow professionals.

TechTools

When you become a school counselor, use the power of technology to maximize your chances of behaving legally and ethically.

- Visit the ACA, ASCA and other professional websites and bookmark their links to ethical codes and standards so that you will have a ready reference of resources and laws at your fingertips to support your work and to help you continue to behave legally and ethically. Grow your library of websites that can help you do your work.
- Reduce the risk of negligent misrepresentation and malpractice by learning to regularly consult specific sites that you might need in your work, such as the NCAA clearinghouse site, the U.S. Department of Education site, and your state department site.
- Advocate that your school district establish an electronic newsletter so that critical, timely legal information can be passed to all interested persons.
- Encourage your school district to subscribe to legal search engines such as Lexis. Sites such as these will allow you to submit key words for topics in which you are interested. Every time a law is passed or a court case is heard that includes those key words, you will be notified via e-mail.
- Selectively and carefully identify and publicize respectable agencies and organizations that offer websites, information dissemination, and chatrooms that can serve as support for students who might not otherwise seek help. For example, there are sites for students wrestling with sexual identity issues such as the Gay, Lesbian and Straight Education Network (GLSEN) website at http://www.glsen.org and the Coming Out-Getting Support section of the Parents, Families and Friends of Lesbians and Gays (PFLAG) website at

http://www.pflag.org/index.php?id=12. To determine which sites are respectable, start with nationally known sites such as GLSEN and inquire under the link called "contact us" as to your specific needs or call local organizations that you know to be respectable and ask them for websites they recommend.

- Audio-visual equipment can heighten professional development activities. Counselors can acquire a library of videotapes, such as tapes about the *Eisel* court case, the *Davis* case, and others, and have teachers check out these tapes for viewing (possibly for a reward such as credit toward certificate renewal).

School Counselor Casebook: *Voices From the Field*

The Scenario Reviewed

One of the three counselors in your school plans to conduct three small groups this semester. The first group will be for students whose parents are newly divorced or are going through a divorce; the second will be for students who are chronic referrals for aggressive or violent behavior; the third will be for students who are not getting their class work or homework completed. Your colleague comes to you and asks your advice on her choice of topics for these groups. She also asks you if she should get written or oral parental permission before beginning any of the groups.

A Practitioner's Approach

Here's how a counselor educator responded to the school scenario:

The ASCA and ACA Code of Ethics and Standards of Practice give us guidance in examining the issue of obtaining permission from parents before allowing students to engage in group counseling. Our ethical codes tell us that "counselors recognize that families are usually important in students' lives and strive to enlist family understanding and involvement as a positive resource, when appropriate." According to *Ethical Standards for School Counselors* (ASCA, 2004) "the professional school counselor respects the inherent rights and responsibilities of parents for their children and endeavors to establish, as appropriate, a collaborative relationship with parents to facilitate the counselee's maximum development." In addition to respecting the rights of parents, "the professional school counselor adheres to laws and local guidelines when assisting parents experiencing family difficulties that interfere with the counselee's effectiveness and welfare." For further direction, the Association for Specialists in Group Work Best Practice Guidelines offers consideration that "group workers obtain the appropriate consent forms for work with minors and other dependent group members."

In answering the question about the appropriateness of topics for small groups, especially when a family's confidentiality may be breached, such as the case with groups for children and divorce, it is important to consider the developmental levels of the students. Developmentally, PK–12 students may not be able to give informed consent, and school counselors must be especially cautious to act in the best interests of students when they decide to place them in a potentially vulnerable position such as becoming a member of a small group.

The school counselor has to assess student readiness and maturity to discuss the sensitive and emotionally laden topic of their parents' divorce in front of other students. It is also important to remember the fact that students repeat information, and topics of discussion may be repeated in classrooms and hallways. The school counselor has to monitor what is being said to protect students from harm in the event that group confidentiality is breached. It is the responsibility of the school counselor who is facilitating a small group to ensure a safe environment for students.

Often school counselors will conduct a needs assessment with teachers or students to find out what topics should be considered for small groups. The school counseling advisory board can assist in supporting the need for groups and the topics selected. The advisory committee might also be aware of community standards or individuals who may oppose offering certain group counseling topics and also suggest alternatives as to how to address important issues that impact students within the school setting.

Dr. Gloria Dansby-Giles is a professor of counselor education at Jackson State University in Jackson, Mississippi. Gloria has served as the Southern Region vice president and ethics chair of the American School Counselor Association. Reprinted with permission by Dr. Gloria Dansby-Giles.

Chapter Summary

Professional Ethics

All school counselors are governed by the American School Counselor Association code of ethics. Ethics are the customs, mores, standards, and accepted practice of a profession. Codes are the ideal to which school counseling professionals should aspire, while laws are the minimum standard society will tolerate.

A Model of Ethical Decision Making

The model of ethical decision making offers a framework within which to grapple with ethical dilemmas. The traditional models of ethical decision making include these steps: examine the facts; review the relevant ethical guidelines; identify the nature and dimensions of the problem; consult or seek supervision; consider possible and probable courses of action; examine the good and bad consequences of various decisions; and implement your course of action. Because of the unique nature of counseling in schools, we must also add these steps: identify your emotional reaction; consider parental rights; consider the setting; and consider the student's chronological and developmental levels.

The Complications of Confidentiality in the Context of Schools

School counselors must consider not only student rights but parental rights when working legally and ethically in schools. Parents are continually vested by our courts with legal rights to guide their children. School boards and administrators adopt policies, which counselors are ethically bound to obey. Teachers, when informed regarding children's special needs and circumstances, are in the best position to impact positively on a child's life during school and often beyond the school day. All of these issues contribute to the complex nature of working with minors in schools.

Students' Rights and Responsibilities

Tension exists between a child's right to privacy and the parents' right to be the guiding voice in their child's life. Generally, the younger the child, the more rights are vested in the parents. Students must avoid unlawful activity, and infractions may result in suspension, expulsion, or financial restitution.

Parents' Rights and Responsibilities

Parents have the right to guide their children's lives in value-laden decisions. FERPA (1973) gives parents the right to talk to teachers and school administrators about their children, to see their children's educational records, and to decide if their children will participate in a questionnaire, survey, or examination regarding a parent's personal beliefs, sex practices, family life, or religion.

Confidentiality and Community Standards

How we address ethical problems will depend in large part on the culture and/or standards of the community. Ethics are situational and depend on the values of the larger community.

Confidentiality and Privileged Communication

All school counselors have a confidentiality responsibility, and in a few states, school counselors are granted partial privilege, which protects students by securing their confidences except when required by a court of law to breach those confidences.

Key Terms

ASCA Code of Ethics and Standards of Practice p. 300
Community standards p. 307
Confidentiality p. 301
Duty of care p. 312
Educational records p. 306
Ethics p. 300
Family Educational Rights and Privacy Act (FERPA) p. 306
in loco parentis p. 311
Informed consent p. 304

Laws p. 300
Multiplicity of responsibility p. 307
Negligence p. 309
Negligent misrepresentation p. 316
Office of Civil Rights p. 322
Privacy rights p. 314
Privileged communication p. 304
Special relationship p. 312
Standard of care p. 301
Suicidal ideation p. 312
Title IX p. 322

Learning Extensions

1. Find the addresses of these websites on the World Wide Web and follow these directions:
   - Print the NBCC Webcounseling Standards.
   - Order online, from the Office of Special Education Programs, the publication *Early Warnings, Timely Response: A Guide to Safe Schools*, and read it.
   - Explore the site for the Office of Special Education Programs (online). Under IDEA 97, find general information and become comfortable with the law. Using all the information you have gathered, discuss the implications for school counselors.
   - Go to the ASCA and ACA websites and read the ethical codes. Discuss the sections of the code that you found to be the most important, the most ambiguous, and the least helpful.

2. Discuss the ethics of academic advising.

3. Study the standards of the community where you hope to be a counselor by interviewing at least five of the following people: local clergy, business owner, parent, teacher, principal, guidance counselor, other educator, public employee, elementary student, middle school student, high-school student, or staff member of a school. Write up a two-page report detailing your perspective of the community standards of the area.

4. A school counselor's responsibilities extend beyond the minor student client to the parents or guardians of that student. In a two- to three-page reaction paper, discuss how the school setting determines our responsibilities to parents and what impact those responsibilities have on the school counselor's work.

5. Prepare a 15-minute staff development presentation appropriate for a faculty meeting highlighting a topic of legal or ethical concern, such as child abuse reporting.

Chapter 12

Career Planning and Student Transitions

Chapter Objectives

By the time you have completed this chapter, you should be able to:

- Understand the importance of career development in every student's education.
- Help students connect student motivation, achievement, and future goals.

- Understand the influence of parents, peers, and economic pressures on career success.
- Identify the career planning elements in your comprehensive school counseling and career guidance program.
- Assess your current career planning practices based on nationally accepted criteria.
- Develop appropriate K–12 strategies for addressing the career development needs of students based on knowledge of the National Career Development Guidelines (National Occupation Information Coordinating Committee, 1989; ACRN, 2004) and the career development components of the ASCA National Model and the National Standards for School Counseling Programs.
- Demonstrate familiarity with assessment tools, resources, technology applications, and other tools to support comprehensive career development.
- Develop strategies to motivate colleagues, school administrators, parents, and members of the community to collaborate to create a bright future for every student.

School Counselor Casebook: Getting Started

The Scenario

Two eighth-grade students stop by your office to request that they be allowed to drop the honors program. They explain that their reason for wanting to drop the program isn't because the work is too difficult; they just don't know why they need the honors program when the regular grade-level courses seem like a perfectly fine option. These students had already talked to their homeroom teacher about dropping the courses and were told that honors classes would further their opportunities for college. However, the teacher could not tell them why. One of the students said to you that because she wants to study computer graphics at the regional Tech Center next year, she doesn't see a need to worry about college.

Both students seem to be completely uninformed about career options, why postsecondary education is important, and what it will take to succeed in high school. You know that very little attention is paid to career and postsecondary awareness in the middle school. What would you do?

Thinking About Solutions

As you read this chapter, think about what you might do as a middle school counselor to help students become better informed about career options and the importance of postsecondary education. When you come to the end of the chapter, you will have the opportunity to see how your ideas compare with a practicing school counselor's approach.

The Global Economy and the Work Force

> Ninety percent of this year's kindergarten students will find themselves in jobs we know nothing about today.
> — *J. D. Hoye, 1998, former director of the National School to Work Office*

Leaving the future of America's youth to happenstance places young people at risk in an increasingly competitive job marketplace. In recent decades, the advancement of technology and increasing demand for highly skilled workers has placed a strong emphasis on the delivery of **career development** and **career guidance** programs in America's schools. Every student needs the motivation to complete high school with the academic preparation to have all options after graduation (Education Trust, 1997), including 2- and 4-year colleges, career and technical schools, and military opportunities. Preparing students to select a career pathway and guiding them to enroll in course work that is appropriate and essential to support their goals is critical to meeting the global and economic challenges of the 21st century.

Business and industry recognized the need for workers to come to the corporate office or to the factory with the affective competence to support employability preparation skills. The National Commission on Excellence in Education (1983), the Carnegie Forum on Education and the Economy (1986), and the U.S. Departments of Education and Labor (1991) reported that our nation's economic future is dependent upon providing students with access and success in higher level educational opportunities, critical thinking and analysis skills, and the development of affective competence.

In 1991 a joint commission was formed, comprising representatives from business, industry, and education. The Secretary of Labor's Commission on Achieving Necessary Skills (SCANS) produced a report entitled *What Work Requires of Schools* (U.S. Department of Labor, 1991). The document emphasized the development of strong affective and academic competence and identified competencies, foundation skills, and personal qualities that are needed for solid performance in the workplace. The five SCANS competencies included the ability to

1. identify, organize, plan, and allocate resources such as time;

2. work with others;

3. acquire and use information;

4. understand complex interrelationships;

5. work with a variety of technologies.

School counselors are instrumental in supporting not only academic success but also the personal-social skills identified by the SCANS report as needed by students for workplace success. The SCANS report encouraged schools to teach higher order thinking skills, while providing opportunities for students to apply selected personal qualities including responsibility, sociability, self-management, integrity, and honesty in a meaningful way. These competencies brought attention to the importance of employability skills, and for the first time, educators were urged to integrate academic and affective education in the areas of basic skills, thinking skills, and personal qualities (Table 12.1)

The skills that are necessary for success in the workplace were no different than the personal-social and character traits that educators desire for students in their classrooms.

The School to Work Opportunities Act (STWOA) (U.S. Department of Education, 1994) encouraged educators to integrate academic and technical knowledge and skills to better prepare graduates of our high schools to meet the needs of both employers and postsecondary institutions (Worthington & Juntunen, 1997). For five years, the STWOA annually funded ten state departments of education to build a model of collaboration involving K–12 educators, business leaders, and higher education leaders that would integrate career awareness and career preparation, and employability skills into the kindergarten through grade 12 curriculum. The STWOA also provided for closer monitoring of at-risk students who would benefit from career and technical education, with the expressed purpose of preventing dropouts who become entrenched in entry-level, low-wage jobs with little opportunity for advancement (Herr, 1997).

A second federal initiative, Tech Prep, created an articulated system of education that created partnerships between the high school and the two year college. Predominantly focusing on career preparation, two plus two programs, i.e., two years of high school plus two years of college would offer a graduate the ability to compete in the global economy. Both initiatives promoted high achievement and the acquisition of employability (SCANS) competencies and emphasized collaboration with business and industry with the ultimate goal of improving labor market preparation.

When students develop a strong sense of self and understand the connection between their studies and future opportunities, they have an easier time learning academic subjects (Sciarra, 2004). School counselors were viewed as key facilitators for STWOA and Tech Prep due to their knowledge and training in career awareness and

Table 12.1

Basic Skills	Thinking Skills	Personal Qualities
Reading	Creativeness	Self Esteem
Writing	Decisiveness	Self Management
Mathematics	Problem Solving	Integrity
Speaking	Reasoning	Sociability
Listening		

SCANS, 1991.

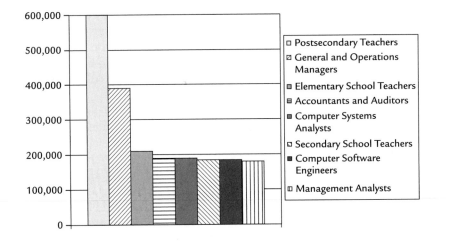

Figure 12.1 Change in Employment, Large Growth, High Paying Occupations, Usually Requiring a Bachelor's Degree or Graduate Degree, Projected Openings 2001-12.

U.S. Department of Labor, Bureau of Labor Statistics, February 2004, *Monthly Labor Review*.

career development (American School Counselor Association [ASCA], 1996) and their ability to motivate and inspire.

The need for higher educated and skilled workers continued to increase faster than the supply of workers, especially with the dramatic fluctuations in the economic outlook. There are more workers than there are jobs that require a only high-school education or less (Postsecondary Education Opportunity, 2000). According to the U.S. Department of Labor (2000, October), 70% of the 30 fastest growing jobs will require an education beyond high school, while 40% of all new jobs will require at least an associate's degree. Figure 12.1 shows the projected numbers of new jobs requiring a 4-year degree or more in the coming years.

The data in Figure 12.2 tell the story: the more you learn the more you earn, and the less likely you are to be unemployed. Increasingly, income is determined by the level of educational attainment. More education leads to higher income, which in turn produces higher standards of living for families. Education continues to pay because employers believe that an educated worker can learn tasks more easily and is better organized.

Several recent studies found that the academic and technical skills of American secondary students were lacking, and thus there is a continued need to provide students with the basic components of STWOA, including career awareness, exploration, and the opportunity for career and technical training (American Youth Policy Forum, 2000; National Commission on the High School Senior Year, Education Trust, 2001a). The National Commission on the High School Senior Year found that American youth are not well prepared for jobs and careers requiring high technical skills and a high-school diploma is no longer enough to achieve success in postsecondary education or

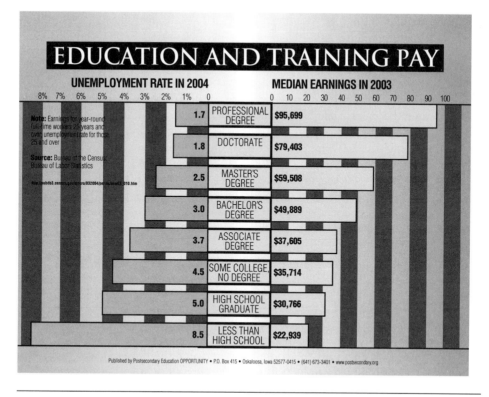

Figure 12.2 Education and Training Pay.

Reprinted with permission by www.postsecondary.org.

the workplace. Math and science course-taking patterns failed to keep pace with the increased demand for workers with advanced technical skills (Jurich & Estes, 2000).

Job instability and a new market outlook require a different work force for the 21st century. As recently as 20 years ago, it was fairly commonplace for a high school or college graduate to take a job with a company and stay with that company throughout his or her working life (U.S. Department of Labor, 2003a). Statistics show that this is no longer a way of life; a person entering the work force will change jobs an average of eight times before retirement (U.S. Department of Labor, 2003a). What's more, the same person will change career paths three or more times (U.S. Department of Labor, 2003a).

Although no one can predict with complete accuracy which jobs will exist in the future and which jobs will become obsolete, it is possible to assess a specific job's outlook. Hoyt (2001) reported that approximately 21 million of the anticipated 50 million new jobs between the years 1996 and 2006 will only require 2 to 3 weeks of short-term, on-the-job training, so it's clear that low-skilled, low-wage jobs abound in the American economy.

Young people leaving school for entry-level jobs do not realize that employment at this level may not provide a living wage. The Gallup Organization (1999) revealed that 69% of working adults reported that if choosing careers again they would get more information about available options than they had previously (Feller & Davies, 2002).

School counselors can guide students to examine opportunities that exist in the field including the average age of the employees in that job title, the number of people in training and preparation programs, the developing technology, and economic and demographic trends. There is a wealth of information available on the Internet, such as the *Occupational Outlook Handbook* (U.S. Department of Labor, 2003a) and a myriad of websites devoted to career guidance.

School counselors are key information brokers, serving as the gateway to curricular development related to career and technical occupational opportunities. Career information support helps students better understand the connection between earning and learning.

There is a substantial earnings differential from the lowest to highest levels of educational attainment (see Figure 12.3). When school counselors help students analyze the correlation between educational attainment and income, it can have a very powerful influence on young people who dream of lifestyles that offer financial independence, advancement, and success. Helping students realize their dreams is a critical and essential component of the work of school counselors. When students discover their passion and see the connection between their dreams and their education, it serves to motivate students to get higher grades, achieve better attendance, and make a stronger commitment to their education.

Demographics also provide key information in preparing the worker of the future. The millennial generation will soon surpass the size of Generation X, and may become as large as the baby-boom generation (Howe & Strauss, 2000). Between 2000 and 2012, the number of employed workers will increase from 146 million to 168 million (*Occupational Outlook Quarterly*, U.S. Department of Labor, 2004).

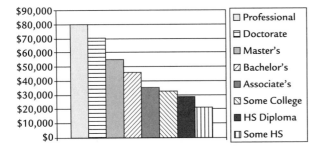

Figure 12.3 Median Earnings for Year-Round, Full Time Workers Ages 25 and Older, by Educational Attainment, 2000.

U.S. Department of Labor, *Occupational Outlook Quarterly*, Spring 2002, p. 52.

Competition will be strong and consumer demands will influence the need for goods and services. The high-tech industry is a prime example. When a product is in high demand, jobs in that industry are generally plentiful. However, unforeseen events, including 9/11 and changes in consumer confidence, are affecting individual occupations or industries in this decade (*Occupational Outlook Quarterly*, U.S. Department of Labor, 2002).

New technology creates obsolescence and opportunity. The dot-com industry, a product of the late 1980s, continues to reinvent and revitalize itself. Company downsizing, due to technological innovation, significantly impacts on the work force, causing many people to lose their jobs and seek new employment and careers (Lawhorn, 2004). Today, technology is changing faster than ever before, which means that the job market changes rapidly (*Occupational Outlook Quarterly*, U.S. Department of Labor, 2004). Students will need to transition to the workplace with the ability to adapt to changing environments and to acquire new knowledge and skills to keep pace with the new work force.

Career Decision Influencers

Erickson (1968) noted that youth are particularly sensitive to the experiences and influences of those who surround and support them. Student experience and familiarity undeniably influence the actions they take about their future. Bandura's (1977) observations remain true today and remind us that social learning can greatly sway aspiration and motivation.

Parents/Caregivers

Parents or caregivers have a profound effect on youth decision making. In *Decisions Without Direction* (Career Institute for Education and Workforce Development, 2002), a national study of high-school juniors and seniors, the results concluded that the students surveyed received little or no career guidance outside of their home (see Figure 12.4). Not surprising, parents are viewed by their children as the primary influence on career decision making. The study also revealed that students do not perceive that they are receiving any career guidance during their high-school years.

Hoyt (2002) reminded us that parental aspirations result in approximately 70% of high-school graduates enrolling in college each fall with the intent to complete a 4-year bachelor's degree. It is estimated that one in four will drop out after the first year, and approximately 35% will achieve a bachelor's degree (National Center for Education Statistics, 2002) (see Figure 12.5).

Parents and students need to be well aware of the myriad options available to them that will result in satisfying career opportunities. Hoyt (2002) encouraged educators to inform both students and parents about postsecondary options and the

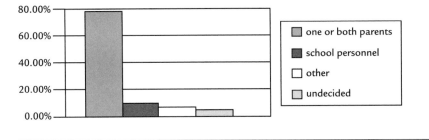

Figure 12.4

Adapted from *Decisions Without Direction*, 2002.

need to acquire high-tech skills, have access to specialized programs, and develop a facility with computer usage. With the job market undergoing rapid change, parents rely on school counselors and career guidance personnel to provide career information and guidance that is aligned with the educational choices that students seek after high school (Schneider & Stevenson, 1999).

Educators

Educators influence career choice. Figure 12.6 demonstrates that teachers have more influence on student career decisions than do school counselors.

Students also reported that teachers have provided advisement on career options or presented options to help further their education. Sixty-eight percent of the students who participated in *Decisions Without Directions* (Career Institute for Education and Workforce Development, 2002) believed that the best jobs and career required, at a minimum, a 4-year degree. Lynch (2000) urged counselors and teachers to bury the fallacy that a 4-year degree is the only option to a rewarding career and help students best match their interests and abilities with their motivation and achievement. However, teachers and school counselors are critical in

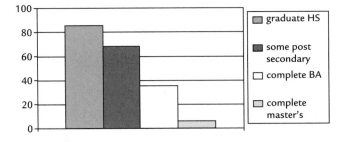

Figure 12.5 Student Completion Rates.

National Center for Education Statistics, 2002.

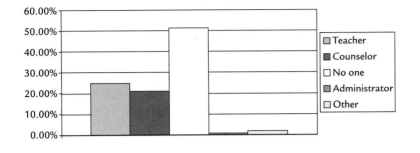

Figure 12.6 School-based Career Influencers.
Decisions Without Directions, 2002.

helping high-school graduates understand that those who do not receive any kind of postsecondary education or training are unlikely to obtain what most persons would describe as a "good" job and one with a "future" (Hoyt, 2001).

Peers

The influence of the culture and of peers on youth's decision-making ability has been the subject of numerous publications (Howe & Strauss, 2000). Youth share interests and perspectives with their peers, but this influence is greater on socialization issues than on career choice (Lesko, 2001). Peer-to-peer influence is focused predominantly on school achievement, substance abuse, and gang involvement, all of which can have a profound impact on a student's ability to successfully complete high school (U.S. Department of Health and Human Services, 2002).

Researchers and data strongly suggest that there is a link between career choice and economic conditions (Bettis, 1998; McLeod, 1995; *Occupational Outlook Quarterly*, U.S. Department of Labor, 2003b). The U.S. Department of Labor (2002) reported that 80.6% of recent high-school graduates who were not attending a 2- or 4-year college were in the labor force.

The remaining 19.4% are potentially unemployed. As the employment-to-population ratio declined from 6.97% in 2000 to 6.38% in 2002, workers with less training found fewer employment opportunities. The demand for college-educated workers has risen faster than the supply since 1979 (U.S. Department of Labor, 2003a).

The data tell the story. As demographics and technology continue to change, students more than ever before need accurate and timely information to help them choose wisely in school and plan for their transition after high school. In 1994, the U.S. General Accounting Office (GAO) reported that 30% of young people aged 16–24 lacked the skills for entry-level employment, and 50% of adults in their late 20s had not found steady jobs. Students struggled then (as many do now) with weak academic preparation, little career guidance, and few workplace experiences.

Theoretical Underpinnings

Major theorists' writings and practice have strongly influenced career development. **Career counseling** is guided by theory which provides a point of reference from which the counselor develops a personal perspective of human growth, development, and behavior (Gladding, 2004). Developmental theory is a strong influence in career counseling, because the life stages and changes impact the counseling. Career maturity is demonstrated by the successful accomplishment of age-appropriate and developmental learning across the life span (Super, 1980). Super's **Life Span–Life Space** approach (1980) suggested that career development evolves along a continuum from birth throughout the life span. These early stages of growth in children addressed fantasy (ages 4–10), interest (11–12), and capacity (13–14), and assisted children in developing an early awareness of the world of work and of their interests. In the exploration stage (ages 15–24), youth and young adults acquire career awareness by discovering skills, talents, motivation, strengths, and weaknesses. They begin to understand that a strong commitment, as well as acquiring coping and resiliency skills, is essential to educational and career success. As young adults evaluate their strengths and weaknesses, career counseling can lead a student to a better understanding of his or her fear of failure, the influence of parents and caregivers, and the individual's willingness to overcome obstacles to achieve his or her goals. This growth in self-concept informs decisions, choices, and eventually career selection. Because Super uses the concept of career maturity as a means of identifying which developmental tasks have been accomplished on the continuum of life development, career success is seen as the result of the congruence of abilities, personality, and aptitude with the choice of career environment.

Using the perception that people are attracted to a given career by their personalities, Holland (1994) proposed that the environment could greatly influence a person's orientation to career choice, personal satisfaction, and stability.

Holland's typology approach to career development is based in self-knowledge and includes four components:

Consistency: Career choice is an expression or extension of one's personality into the world of work.

Differentiation: Individuals who match a personality type will demonstrate little resemblance to other types.

Identity: Individuals can acquire a clear and stable picture of their interests, goals, and talents.

Congruence: The individual's personality type is in harmony with the choice of work environment.

The *Self-Directed Search* (Holland, Fritzsche, & Powell, 1994), an assessment tool, is based on the theory of career typology and is the basis for most of the career inventories in use today. The typology categorizes the relationship of personality to the work environments with respect to six types of personality orientations. Known as the "Holland Codes," these factors of influence on career choice are briefly described below:

Realistic. Individuals show an interest in working with objects such as tools and machines. Mechanical creativity and physical dexterity are important skills for this area. Individuals who score high on this theme prefer dealing with things rather than with ideas or people.

Investigative. Individuals display an interest in science, theories, ideas, and data. Analytical skills are important, and a high score in this theme is indicative of someone who is creative, prefers to think through problems, and enjoys challenges.

Artistic. Individuals are concerned with self-expression and art appreciation. High scorers have artistically oriented interests and a greater need for individual expression, and generally describe themselves as original, expressive, and unconventional.

Social. Individuals prefer to work with people in areas such as human welfare and community service. People skills, such as listening and showing understanding, are very important for this category. Someone who scores high in this category tends to be sociable, humanistic, and gets along well with others.

Enterprising. Individuals have an interest in business and leadership roles. Communicating with others and an ability to motivate and direct others are important skills for these occupations. Those who score high in this theme are often described as ambitious and enthusiastic. They tend to prefer social environments in which they can assume leadership and enjoy persuading others to their viewpoints.

Conventional. Individuals have an interest in organization, data, and finance. A high score in this theme indicates that an individual is most effective when dealing with well-defined tasks. In addition, these individuals prefer to know precisely what is expected of them and could be described as orderly and dependable.

Personality descriptions can help one to better understand how individual skills and interests relate to career choice and help to find the careers that best match interests and abilities (Holland, Daiger, & Power, 1980). Cognitive-behavioral theory (Krumboltz, Mitchell, & Jones, 1976) stressed that each individual's learning experiences, such as generalization of self, sets of developed skills, and career entry behavior, influence an individual's career choice. The process of career development involves four factors: genetic endowments and career opportunities; environmental conditions and events; learning experiences; and task approach skills. Because career decision making is a lifelong process, it is a critical skill to be taught to students at an early age.

More recently, Mitchell, Levin, and Krumboltz (1999) have proposed that career success often results from "planned happenstance"; that is, the individual creates and/or transforms an unplanned event into a life opportunity. Although individuals will admit that unplanned life events influenced or impacted their career path, many see these as happenstance. Krumboltz suggests that individuals often overlook the intent of their actions. Thus they may not take the time to get to know those who significantly influenced their lives or the purposeful actions that were taken and not serendipitous.

The confidence and self-efficacy level of individuals can also influence career development. Bandura's concept of self-efficacy (1993) suggests that an individual's concept of his or her confidence in performing tasks creates the balance between what the individual knows and the resulting action. An individual's beliefs about his or her ability to accomplish a task may be more influential than the actual ability to complete a given task. Turner and Lapan (2002) applied Social Cognitive Career Theory (Bandura, 1986; Lent, Brown, & Hackett, 1996) and examined the influence of perceived parental support to career self-efficacy. It was reported that parental support accounted for as much as one third to almost one half of their adolescents' career task related confidence. Once again we are reminded of the influence of parents on youth's decisions about future career choices.

These four approaches, Super, Holland, Krumboltz, and Bandura, offer school counselors a philosophical and theoretical knowledge foundation to construct age-appropriate career oriented systems that consider developmental life stages, personality influence, learning experiences, and self-confidence to best prepare today's youth for the careers of tomorrow.

Career Development and the Transformed School Counselor

Without the commitment of school counselors and other educators taking a leadership role and assuming the responsibility for designing and implementing a sequential and integrated career development program, many students will receive little or no career guidance support (Ettinger & Rudolph, 1994; Feller & Davies, 2002). The American School Counselor Association (ASCA) strongly urges school counselors to provide a balance of academic, career, and personal-social development as the foundation of the comprehensive school counseling program (ASCA, 2003; Campbell and Dahir, 1997).

Career development is considered an equal domain in the comprehensive model (ASCA, 2003). Data present a strong case to provide career development for every student. The foundation of school counseling is strongly grounded in vocational guidance, which emerged in the late 1890s and has been a consistent focus of attention since the origins of the profession. Career counseling assists students in acquiring a greater understanding that they have choices and the realization that their behaviors impact decisions. Counseling helps students understand the importance of self-efficacy as they establish a sense of who they are, and initiate the necessary and essential changes to help them achieve their career goals.

At the elementary level, career counseling helps students find their voice and practice decision-making skills. Young students can commit to preferences and separate their likes from their dislikes. At the secondary level, students actively participate in making decisions that affect attitudes and behaviors and ultimately impact future choices.

Using a Systemic Approach to Career Development

Career development is the sum of all of the processes and factors that influence, inform, and impact career choice and career success over one's lifetime. School counselors are committed to ensuring that each student is prepared to move forward to the next step of life, from grade level to grade level, and to life after high school. Career development provides the pathway.

Niles and Harris-Bowlsbey (2002) define career development as "the lifelong psychological and behavioral process as well as the contextual influences shaping one's career over the lifespan" (p. 7). According to Maddy-Bernstein (2000) career development is "the total constellation of psychological, sociological education, physical, economic, and chance factors that combine to influence the nature and significance of work in the total lifespan of any given individual" (p. 2). Theorists have acknowledged that career development is intertwined with personal development (Niles & Goodnough, 1996; Super, Savickas, & Super, 1996).

The career development process crosses the life span and informs and influences various stages of a person's education and personal growth as they seek career satisfaction. Preparing students to select a career goal and guiding them to enroll in the appropriate course work that will lead them to achieve their career goals is essential to their success in a 21st-century world. School counselors provide every student with the necessary help and direction to be successful in school and, ultimately, in life (Cunanan & Maddy-Bernstein, 2000). The need for career development knows no boundaries. Young people growing up in poverty perceive career options differently than more privileged youngsters (Education Trust, 2001a).

Students of privilege may envision themselves in a prestigious 4-year college, while impoverished youth might see themselves thrust into the workplace as soon as they graduate from high school. Cultural norms and family expectations also can influence career goals. School counselors must be knowledgeable of the cultural traditions that could potentially limit a student's choice of options after high school or create a discord between the student and his or her parents or caregiver.

Students with learning and other disabilities are at a higher risk for not completing high school. During the 1999–2000 school year, only 25.5% of students with disabilities graduated from high school with a standard diploma (Office of Special Education Programs, 2000). The graduation rate of course varies by the type of disability, but the data explain that students with any type of disability are limited in their ability to seek a successful career pathway due to a lack of educational opportunities. Research also shows that many high-school students and young adults lacked a clear understanding of their disability and its impact both on career choices and ability to perform a job (Hitchings & Retish, 2000). Students with disabilities found their opportunities restricted at an early age and experienced academic failure, which in turn led to low self-esteem and limited self-knowledge (Michaels, 1997). Despite mandates at the federal and state levels to ensure that all disabled students would participate in career and transition planning, a large number of disabled students were not actively engaged in career development. Many believed they had little control over career decisions and as a result were more likely to drop out (Blackorby & Wagner, 1997). Even those with realistic ambitions seldom were guided to acquire the education or training that would prepare them for appropriate jobs (Kortering & Braziel, 2000).

Every student, regardless of race, culture, socioeconomic status, or learning ability or disability can benefit from a career guidance and counseling program. Educators, teachers, school counselors, and school administrators in partnership with parents or caregivers have a responsibility to support students to ensure that they have all options after high school and find meaningful paths to careers. *Breaking Ranks* (National Association of Secondary School Principals, 1996, 2004) encouraged schools to provide every student with a transitional experience to prepare for life after high school, and recognized the ultimate need for each student to become a contributing member of the community.

The ASCA Model and Career Guidance

Practicing school counselors use the comprehensive school counseling program model to incorporate and integrate career guidance strategies throughout academic, career, and personal-social development. The ASCA model demonstrates that counselors are providing career development and career guidance activities to students, parents, and staff in all four program components: the guidance curriculum, individual student planning, responsive services, and system support (ASCA, 2003).

According to Myrick (2000) career guidance is the constellation of services that focus on personal and career growth and school adjustment. Vocational guidance is the process to assist an individual to choose, enter and/or progress in an occupation. "Guidance is an instructional process in which a student is given information and told how to move progressively toward a personal goal" (Myrick, 1997, pp. 2–3). In a school setting, we use career guidance strategies to involve students at developmentally appropriate stages in career development. These strategies include career awareness, exploration, assessment, and career counseling.

Career awareness   helps students identify the world of options and opportunities that await them. For many students, familiarity with the world of work is limited to the experiences of parents and family members or what awareness they have acquired from television and media. Career awareness helps students connect self-knowledge and information gathering and helps them to see a world of opportunity as they begin to think about their personal and professional futures.

Career exploration offers students opportunities in the context of real-life and hands-on experiences to supplement traditional classroom instruction. Experiences such as connecting school learning with part-time work, as well as project-based learning; career and technical education; mentoring and shadowing experiences; service learning; apprenticeships; internships; and co-op education are motivational and help students become more aware of the world of possibilities.

Career assessment helps students use the information they gain from appraisal of skills, abilities, achievement, and interests to better understand who they are, where are they going, and how they will get there (see Figure 12.7).

School counselors use a variety of achievement, interest, and ability assessments to consult with students, parents, and teachers and help all involved to understand the outcomes of the results and how to use the information in meaningful ways. Assessments can be as simple as a one-page interest survey or as complex as the Armed Services Vocational Aptitude Battery (ASVAB) which takes several hours for a student to complete. Many interest inventories (**Self Directed Search**, the Strong Interest Inventory) and Computer Assisted Career Guidance Systems (Discover, Choices, SIGI-PLUS) are based on Holland's theory and help students identify the relationship between personality type and career preference.

The **Myers-Briggs Type Indicator** (MBTI) is a widely used personality assessment for high-school students, providing feedback about an individual's patterns of behavior. Based on the theory of psychological types by Carl Jung, the MBTI can help students understand their preference in making decisions, organizing one's life, and acquiring information. The MBTI uses four categories of behavior that address the focus of a person's orientation (extraversion or introversion); the way a person gathers information (sensing or by intuition); the way a person makes decisions (by thinking or by feeling); and how a person deals with the outer world (judging or perceiving). The MBTI also helps the student understand personal preferences in relationship to the outer world of people and things or to the inner world of ideas, and this understanding is articulated with career environments that may be best

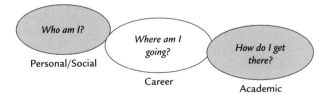

Figure 12.7 Career Assessment.

suited to his or her personality. After the student gathers information, participates in assessments, and engages in exploratory experiences, he or she is ready to create a career plan.

Career planning is an important component of national and state legislative initiatives, such as the School to Work Opportunities Act (U.S. Department of Education, 1994c), and is an important component of state-developed career development standards. The School to Work Opportunities Act recognized that students should begin the career planning process as early as elementary school and encouraged all stakeholders to help students acquire the skills needed to transition from grade level to grade level, and from high school to quality postsecondary and career opportunities. A career plan helps the student establish a focus and a motivation for achievement and can identify the strategies and tasks necessary to accomplish future goals. It guides the student to make decisions about academic preparation, work experience, and the education and training necessary after high school to make successful transitions to the career path of his or her choice.

A career plan can document the results of the assessments in terms of the aptitudes, skills, interests, and personal preferences achieved by each student throughout his or her elementary, middle, and high-school experiences. As part of an annual process to review educational and career goals, students can make necessary adjustments as knowledge and skills are attained and/or interests change.

As the cornerstone of a comprehensive school counseling and career guidance program, the career plan helps school counselors to demonstrate student achievement of the competencies in the National Standards for School Counseling Programs (ASCA, 1997) and/or those in the **National Career Development Guidelines** (1989, 2004). Students, teachers, and parents are even more aware of the knowledge and skills acquired as a result of participating in a school counseling program.

New and emerging technology continues to develop **Computer Assisted Career Guidance Systems** (CACGS) to deliver career awareness, exploration, and career planning across a broad range of student activities and experiences. Computerized systems offer students and adults the ability to explore the world of work, gather information, participate in interest surveys and other career assessments, and help clients with career decision making (Gati, 1996). CACGS assist individuals in making current career decisions as well as improve their capacity to make effective career decisions in the future (Sampson, 1997, p. 6).

Many CACGS use an Internet platform, which offers the ability to easily update materials, immediate feedback, interactive simulations, and data storage (Gore & Leuwerke, 2000).

Getting Started in Career Planning

Resources abound to help school counselors in their career planning work with elementary, middle, and high-school students. Planning for Life, a career planning initiative, was a collaboration between the United States Army and the American

Counselors Making a Difference

Meet the School Counselors of Charleston County

A Career Planning Commitment to Improve Student Success

Throughout our school district, the administration and interpretation of a battery of career assessment instruments for all eighth graders helps students, counselors, teachers, and parents identify strengths and weaknesses and areas of career interests. Teachers are better able to align lesson plans with students' interests based on this assessment. School counselors use this assessment to help each student select the appropriate high-school courses for the career/educational 4-year plan. Parental involvement is encouraged through evening workshops, PTA meetings, and individual conferences.

Students have made the connection between school and work. Eighty-two percent of the seniors surveyed in 2001–2002 felt that work-based learning experiences should be a part of the curriculum. Over the past 3 years, the percentage of students participating in work-based learning experiences such as apprenticeships, cooperative education, internships, and job shadowing has increased. In 1999–2000, 51.5% of the seniors participated in a work-based learning experience; in 2000–2001, 62.1%, and in 2001–2002, 70%. Students who have enrolled in the appropriate academic courses as well as in elective courses that lead to a definitive career pathway are more likely to remain in school, attend school on a regular basis, and see the importance of continuing their education after high school.

The student success rate can be measured in how well the students feel they are prepared for their postsecondary plans. Each year in May, seniors complete the *Annual Survey for Graduating Seniors*. Over the past 3 years the percentage of students who felt they were prepared for their postsecondary plans has risen from 43.3% (2000) to 47.4% (2001) to 51.8% (2002). In 2000, 71.7% of the students planned to continue their education in some type of school or training program, whereas that number increased in 2001 to 88.3% and again increased in 2002 to 91.9%.

Through career planning, our commitment to accountability and school improvement is significant. By ninth grade, each student must identify a career cluster, which emphasizes both academic and applied skills. This structure supports accountability and makes learning relevant. The curriculum will be aligned with current workplace needs to include academic, social, and applied content, and will be appropriate to all educational institutions. Because each student's career plan is individualized, it helps to guide course-work selection, motivates learning, aligns postsecondary planning with educational goals, and ultimately prepares students for career success. The school counselors in the Charleston County School District, working collaboratively with teachers, administrators, parents, and community members, ensure that "no child is left behind."

From *Planning for Life: A Resource Guide for Counselors*, (2001). Reprinted with permission by Mary Zilko.

School Counselor Association to promote the involvement of students, families, business, labor, and educators in partnerships to enable youth to seek successful futures. Planning for Life resource guide (Dahir, 2001) was promoted by the American School Counselor Association as a model comprehensive career planning system. The six essential elements are vision, commitment, comprehensiveness, collaboration, program management, and program evaluation.

Vision describes what students will accomplish as a result of an effective career guidance and planning program and how it contributes to the school's mission.

It is important that school and community members participate in the creation of the vision statement and that it is communicated to all stakeholders.

Commitment is essential to gather the necessary resources and supports for the career guidance and planning program by the school district, family, and community. The entire school faculty is supportive in integrating the career guidance and planning process in curriculum initiatives. Business community members can participate in a variety of activities such as advisory boards, career fairs, and in mentoring and shadowing opportunities. Parents and caregivers are also critical to the success of their children's career planning, but the most important commitment must come from the students themselves as they take ownership of their career plans.

Comprehensiveness is the degree to which every student participates in the career planning process as part of the school counseling and career guidance program.

A comprehensive school counseling program will include a career planning process that involves every student and will be based on a comprehensive set of outcomes or competencies. Career planning activities are conducted at all grade levels and are explored without limitations for all students regardless of gender, race, or physical condition. A variety of formal and informal individual assessments will help students gather accurate information about their interests, abilities, and achievement. Most important, each student has a written career plan.

Collaboration is shared ownership by stakeholders in the career planning process and demonstrates the participation of all stakeholders. The roles for each partner are defined to clearly present everyone's contribution in the career planning process. Developing an advisory committee that includes all stakeholders can help to review and revise the career planning program. Administrative support will ensure that career guidance activities are integrated into curricula and other school activities. Partnerships with business and community agencies can enhance student opportunities for career exploration and present opportunities are available for parents and caregivers to review and discuss their child's career plan.

Program management is an organizational tool that ensures the effective use of resources in the coordination, articulation, and transition of the program from one grade level to the next. There should be a description of the management procedures to determine who is ultimately responsible for implementing each aspect of the career guidance and career planning program. Annual program revisions are made in the program based on needs assessments and feedback. Stakeholders are regularly informed of the status of the program through various forms of communication.

Program evaluation   is the degree to which the program provides evidence of success. Program evaluation ensures that the program has accomplished what it has intended to do. There should be evidence of feedback and an ongoing process for revisions to ensure the quality of the career planning program. The evaluation of student achievement of specific competencies is based on documentation and evidence. There is a process in place to revise the program annually based on evaluation results.

Connecting With Standards and Competencies

Student attitudes, skills, and knowledge are the foundation for the comprehensive model (ASCA, 2003). The majority of career development and career guidance programs use either the National Career Development Guidelines (1989; 2004) or the National Standards for School Counseling Programs (1997) to select the competencies that define what students should know and be able to do.

The National Career Development Guidelines

Recognizing the benefits of a systematic career guidance program across the life span, the National Occupational Information Coordinating Committee (NOICC) designed the National Career Development Guidelines (NOICC, 1989). These guidelines offered the counseling and career guidance community a framework to help students and adults acquire the skills necessary for success in the workplace. Through a developmental and organized process, adults and students could explore their interests, apply acquired skills and abilities, discover the many educational and occupational opportunities and options available, become aware of the education and training required for their career choice, and begin to develop and manage their career pathway. The National Career Development Guidelines help students and adults to

- understand the relationship between educational achievement and career planning;
- understand the need for positive attitudes toward work and learning;
- acquire skills to locate, evaluate, and interpret career information;

- acquire skills to prepare to seek, obtain, maintain, and change jobs;
- understand how societal needs and functions influence the nature and structure of work.

(NOICC, 1989/2004)

The guidelines address three major competency areas: self-knowledge, educational and occupational exploration, and career planning.

Self-knowledge   guides students to become competent in their knowledge and understanding of self-concept, acquire skills to interact with others, and to recognize and understand the importance of growth and change. As students transition into adulthood, they learn and apply these skills to maintain a positive self-concept and demonstrate behaviors that are effective at home and in the workplace.

Educational and occupational exploration   helps students to acquire competency in making connections between educational achievement and career planning. Students acquire skills in locating, evaluating, and interpreting career information, and learn to apply this information to seeking, obtaining, maintaining, and changing jobs.

Career planning   provides students with knowledge of the career planning process as well as support to make the decisions that align their educational goals with career goals. Students combine what they have learned about self-knowledge and the results of their educational and occupational exploration to develop a plan that will help them make informed decisions about their present and the future. Students begin to understand the influence of affective and academic skill development in the context of life-career choices.

The National Career Development Guidelines (1989) were carefully examined for their applicability and relationship during the development stages of the National Standards for School Counseling Programs (ASCA, 1997). The guidelines offered a strong foundation for the academic, career, and personal-social domains.

The Career Development Domain of the National Standards for School Counseling Programs

Comprehensive, developmental national standards–based school counseling programs employ strategies to support student achievement and success, provide career awareness, open doors to opportunities, encourage self-awareness, foster interpersonal skills, and help all students acquire skills for life. "The standards assist students in acquiring and using life-long skills through the development of academic, career, self awareness and interpersonal skills" (Campbell & Dahir, 1997, p. 9).

The three national standards for career development guide school counselors to implement school counseling program strategies and activities that will help students

Box 12.1

Self-Knowledge

Elementary

- Knowledge of the importance of self-concept
- Skills to interact with others
- Awareness of the importance of growth and change

Middle/Junior High School

- Knowledge of the influence of a positive self-concept
- Skills to interact with others
- Knowledge of the importance of growth and change

High School

- Understanding the influence of a positive self-concept
- Skills to interact positively with others
- Understanding the impact of growth and development

Adult

- Skills to maintain a positive self-concept
- Skills to maintain effective behaviors
- Understanding developmental changes and transitions

Educational and Occupational Exploration

Elementary

- Awareness of the benefits of educational achievement
- Awareness of the relationship between work and learning
- Skills to understand and use career information
- Awareness of the importance of personal responsibility and good work habits
- Awareness of how work relates to the needs and functions of society

(continued)

Box 12.1 continued

Middle/Junior High School

- Knowledge of the benefits of educational achievement to career opportunities
- Understanding the relationship between work and learning
- Skills to locate, understand, and use career information
- Knowledge of skills necessary to seek and obtain jobs
- Understanding how work relates to the needs and functions of the economy and society

High School

- Understanding the relationship between educational achievement and career planning
- Understanding the need for positive attitudes toward work and learning
- Skills to locate, evaluate, and interpret career information
- Skills to prepare to seek, obtain, maintain, and change jobs
- Understanding how societal needs and functions influence the nature and structure of work

Adult

- Skills to enter and participate in education and training
- Skills to participate in work and lifelong learning
- Skills to locate, evaluate, and interpret career information
- Skills to prepare to seek, obtain, maintain, and change jobs
- Understanding how the needs and functions of society influence the nature and structure of work

Career Planning

Elementary

- Understanding how to make decisions
- Awareness of the interrelationship of life roles
- Awareness of different occupations and changing male/female roles
- Awareness of the career planning process

Middle/Junior High School

- Skills to make decisions
- Knowledge of the interrelationship of life roles

Box 12.1 continued

- Knowledge of different occupations and changing male/female roles
- Understanding the process of career planning

High School

- Skills to make decisions
- Understanding the interrelationship of life roles
- Understanding the continuous changes in male/female roles
- Skills in career planning

Adult

- Skills to make decisions
- Understanding the impact of work on individual and family life
- Understanding the continuing changes in male/female roles
- Skills to make career transitions

National Occupational Information Coordinating Committee (NOICC), U.S. Department of Labor (1989/2004)

acquire attitudes, knowledge, and skills to successfully transition from grade to grade, from school to postsecondary education, and ultimately to the world of work. Career development activities include the employment of strategies to achieve future career success and job satisfaction, as well as fostering understanding of the relationship between personal qualities, education and training, and future career goals. The three career development standards are:

Standard A.   Students will acquire the skills to investigate the world of work in relation to knowledge of self and to make informed career decisions.

Standard B.   Students will employ strategies to achieve future career success and satisfaction.

Standard C.   Students will understand the relationship between personal qualities, education and training, and the world of work (ASCA, 1997).

School counselors are encouraged to identify competencies for their students that will help them developmentally acquire the attitudes, knowledge, and skills that are integral to a career development program. The standards and competencies encourage students to participate in a series of structured activities that result in applying decision-making and planning skills in building their futures. The competencies selected should involve students in all aspects of a comprehensive career guidance system, which includes career awareness, exploration, assessment, counseling, and planning.

Thus, by the time a student graduates from high school, she or he should be able to formulate and bring into focus tentative career goals, select the appropriate academic and career/technical postsecondary options, and identify the levels of competence, certification and/or achievement necessary to reach her or his goals.

Applying School Counseling Skills to Career Development

Career development is often the component of the school counseling program that receives the least attention. Every child dreams of success; school counselors are ethically obligated to focus our energies and help every child identify the path to success to realize their dreams (Schwallie-Giddis & Kobylarz, 2000). Transformed school counselors use leadership, advocacy, teaming and collaboration, the use of data, and integrating technology in a meaningful context (Education Trust, 1997).

School counselors using their leadership skills ensure that all students acquire the career awareness and career planning skills to make the connection between today's success in school and ensuring all options after high school.

There is an endless array of career development and career guidance options and opportunities available to school counselors to motivate students to strive to reach their future goals. Oftentimes, it is hard for counselors to understand why some students just don't seem to "get it"! Why can't they see the connection between education and future success? Cultural traditions can impact students' selection of options and opportunities. Gender matters, whether in breaking down parental or community biases or working closely with a student needing support to choose a nontraditional career path. Parents, peer pressure, and how confident a child is about his/her ability to be successful significantly influence an individual's career choice.

Making connections is the key to impacting future choice between and among students, their counselors, teachers, peers, and family, and most important, in helping students see the relevance of school to their dreams and aspirations. School is a place for youth to exert their influence and establish an identity. School is a place to explore, learn, apply, and acquire academic and affective attitudes, knowledge, and skills. School counselors face the challenge of helping students meet expectations of the higher academic standards and simultaneously assist students to successfully be prepared to become productive and contributing members of our society. Career motivation contributes strongly to a student's willingness to work a little harder, put forth a little more effort, and better understand the relevance of school to future opportunity. Comprehensive school counseling programs that include a strong career development and career guidance component will help our students to

- understand who they are, their interests, motivation, and ability;
- develop skills in the career planning process;
- establish career goals;

- become involved in career awareness and career exploration activities;
- visualize a positive future;
- make connections between personal qualities, achievement, the motivation to get an education, and dreams of success.

Career development can no longer be put on the back burner. According to the national standards, it is equally as important as academic and personal social development in the work of school counselors with students. School counselors who motivate students to discover their passions and work with them to develop goals and strategies invaluably contribute to helping students realize their dreams.

TechTools

When you become a school counselor, use the power of technology to maximize the efficiency and effectiveness of career planning.

- Use the Internet to demonstrate to students and parents the wealth of career awareness and career development information available on the World Wide Web.
- There are many free career exploration tools, such as www.Careerzone.net, that are appropriate in your work with students. Identify your state department of labor's website; this is often a good place to start.
- If your school does not have the resources to build a career center, consider creating a virtual career center. Link this to the school counseling department website.
- When you enter the field of school counseling, you can stay current in your research by visiting electronic journals such as *The Journal of Technology in Counseling, 1*(1). Available online: http://jtc.colstate.edu/vol1_1/advocacy.htm
- Design an electronic newsletter about career planning for parents and students.
- Look on the NACAC website for resources to help you prepare and present a multimedia presentation on career or college planning to an audience of students, or parents, or faculty. The National Association of College Admissions Counseling (NACAC) can be found at http://www.nacac.com

Internet Resources

Bureau of Labor Statistics: http://stats.bls.gov/opub/rylf/rylfhome.htm

My eCareers 101: http://www.MyeCareers101.com

U.S. Department of Labor: http://www.dol.gov

ACT: Information for Life's Transitions: http://www.act.org/

Into Careers: http://www.Intocareers.com

College Xpress: www.collegeexpress.com

Focus: http://focuscareer.com/

Hobson's Collegeview: http://www.collegeview.com/

Journal of Technology and Counseling: http://jtc.colstate.edu

My Future: http://myfuture.com/

National Career Development Association: http://ncda.org/about/polccc.html

Next Steps: http://www.nextsteps.org/

SIGI Plus: http://www.ets.org/

U.S. News and World Report: http://www.usnews.com/usnews/edu/eduhome.htm

School Counselor Casebook: Voices From the Field

The Scenario Reviewed

Two eighth-grade students stop by your office to request that they be allowed to drop the honors program. They explain that their reason for wanting to drop the program isn't because the work is too difficult; they just don't know why they need the honors program when the regular grade-level courses seem like a perfectly fine option. These students had already talked to their homeroom teacher about dropping the courses and were told that honors classes would further their opportunities for college. However, the teacher could not tell them why. One of the students said to you that because she wants to study computer graphics at the regional Tech Center next year, she doesn't see a need to worry about college.

Both students seem to be completely uninformed about career options, why postsecondary education is important, and what it will take to succeed in high school. You know that very little attention is paid to career and postsecondary awareness in the middle school. What would you do?

A Practitioner's Approach

Here's how a practicing school counselor responded to the school counselor casebook challenge:

Students, regardless of grade level, need to have a sense of where they're going, and what the outcome of their labors will provide. Apparently, a career component of their educational studies is lacking. After listening to them carefully, I would ask them about their goals in life. I would offer them (and their classmates) a career assessment, via the technology department. If my school didn't have a specific career assessment tool in place, I would use one of the many free career assessment programs on the Internet. If the students did not have a career profile in their permanent files, I would talk with my colleagues immediately to put a formalized career program into place for the whole building. I would work toward having each and every student create a career portfolio, which would identify every student's strengths, interests, and abilities, with the goal of eventually providing them with a list of career choices and college opportunities.

Because so many of the students' classmates also seem to be confused about the reasons for being accelerated, I would ask the classroom teachers if I could utilize a class period in order to make a presentation. It would be a "4 years and beyond" program, in order to let the students know where their studies will lead them. I would utilize a PowerPoint presentation to help the students to see how, if they continue in their course of study, they will eventually be eligible for AP courses. I would stress the benefits of taking college courses at the high-school level, including issues of cost benefits, and also discuss the whole college process, an explanation of GPA, and weighted class rank.

Additionally, I would organize an evening group meeting for students and parents of accelerated/honors students, in order to explain the benefits of an accelerated program. I would invite their teachers to attend. I would present the same information to the parents that I offered to the students in class.

I would ask teachers to integrate a college/career component into their program. For example, based on the outcome of their career assessments, I would ask English teachers to incorporate a graded assignment on possible career opportunities within their targeted areas of abilities and interests. I would ask math teachers to assign a project on calculating the salary schedules of various career choices. I would ask technology teachers to incorporate career and college searches into the curriculum, and/or allow the counselors to present websites and college/career information in their classes. This information would be printed out and placed in each student's career portfolio.

During annual student-parent conferences, I would review the career information in the student's file. I would ask the students and parents to complete a "brag sheet," focusing on perceived strengths, interests, and abilities. I would encourage parents to talk to their children about college and career choices.

I would orchestrate a business advisory group, with business and community members, to work closely with staff in order to provide shadowing, mentoring, internship, and paid work experience in the workplace. This group would be charged with running an annual career fair for all students. Career fair participants would receive certificates of appreciation for their efforts. Alumni of the school would be the target group to represent various career paths; however, anyone willing to present would be encouraged to attend.

Furthermore, I would run a voluntary lunchtime group called "Career Exploration." Stressing that careers can happen by choice or by chance, I would encourage students to take charge of their futures by making informed choices. The lunch groups would run in 8-week sessions, with a culminating pizza party, or the food of their choice.

Collaboration is key to the success of making this happen. I would consult with all of the counselors throughout the district and make plans to facilitate a districtwide plan to incorporate college and career lessons on every grade level and get the teachers actively involved. A career portfolio would follow the students throughout their school career and would be examined and reassessed each year during our annual parent-student conferences.

The ultimate goal is to help students realize what their dreams are, what they need to do in order to get there, and how this will assist them in enjoying success in their lives.

Mary Zilko is the school counseling coordinator in the Amityville School District on Long Island. She has served as school counselor at the middle and high-school levels, and has worked at the college level as director of student services. She is certified by New York State in school counseling and school district administration and is a National Board Certified Counselor.

Chapter Summary

The Global Economy and the Work Force

Increased academic expectations, pressures from the global economy, changing technology, and the continuous shifts in societal issues and values impact and influence today's schools. Preparing students to select career goals and guiding them to enroll in the appropriate course work that will lead them to achieve their career goals is essential to their success in a 21st-century world.

Although no one can predict with complete accuracy which jobs will exist in the future and which will not, school counselors can communicate to students that jobs with a prediction of decline will need workers to replace those who leave the labor force through attrition and retirement. Data also strongly suggest that education pays.

Career Decision Influencers

Youth are particularly sensitive to the experiences of those who surround and support them. The circumstances and influences that students face undeniably influences the actions they take about their future. Key influencers include parents, educators, and peers.

Many students struggle with weak academic preparation, little career guidance, and few workplace experiences. Without the commitment of school counselors and other educators to their responsibility to design and implement sequential and integrated career development programs, many students will receive little or no career guidance support.

Theoretical Underpinnings

Career counseling is guided by theory, which provides a point of reference from which the counselor develops a personal perspective of human growth, development, and behavior. Career counselors also recognize and choose the appropriate orientations, strategies, theories, and approaches according to the models applied and the assistance that a student needs.

Career Development and the Transformed School Counselor

School counselors can take a leadership role and assume the responsibility for designing and implementing a sequential and integrated career development program. The American School Counselor Association urges school counselors to provide a balance of academic, career, and personal-social development as the foundation of the comprehensive school counseling program.

Using a Systemic Approach to Career Development

All educators have a responsibility to support students to ensure that they have explored all options available after high school and that they identify meaningful paths to careers. School counselors can provide every student with a comprehensive transitional experience, and recognize the ultimate need for each student to become a contributing member of the community.

The ASCA Model and Career Guidance

Practicing school counselors use a comprehensive school counseling program model to incorporate and integrate career guidance strategies into academic, career, and personal-social development. Career awareness, exploration, assessment, planning, and counseling are strategies used to deliver career guidance in a comprehensive and systematic manner.

Getting Started in Career Planning

It takes the commitment of the entire school community to value the important role that career planning plays in academic and affective development. Career development is a life skill that must be valued as part of the lifelong learning process. Involving all stakeholders shows community commitment and support to prepare today's students for an ever-changing and complex world.

Connecting With Standards and Competencies

The majority of school counseling programs use the National Career Development Guidelines (1989, 2004) or the National Standards for School Counseling Programs (1997) to identify specific competencies for student career awareness and development.

Applying School Counseling Skills to Career Development

Leadership, advocacy, teaming and collaboration, the use of data, and integrating technology are essential skills to every aspect of the school counseling program. School counselors face the challenge of helping students meet the expectations of higher academic standards and simultaneously assist students to become productive and contributing members of our society.

Key Terms

Computer Assisted Career Guidance Systems p. 346
Career awareness p. 344
Career counseling p. 340
Career development p. 332
Career guidance p. 332
Career planning p. 345
Life Span–Life Space p. 340
Myers-Briggs Type Indicator p. 345
National Career Development Guidelines p. 346
Self Directed Search p. 345

Learning Extensions

1. What career project might you engage your high-school students in that would help them identify what they want to be doing 2 years from now, 5 years from now, and 10 years from now?

2. What attitudes, knowledge, and skills are essential for your students to acquire in order to achieve their educational and career plans?

3. Your school is situated in a suburban community, in the shadow of a large metropolitan area. You ask your fourth graders what they know about the differences between working in the city and working in the suburbs. You find out that they know very little except the fact that many of their parents work in the city. How can you use this information to help them understand the influence of lifestyle on career choice?

4. Your principal asked you to attend a local community partnership meeting. As you look around the table you begin to realize the diversity of professional and technical skill represented at the meeting. You are thinking how your elementary students would benefit from exposure to the bigger picture of the world of work. What will you do?

5. Your school is located in a small town in a rural community. Main Street is only 4 blocks long, yet there is quite a good variety of shops and services represented there. How can you use your community resources to help your seventh graders become more aware of career opportunities?

6. Service learning can have a strong influence on building character. How can it also influence career choice?

7. Your district has asked the school counselor to develop a career plan. You need to decide if you want to develop a plan that will work from K to 12 or if you want to create a different plan for each grade level. What are the key elements that need to be included? There are many samples for you to look at on the World Wide Web; there is no reason not to investigate what career plans exist and how they may inform your thinking. Draft a career plan and present it to your colleagues.

8. Identify and write a descriptive summary for eight websites that can be used for career guidance and career planning for the grade level you want to work with. To support your career guidance program, make sure that you look at and research these four categories: career awareness, career exploration, career assessment, and career counseling.

Chapter 13

Promoting a Safe and Respectful Learning Environment

Chapter Objectives

By the time you have completed this chapter, you should be able to:

- Understand safe school concerns facing educators today.
- Discuss techniques for preventing or de-escalating violent situation in schools.
- Discuss behaviors within a developmental and social context that are early warning signs of potential violence or other troubling behaviors in children.

- Understand the value of conflict mediation and resolution programs for students.
- Discuss strategies to prevent or de-escalate bullying in the school environment.
- Become familiar with the legal issues that impact school safety and a respectful environment.
- Explore ways of integrating character education.
- Develop strategies to create a safe and respectful school environment.

School Counselor Casebook: Getting Started

The Scenario

The conversation at today's team meeting focused on a small group of disengaged students. Two of the teachers commented that the students were in different classes and that they were antisocial except with their group. None of the teachers noticed any gang indicia or color display. The social studies teacher spoke up to say that even though she does not have specifics, she is certain she overheard a conversation in the cafeteria in which a few of these disengaged students were "threatening" other students. She turns to you, the school counselor, and asks, "What should we do about this?"

Thinking About Solutions

As you read this chapter, imagine yourself as the school counselor in this situation and think about how you might answer that question. Keep the following questions in mind: Are the students described as disengaged by their teachers a reason for concern? What kind of investigation would this "overheard" conversation warrant? What ethical and legal obligations would you have to investigate? When you come to the end of the chapter, you will have the opportunity to see how your ideas compare with a practicing school counselor's approach.

Seeking a Safer Learning Environment

Nationwide, there have been 32 targeted acts of **school violence** resulting in homicide since 1985 (U.S. Department of Education & U.S. Secret Service, 2002a). Violence in America's schools cuts across all neighborhoods (U.S. Department of Education & U.S. Secret Service, 2002b). Although media attention on school violence often portrays violence as the reflection of inner-city norms, this is Hollywood's interpretation. Of the 28 reported cases of school shootings between 1982 and 2001, all but one occurred in a rural or suburban school setting (Kimmel, 2003). Schools nationwide seek assurances that targeted incidents will not occur in their community, whether urban, rural, or suburban.

Although public perception is that schools are no longer safe—and the media often present a picture that would indicate violence is on the rise—the fact is that targeted acts of violence are the exception to the rule and have been decreasing in number (U.S. Department of Education Office of Safe and Drug-Free Schools, 2003; U.S. Department of Education & U.S. Secret Service, 2002a).

The *Annual Report on School Safety* (U.S. Department of Education & U.S. Department of Justice, 2003) has declared that incidents of violence in schools are declining. In 2002, 90% of the nation's schools reported no serious violent crime, while 43% stated that they experienced no crime at all (U.S. Departments of Education & Justice, 2003).

Nevertheless, public policymakers, police officials, school administrators, and parents continue to search for explanations about violence in schools. The locations in which high-profile school shootings have occurred are generally perceived as those in which young people are given inadequate support in finding their own way in a difficult world (U.S. Department of Education & U.S. Secret Service, 2002a). Schools do not always present themselves as compassionate institutions. When parents become less stringent about discipline at home and in the school, the standards bar is lowered on "acceptable" moral and social behavior; this results in attitudinal and behavioral differences in children and youth (Shafii & Shafii, 2001).

The Challenge for Educators

The Challenge: All children need a safe environment in which to learn and achieve; one free of fear and intimidation, for teachers as well as children.

The Solution: Ensure a safe and orderly school by implementing programs that protect students and teachers, encourage discipline and personal responsibility, and combat illegal drugs.
— *U.S. Department of Education Office of Safe and Drug-Free Schools, 2002*

Goal 4 of the No Child Left Behind Act (2001) reminds educators that every school needs to be safe and drug free. Character education programs are an important component of the implementation of No Child Left Behind (NCLB) and have become part of the solution for addressing concerns about **school climate**. The act encourages laws to be aggressively enforced and states that the first job of government is to protect its citizens. It further requires states departments of education and public schools to report on school safety to the public; provide protection to teachers and educators so they can teach and maintain order; and anticipate the potential for violence (NCLB, 2001).

Educators and communities have been working diligently to ensure that their schools are an emotionally and physically safe haven for students. A growing interest in character education is an acknowledgment that schools also believe that principles such as responsibility, integrity, trustworthiness, care, kindness, and respect are foundational to creating positive school climate and reducing incidents of aggression (Likona, 2004). The personal-social development standards complement character education efforts and emphasize respect for self and others, taking responsibility, and personal safety. School counselors, as part of this collaborative effort, play a vital role in both prevention and intervention efforts.

School Violence Defined

School violence can be defined as encompassing a wide range of activities, including assaults with or without weapons; physical fights; threats or destructive acts other than physical fights; robbery; harassment; dating violence; molestation; rape; bullying; hostile or threatening remarks between groups of students; and gang violence (Fischer & Kettl, 2001). **Bullying,** the most common form of school violence, is on the rise (U.S. Department of Education, 2002).

One quarter of all middle school children were either victims or perpetrators (sometimes both) of chronic bullying that included threatening, name-calling, punching, slapping, sneering, and jeering (U.S. Department of Health and Human Services, 2002). Experts in aggressive behavior believe there is no easy way to stamp out bullying (Beale & Scott, 2001).

Sexual harassment has become an issue of national attention as a result of survey research that revealed that 81% of the students, both girls and boys, had received unwanted sexual attention in school (American Association of University Women, 1993). The updated *Hostile Hallways* study (American Association of University Women, 2001) concurred that the problem continues to be pervasive, with 83% of the girls and 79% of the boys reporting that they were victims of sexual harassment. In 1986, the Equal Employment Opportunity Commission (EEOC) extended the definition of sexual harassment from Title IX legislation (1972) to include sexual advances, request for sexual favors, verbal or physical conduct of a sexual nature when submission to such conduct is a term or condition of an individual's academic advancement, or creating an environment that is intimidating, hostile, or offensive, impacting the academic environment (EEOC, 1986).

This definition has been extended by the Office for Civil Rights (1997) to include a hostile environment that is severe or pervasive enough to interfere with a student's education. The implications of sexual harassment provide school counselors with the legal muscle to bring the problem to the forefront of a school's attention. The Supreme Court decision in *Davis v. Monroe County Board of Education,* (1999) found the school district liable for severe, persistent, and pervasive incidences of sexual harassment if there is deliberate indifference. The Office of Civil

Rights (OCR) requires that each school district, as part of Title IX compliance, have in place specific policies and procedure to address sexual harassment (OCR, 2001).

Educators and school counselors have a responsibility to understand youth behavior and establish a context that separates the healthy, normal growing-up behaviors from those that are deviant, that defy school policies or the law, and that can result in a threatening situation. Educators and parents are often challenged to differentiate between students' experimentation in their attempt to establish a personal identity and the demonstration of truly risky behavior that can lead to antisocial and violent action. For example, should adults respond differently to the student who has a "short fuse" and "hangs out" with known substance users than they respond to the student who is academically on track and active in school events but has dyed his hair and pierced his tongue?

Experimentation is a natural part of growing up, and seeking independence is a normal developmental stage for adolescents. When a teen's interests and styles reflect popular peer-group standards, it is usually not a cause for alarm. When combined with falling grades, truancy, alcohol consumption, or other aberrant behaviors, the student's adoption of tattoos, body piercing, and bizarre clothing can be a call for help. Teachers, administrators, parents, and school counselors address inappropriate behavior every day. As with every preceding generation, behavior and appearances that vary from the norm can be seen as incongruous, and oftentimes the typical response is to punish and exclude students (Skiba & Peterson, 1999).

It is equally important to differentiate between a **disruptive student** and a violent student. A disruptive student is one who interferes with the educational process or a teacher's authority over the students in the classroom (U.S. Department of Education & U.S. Department of Justice, 2003). Behaviors can range from the more innocent disruptions, such as frequently strolling into class late, or arguing with the teacher, or constantly shouting out. In contrast, the student who is violent commits an intentional act of aggression against a teacher, another school employee, or another student. The violent student may possess or threaten to use a gun, knife, or other dangerous weapon, to damage or destroy school district or personal property (U.S. Departments of Education & Justice, 2003). Both situations require the intervention of school personnel, including school counselors. Intervention is necessary to maintain the school as a peaceful learning environment and to keep students out of harm's way (Dwyer, Osher, & Warger, 1998).

The Etiology of School Violence

Schools can successfully identify students at risk of violent behaviors when effective prevention measures are put in place (U.S. Department of Education & U.S. Department of Justice, 2003). Research has shown that the first steps toward preventing violence are to identify and understand the factors that place youth at risk for violent victimization and perpetration (National Center for Injury Prevention and Control, 2002).

Table 13.1 Factors Contributing to Youths at Risk of Violent Behavior

Individual	Family	Peer/School	Neighborhood
History of early aggression; beliefs supportive of violence; social-cognitive deficits; hyperactivity, restlessness, risk taking; beliefs and attitudes favorable to deviant or antisocial behavior.	Poor monitoring or supervision of children; exposure to violence; parental drug/alcohol abuse; poor emotional attachment to parents or caregivers; child maltreatment; parent criminality.	Associate with peers engaged in high-risk or problem behavior; low commitment to school; academic failure; frequent school transitions; truancy and/or dropping out; gang membership.	Poverty and diminished economic opportunity; high levels of transiency and family disruption; exposure to violence; availability of drugs and firearms.

Source: National Center for Injury Prevention and Control (2002).

The greater the number of **risk factors** to which an individual is exposed, the greater is the probability that the individual will engage in violent behavior (Hawkins et al., 2000). These contributing factors are translated into the attitudes and behaviors of students that are considered antisocial and impact school climate. Risk factors include these:

Alienation   Students who feel alienated usually perceive a lack of genuine love from significant others in their lives (Pollack, 1998). Alienated students may turn to gang involvement to provide an environment of "belonging" (Goldstein & Kodluboy, 1998).

Depression and Anxiety   Children who are consistently sad, anxious, moody or negative may be experiencing the symptoms of an emotional problem (Shafii & Shafii, 1992). Suicide is one of the leading causes of death among adolescents.

Destructive Behavior   When a child hurts himself or others, it's a red flag that she or he needs help. Destructive behavior includes violent temper tantrums, fighting, threats, hurting animals, vandalism, setting fires, and being fascinated with weapons (Lowry, Powell, Kann, Collins, Kolbe, 1998).

Gang Involvement   Adolescents and teens seek gang membership for affiliation and a sense of belonging. However, the community views gangs as engaging in activities that are intolerable, illegitimate, criminal, or a combination thereof (Goldstein & Kodluboy, 1998).

Manipulative Behavior   Children who have the ability to manipulate a situation know what to say, and when and where to say it. Respect is selective, and although students may appear to be obedient to authority figures, they are poised to intimidate the weak and powerless (Sandhu, 2000).

Peer Problems Normal teens focus on their friends. In fact, their peer group often becomes more important than their family. When a teenager is a loner, it may be a sign that something is seriously amiss (Bluestein, 2001).

Bias and Prejudice Attitudes of bias or prejudice may lead to involvement in hateful behaviors. Hate-induced activities can lead to violence that threatens and intimidates all students. Hate may be directed at ethnic minorities or people with disabilities, may surface in religious discrimination or gender-based bias, or may target sexual minorities who are gay or lesbian (Teaching Tolerance, 2003).

Use of Drugs Over the past two decades, researchers have tried to identify the factors that differentiate those who use drugs from those who do not. Prevention of

Table 13.2 Early and Imminent Warning Signs of Violent Behavior

Early Warning Signs	*Imminent Warning Signs*
Social withdrawal	Serious physical fighting with peers or family members
Excessive feelings of isolation and being alone	Severe destruction of property
Excessive feelings of rejection	Severe rage for seemingly minor reasons
Being a victim of violence	Detailed threats of lethal violence
Feelings of being picked on and persecuted	Possession and/or use of firearms and other weapons
Low school interest and poor academic performance	Other self-injurious behaviors or threats of suicide
Expression of violence in writings and drawings	Has a detailed plan to harm others
Uncontrolled anger	
Patterns of impulsive and chronic hitting, intimidating, and bullying behavior	
History of discipline problems	
Past history of violent and aggressive behavior	
Intolerance for differences and prejudicial attitudes	
Drug use and alcohol use	
Affiliation with gangs	
Inappropriate access to, possession of, and use of firearms	
Serious threats of violence	

Source: Early Warning, Timely Response: A Guide to Safe Schools (U.S. Department of Education, 1998).

drug use, which is related to violent behavior, is based on identifying and reducing risk factors and strengthening protective factors. Risk factors are associated with greater inclination toward drug use; protective factors are associated with lessened inclination for drug use. Protective factors include bonding, healthy beliefs, and clear standards (National Institute on Drug Abuse, 1997). The individual who possesses the protective factors will be more resilient, prevent problems, and promote a healthy lifestyle (Hawkins et al., 2000).

Educators are better prepared to act with purpose to create a safer environment when they have a better sense of the warning signs that can place students at risk for potentially engaging in violent victimization and perpetration. Research confirms that most children who are troubled show multiple **early warning signs** (Hawkins, Farrington, & Catalano, 1998). Factors such as low educational achievement, low interest in education, dropping out of school, and truancy are seen as potential contributors to criminal and violent behavior (National Center for Injury Prevention and Control, 2002).

Early Warning, Timely Response: A Guide to Safe Schools (U.S. Department of Education, 1998) heightens the awareness of educators to the behaviors and attitudes that students at risk of violent behavior present. The early and **imminent warning signs** are research based and offer guidance to educators and stakeholders to identify the factors that can negatively impact individuals and/or groups of students and school climate.

Contributing to a Safe and Respectful School Environment

Educators and communities need to work diligently to ensure that their schools are an emotionally and physically safe haven for students. A growing interest in character education is an acknowledgment that schools also believe that principles such as responsibility, integrity, trustworthiness, care, kindness, and respect are foundational to creating positive school climate and reducing incidents of aggression (Likona, 2004). The personal-social development standards complement character education efforts and emphasize respect for self and others, taking responsibility, and personal safety. School counselors, as part of this collaborative effort, play a vital role in both prevention and intervention efforts.

School counselors as leaders and advocates can motivate and collaborate and are called upon to join their fellow educators in creating and maintaining a safe and respectful school environment. Sandhu (2000) offered school counselors suggestions within their realm of influence to contribute to developing and maintaining a safe and respectful environment:

- Proactively reach out to all students for primary prevention and to maximize every student's development.
- Collaborate and team with teachers to develop sensitivities about students who appear alienated or disaffected.

- Consult with teachers on the characteristics of the warning signs of troubled students and lend support to teachers to help them cope with difficult students in their classrooms.
- Engage all stakeholders in the process to comprehensively address the problem.
- Develop strong relationships with students who have been victims of violence themselves or who inflicted violence on others.

Glasser (2000b) reminds us that students who are alienated can be disruptive or violent. Sandhu's (2000) suggestions are designed to reduce this alienation. Unhappy individuals carry within them the potential to do harm, to themselves or to others, as do those who can motivate others to strike out in self-defense or as a result of peer pressure. School counselors often are the first personnel in a school building to be aware of individual student issues, interactions among groups of students, and changes in the school climate and environment. This positions counselors to play a vital role in bringing issues to the forefront of the faculty's attention (Capuzzi & Gross, 2000). Faculty can be advised to do these things:

- Establish a caring and supportive relationship with children and youth.
- Get to know needs, feelings, attitudes, and behavior patterns of students.
- Review school records with the school counselors to identify patterns of behaviors or sudden changes in behavior.
- "Do no harm" by making sure that the early warning signs are not used as rationale to isolate, exclude, or punish a child.
- Understand violence and aggression within a context that realizes that many factors can contribute to aggressive behavior. Some children may act out if stress becomes too great, if they lack positive coping skills, and if they have learned to react with aggression.
- Avoid stereotyping and be aware of false cues including race, socioeconomic status, cognitive or academic ability, or physical appearance. In fact, such stereotypes can unfairly harm children, especially when the school community acts upon them.
- View warning signs within a developmental context due to children's different levels of social and emotional capabilities.
- Understand that children typically exhibit multiple warning signs.

Source: Early Warning, Timely Response (U.S. Department of Education, 1998).

As leaders and advocates, school counselors can publicly acknowledge the issues, be catalysts to seek solutions, and collaborate with colleagues to set in motion proactive prevention programs such as peer mediation and character education to address climate and relational issues.

School violence prevention is a challenging problem that requires a multifaceted response and utilizes services that link schools to the community. Research has shown that harsh measures and a repressive environment have not proven sufficient to create a school climate immune from disruption or acts of violence (U.S. Department of Education & U.S. Secret Service, 2002b). Zero tolerance policies have become the norm, punishing minor and major infractions and sending a message that certain behaviors will not be tolerated (Skiba & Peterson, 1999). Student codes of conduct can more clearly delineate student rights and responsibilities while additionally assuring consistency in the administration of consequences (New York State Center for School Safety, 2001).

Subtle or overt signs of aggression in parks, playing fields, the mall, and street corners are spilling into the schools' hallways and also impacting the schools' climate. The basis for the hostility or confrontational acts has as much to do with communities and families as it does with schools (Leinhardt & Willert, 2002). Sports rage, for example, is a common way in which parents model unacceptable behavior to their children. Parents must be mindful of the example they set and the expectations that they hold for their children. Playing fields are not the place for targeted or directed frustration, anger, or violence in the name of competition. Children watch their parents and react accordingly (Barth, Heinzmann, Casey-Doecke, & Kahan, 2003; Heinzmann, 2002).

Characteristics and Actions of Successful Programs

The U.S. Department of Education Safe and Drug-Free Schools Program (2002) has identified common characteristics and actions of programs that have been successful in creating a positive climate and reducing acts of violence. Successful drug-free schools share characteristics that include

1. an early start and a long-term commitment that focuses on young children and sustains interventions K–12;

2. strong administrative leadership that ensures consistent, clear disciplinary policies, as well as staff development training to help teachers and staff appropriately work with disruptive students, mediate conflict, and proactively incorporate prevention strategies;

3. parental involvement and training to alert them to the early warning signs of violence and to engage them to serve as volunteers in school violence-prevention programs;

4. interagency partnerships and community linkages to develop collaborative agreements for school personnel, local businesses, law enforcement officers, and social service agencies to work together to address the multiple causes of violence in schools and in the community.

According to the U.S. Department of Education & U.S. Department of Justice (2002) schools that are successful in creating a positive climate and reducing acts of violence employ actions that include these:

1. Build a solid foundation for all children, which includes supporting positive discipline, academic success, and mental and emotional wellness by creating a caring school environment; teaching students appropriate behaviors and problem-solving skills; positive behavioral support; and appropriate academic instruction with engaging curricula and effective teaching practices.

2. Identify students at risk for severe academic or behavioral difficulties early on. Create services and supports that address risk factors and build protective factors for the students. Approximately 10% to 15% of students exhibit problem behaviors, indicating a need for such early intervention. It is important that staff be trained to recognize early warning signs and make appropriate referrals.

3. Provide intensive interventions for children who are experiencing significant emotional and behavioral problems. This involves providing coordinated, comprehensive, intensive, sustained, culturally appropriate, child- and family-focused services and supports. Such interventions might include day treatment programs that provide students and families with intensive mental health and special education services; multisystemic therapy, focusing on the individual youth and his or her family, the peer context, school/vocational performance, and neighborhood/community supports; or treatment foster care, an intensive, family-focused intervention for youth whose delinquency or emotional problems are so serious and so chronic that the youth are no longer permitted to live at home.

4. Pull together with the community to determine and implement strategies essential to creating a safe school environment. Effectiveness generally requires the collaboration of schools, social services, mental health providers, and law enforcement and juvenile justice authorities. Because school violence mirrors the culture, norms, and behaviors of our communities and neighborhoods, schools are most successful in confronting school violence when the community around them is proactively involved.

5. Consider integrating the principles of character education across the content areas (Likona, Schaps, & Lewis, 2000). Character education can address anger management, empathy, perspective taking, social problem solving, communication, general social skills, and peace building. Students develop empathy and learn acceptable ways to express thoughts and feelings.

Implementing a Respectful Environment

RESPECT is an acronym that stands for **R**eflect, **E**ducate, **S**ecure, **P**repare, **E**xamine, **C**ooperate, and **T**ransform. These verbs denote steps in a procedure for establishing a respectful school climate. RESPECT can act as a blueprint for the leadership team in developing an action plan, and also can be applied to any number of situations to increase the potential for a safe and respectful school climate.

More fully, RESPECT means

- Reflect on the current climate;
- Educate the faculty;
- Secure a commitment;
- Prepare for the unexpected;
- Examine data;
- Cooperate across all the content areas;
- Transform the school culture and climate.

We will use the story of Main Street Middle School, a fictitious school representative of many large suburban middle schools, to illustrate RESPECT in action.

Reflect on the Current Climate

Last year, the Main Street School leadership team was asked to develop an action plan to improve climate and help students acquire the attitudes, knowledge, and skills needed to resist violent acts, drugs, and alcohol, and to reduce other risky behaviors.

Using the U.S. Department of Education Safe and Drug-Free Schools Program (2002) as a guide, the school leadership team (including the school counselor) committed to the challenge of creating a school in which respect is the cornerstone. Everyone in the school community, both internal and external to the school, would be involved in the process. The leadership team surveyed faculty perceptions toward student behavior, discipline, drug and alcohol use, and related behaviors. Additionally a "town meeting" was held to discuss the concerns, needs, and problems of the school with the entire community.

Information gathered from the survey and the town meeting were used to develop a prevention plan to create a safe, respectful environment. Findings pointed to the controversy surrounding zero tolerance policies. While faculty believed that well-defined discipline policies and school security were necessary to maintain order and a safe climate, students viewed the newly instituted zero tolerance policy as restrictive, unfair, and punitive. The data revealed that as a result of its enforcement, the student suspension rate increased. The students asked for the discipline policy to be replaced by a code of conduct. The faculty acknowledged that a code of conduct could address student rights and responsibilities, and could become the cornerstone for a character education program.

The survey and town meeting results helped the leadership team identify community stressors, discipline incidents, and places where bullying was occurring. It placed the team in a better position to reflect on the current situation and begin to consider measures to positively improve climate.

Educate the Faculty

Creating a safe and respectful environment requires that educators ensure that no child will go unnoticed, unattended, or unconnected. Youth who have positive and caring role models in their lives are less prone to engage in risky behaviors.

Educators who establish clear standards for acceptable behavior for themselves and others can be a powerful influence (New York State Center for School Safety, 2001). Students who feel "school connected" are less likely to engage in violent behavior, use substances, or experience emotional distress (McNeely & Blum, 2002). Implementing these protective factors will serve to reduce the potential of risk factors associated with acts of violence and aggressive behavior (New York State Office of Mental Health, 2000). Classroom discussions and activities help raise students' awareness of what constitutes bullying and victimizing, and will help students develop appropriate actions that they can take when they witness or experience incidents of bullying (U.S. Department of Education, 2002). To secure a safe environment, faculty can encourage students to

- seek immediate help from an adult when they are being victimized;
- use words of kindness or condolence to privately support those being hurt;
- express disapproval of bullying behavior by not joining in the laughter, teasing, or spreading rumors or gossip;
- speak up and offer support to victims when they see them being bullied;
- report bullying/victimization incidents to school personnel.

As its next step, the Main Street leadership team requested 20 minutes to deliver an in-service at the next faculty meeting in order to educate the staff and faculty. At the meeting, each member of the faculty received a copy of *Early Warning, Timely Response* (U.S. Department of Education, 1998), which summarizes the early and imminent warning signs. Faculty was encouraged to become keenly aware of students who are at risk and who consequently put others at risk. The in-service closed with faculty members sharing their personal concerns about observed student behavior. Faculty and staff agreed that the process of educating them about early warning signs, the factors contributing to violence, and the ways to prevent problems was a positive step toward establishing a safe environment.

Secure a Commitment

To secure a safe environment, the leadership team at Main Street worked to obtain a commitment from every member of the school community, from students to principal, to pay close attention to what goes on among the student body. The team proposed that every member of the faculty establish a connection with a student who is isolated and troubled. Additionally, the leadership team suggested that the faculty establish clear standards for behavior, encourage character development, and motivate students to contribute to a safe and respectful learning environment.

The team believed that students and faculty could pull together with the common goal of creating an environment that is safe and respectful. By involving students in the process, the team offers the opportunity for them to assume responsibility and take ownership for contributing to the climate of their school, where they spend as much time as they do in their homes. Students rise to the occasion when presented with opportunities to help create fair and respectful classrooms. School personnel organized programs that increased student confidence, knowledge, responsibility, and skills, such as volunteering to be peer facilitators, tutors, and mentors to younger students.

Prepare for the Unexpected

Understanding that crisis and tragedy can strike at any time, from within or from outside of the school setting, the Main Street team was determined to assess the school's preparedness. The No Child Left Behind (2001) imperative requires schools to anticipate acts of violence and be prepared to work through and manage crisis.

No school is protected from tragic occurrences such as the death of a faculty member or student, car accidents, tornado destruction, kidnapping, suicide, or an event of terrorism such as 9/11. Crises can range in scope and severity from incidents that affect a single student to those that can wreak havoc on an entire community. Events such as 9/11 severely affected staff and students, leaving the nation feeling vulnerable and unprepared for tragedies of this magnitude (Dahir, 2001).

Tragedy leaves a permanent imprint on each one of us; grief and loss know no boundaries. Every school member, from student to counselor, need to be aware of the protocols and procedures to follow for any crisis (U.S. Department of Education & U.S. Secret Service, 2002b).

Crisis management plans have specific components mandated by state education regulations, legislation, and/or local school board policy. According to the U.S. Department of Education, U.S. Department of Justice, and American Institute of Research (2002), these can include but are not limited to

- the chain of command to implement procedures;
- clearly defined roles and responsibilities for every staff member;
- specific assignments for school personnel to monitor indoor or outdoor school areas and/or groups of students;
- guidance for scheduled and unscheduled emergency preparedness drills;
- internal and external communication guidelines;
- collaborative procedures for working with police officers, firefighters, emergency medical technicians, bomb squads, parents, community agencies, and local officials;
- guidelines for working with the media;
- follow-up practices for the aftermath

A crisis response plan addresses the personal and the human side of trauma, loss, injury, and grief. Key to providing immediate response is a well-trained crisis response team that meets periodically to update skills and retool each member's preparedness

(Dorn, 2002). Crisis response teams often include school counselors, student services school personnel, and community-based mental health professionals. School counselors and student services personnel, including school psychologists, social workers, and nurses are especially trained to attend to student and staff well-being so that they do not become overwhelmed or traumatized. Crisis response teams can offer support and structure for students, staff, and families to express their grief and sense of loss, while also identifying the interventions and resources necessary for those who may be in need of regularly scheduled counseling or therapy.

At Main Street Middle School, the leadership team desired to assure students that the adults of their environment will protect them. Routine evacuation drills were implemented, with each school professional accepting the responsibilities and accountability for student safety. Police officers, firefighters, emergency medical technicians, and other community members partnered with school personnel to provide students with peace of mind that they will be protected (U.S. Department of Education Office of Safe and Drug-Free Schools, 2003).

Training was provided so that school personnel would know how to not only help their students through a crisis, but to help them to return home safely. The leadership team used the suggestions from the U.S. Department of Education to design both a crisis management plan and a crisis response plan. Every detail was addressed, from the process for emergency exiting to updating classroom and office locations and room assignments. Changes to any aspect of the plan will be communicated to all team and faculty members, and a formal opportunity to review and evaluate the plan will be scheduled at least once a year.

Solid preparation for response and management of the critical incidents can save lives, impact the recovery and healing period, build bridges between school and community, and desensationalize media attention. Here we recount one school's readiness to respond to a tragic event that was beyond the scope of anyone's imagination.

Counselors Making a Difference

Meet the Staff of the High School of Leadership & Public Service

Neighbors to the World Trade Center

"How have we all become important in one day?" asked the social studies teacher of his colleagues at the High School of Leadership & Public Service, two blocks from the Trade Center. His purpose just three days after 9/11 was to help everyone gathered in the room put the World Trade Center tragedy in a different context so they in turn could help their students regain a sense of empowerment, purpose, and hope. It was a way to begin the healing process. The counselor and teachers wanted to help their students escape from the feelings of powerlessness and despair.

This, the first faculty gathering since they had to evacuate to Battery Park, was a time to tell the stories of that day. The heroism of these 70 adults in the midst of the crisis spoke to their preparedness to move students to safety and to set into motion a series of decisions that would protect and guard the students' emotional and physical safety to the extent possible.

Ada Rosario Dolch, the principal, related the chronology of events that took place that morning. Within seconds after the first plane exploded into the World Trade Center, the security agents came rushing into her office and told her that everyone had to evacuate the building, a decision Principal Dolch had already made. It took only a second for the magnitude to sink in, and then Ada quickly made an announcement directing everyone to go to the park. Go they did. All of those drills and practices now became a reality. Students and faculty walking together, scared but moving quickly. In as orderly a fashion as possible, they made their way to Battery Park through the wave of anxious humanity that clogged the streets of lower Manhattan. Seven hundred students and their teachers protected and encouraged each other. They supported each other and helped the others who crossed their path, taking special care of the children in wheelchairs and those who were disabled or blind. They all left behind their pocketbooks and keys, bank cards and credit cards, briefcases, lesson plans, backpacks, and books—all of the ordinary trappings of an ordinary day in the life of high-school teachers and students.

Seven hundred students were taken to safety, protected by the compassion and caring of their school family. The staff protected their students as best they could, watching the horror intensify with the second explosion. It was like a tsunami wave that rolled over the lower part of Manhattan, descending on the crowds with debris, dust, paper, and rubble. As students reached out to each other, they also helped strangers. One rushed to rescue an older woman who was getting trampled and pushed up against the fence.

As the teachers shared their experiences, they conveyed a spirit of hope and optimism about the future. They talked about how to take a message from this crisis to their students: all people are important. With uncertainty about the future but with determination, they talked about how to help the students return to school and how to provide the structure of instruction and opportunities to talk.

"We will do our best," one teacher said. "We have all become important in one day, more so than any of us could have imagined on the first day of school. We will contribute to this effort to rebuild our lives, our families, our school, our neighborhood, our city, our hopes and dreams. We will make this world a better place. That's why we are here. We are survivors, not victims."

Dahir, C. (NYSSCA, 2002). Reprinted with permission by the New York State School Counselor Association and Ada Rosario-Doch.

Schools are never emotionally prepared for violence, grief, and trauma. A structured crisis management plan helps all school personnel and students to better deal with the trauma and stress of the unexpected or unforeseen. The school counselor's ultimate goal, as part of the crisis response team, is to help the school community return to a semblance of normalcy as quickly as possible. ASCA reminds us that the professional school counselor's role is to respond to and advocate for the emotional needs of all persons affected by this crisis (ASCA, 2002). Putting structure and the normal routine back in place will help students and staff regain a sense of safety and security.

School counselors cannot easily separate their involvement on the crisis response or management team from the proactive commitment to ensure that every student will acquire safety and survival skills (ASCA, 1997). School counselor initiative will help students function appropriately in an emergency situation; more important students can acquire the coping and resiliency skills to successfully emerge from crisis, grief, loss, and tragedy.

Examine Data

Student success data can be collected and analyzed systematically to inform and guide the development and implementation of a safe schools program. The use of demographic and performance data makes it possible for counselors to determine how policies and practices are affecting issues of equity and climate (Stone & Dahir, 2004). School report card data tell the story about attendance, suspension, and graduation rates, which have a significant impact on school climate. Collecting and disaggregating data is the critical first step in the school safety process (Forsyth, 1999) and provides a baseline for consistency in data-driven decision making.

At Main Street Middle School, several sixth graders had reported "getting picked on" and "being pushed around," and the leadership team agreed that there were patterns of "bullying" that had been previously reported and warranted investigating.

The leadership team agreed that data collection should be systematic and consistent and that was of the utmost importance to examine the disaggregated data in a variety of ways. The data might provoke some new questions, such as "Is there a relationship between attendance and bullying?" "What are the underlying contributors to suspensions or to hallway tussles?" A careful data analysis of discipline incidents could offer insight about the nature of the recent complaints of the sixth graders and help to identify the specific cause-and-effect relationships that contribute to school safety and to building a safe and respectful school environment.

The leadership team examined all of the variables that contributed to discipline referrals. The monthly data reports revealed the sixth-grade discipline referrals since September. The incident reports showed that 75% of the incidents involved verbal harassment and physical confrontation. Eighty-five percent of these incidents took place in the hallways, lunchroom, and/or on the bus. Almost 40% of the referrals involved the same 25 students, 17 of whom were boys. Would further data disaggregation reveal any connection of these to "bullying"? Has this physical and verbal harassment reduced the achievement of the students who have been victimized? The leadership team realized the value and importance of digging deep to uncover the roots of the problem and consider systemic implications.

Had this conversation and further investigation not taken place, the complaints of the sixth graders may have been dismissed as isolated incidents. Data collection and analysis is necessary to transforming the culture and creating a positive climate by helping to identify the cause and effect of inappropriate behavior as well as develop proactive prevention and remediation strategies. If students do not feel safe in the school environment, they will not learn to the best of their ability (Bluestein, 2001). Student fear and concern for personal safety impact a classroom teacher's ability to engage students in successful achievement (McNeely & Blum, 2002). Specific strategies to eliminate this negative behavior would improve the school's climate and enhance the learning environment for the sixth grade.

Cooperate Across All the Content Areas

Random events and assemblies or occasional thematic days on safety and respect are not enough to change the climate and culture of a school. Basic concerns of the faculty and stakeholders, such as helping students cope with anger, resolve and mediate conflict, develop friendships, acquire a respect for self and others, and understand personal safety could be addressed in teachable moments across the academic areas (Dahir & Stone, 2004). This would require cooperation among all school professionals. When youth feel valued, are involved in positive relationships, and have external and internal guides, they perform better in school (Search Institute, 1998). Building character protects young people from many different "risky behaviors" and promotes positive attitudes (Search Institute, 1998). Students who demonstrate values and skills that make them less likely to engage in risky behavior tend to be more successful in school and in life (Benson, Scales, Effort, & Roehikeepartain, 1999; Scales & Taccogna, 2000).

The Search Institute (1998) promoted asset acquisition for students to help build youth of character, compassion, and commitment. The external assets are the relationships and supports that guide students to behave in healthy ways and make good choices, while the internal assets are the competencies, values, and self-perceptions that guide a young person's ability to self-regulate his or her behavior (Scales & Taccogna, 2000). Looking at student growth and development through an assets lens positively impacts teaching, learning, relationships, and of course, school climate; high-risk patterns of behavior diminish as students increase their acquisition of "assets" (Scales & Taccogna, 2000).

The Developmental Assets (Search Institute, 1998) and the three personal-social development standards offer guidance to develop competencies, which are the outcomes for what students should know and be able to do. Undertaking asset building across the content areas will aid in the design of a proactive safe schools action plan that has student needs at its core and impacts the school climate in positive ways. The personal-social development standards will help students to acquire attitudes, knowledge, and skills to support both affective and academic development. The faculty's buy-in is revealed through beliefs and behaviors. Caring beyond the classroom and creating a positive moral culture in every school building are two of the many ways in which a whole-school effort can focus on youth development.

The Main Street leadership team acknowledged the importance of securing the buy-in and the full cooperation of the faculty and staff. To start the process, several

Box 13.1

Main Street Leadership Team Belief Statement #1

To create a school climate of caring and respect, we the faculty of Main Street Middle School, believe we can:

a. Create a positive and collaborative classroom climate by looking at what we teach, how we teach, and what we ask students to do considering their point of view.

b. Listen to students and give them opportunities to share their concerns, whether it's about why they failed a test, didn't do their homework, or to reflect on what the particular lesson meant to them on a personal basis.

c. Give students choices and responsibilities in rule-making within the classroom and within the structure of the school environment.

d. Look at each situation as a challenge for resolution rather than an action to be disciplined, and think about how to problem-solve rather than punish.

e. Connect with the students and actively listen to their concerns.

f. Use teachable moments to connect the academic curriculum with affective development. For example, many of the required novels that students read address conflict in the plot. Additionally, many social studies teachers facilitate classroom discussions around conflict and peaceful resolutions. Literature can become a venue for connecting academic content with character building.

g. Make a commitment to use culturally sensitive and developmentally appropriate materials.

h. Help students acquire coping and resiliency skills (Dorsey, 2000).

sample belief statements were developed to gain support for the safe and respectful school-wide action plan. These draft statements were the result of research, observations, and faculty room and community conversations. At the next faculty meeting, the draft belief statements were presented and served as a basis for discussion.

Faculty commitment to positive climate and culture protects young people from many different "risky behaviors" and promotes positive attitudes (Search Institute, 1998). Students who demonstrate values and skills that make them less likely to engage in risky behavior, tend to be more successful in school, and in life (Benson et al., 1999).

Cooperation among faculty, administration, and staff will improve school climate and help students acquire the attitudes, knowledge, and skills needed to resist violent acts, drugs, and alcohol, and to reduce risky behaviors. School personnel who hold student needs at the core of their belief systems create safe and dynamic learning communities (Stein, Richin, Banyon, Banyon, & Stein, 2001).

Transform the School Culture and Climate

Ensuring a safe and respectful school environment requires close attention to students' social and emotional lives, the dynamics of relationships, and the environment in which students thrive and grow. Peer pressure, concerns for safety and well-being, harassment, and bullying are some of the challenges that students face every day in hallways that can be hostile or friendly. For some students, issues of personal safety and emotional balance are more important than is meeting academic standards. Does the school faculty project an image of caring and concern? Or do students look elsewhere for support and personal, social, and emotional growth?

Schools and communities together have transformed the school culture and created climates of respect by developing comprehensive, integrated plans that embrace key sectors of the community—the schools, social services, mental health providers, and law enforcement and juvenile justice authorities (U.S. Department of Education, U.S. Department of Justice, & American Institute of Research, 2002).

When the Main Street Middle School prevention and intervention action plan was close to completion and ready for faculty review, the leadership team recognized that it was only part of the long journey ahead. To transform the climate and culture of the school would be a complex process that requires a commitment of time and a willingness to thoroughly examine policies, practices, and behaviors that stratify student opportunities. Transforming the school culture is a responsibility that resides not only with the adults; students too must assume responsibility for contributing to a system that is safe, secure, and respectful. The team acknowledged that although every act of hostility or aggression may not be eradicated, implementing the RESPECT strategies can make a difference with teachers, counselors, administrators, students, and community pulling together.

Planning for success was Main Street's first step in the journey. RESPECT, while far from a perfect design, provided a starting point.

Personalizing the School Experience: Advisory Programs

Schools and society put much pressure on youth to grow up in perfect compliance and conformance with rules and structure that will lead to wonderfully, perfectly successful lives. However, the mechanisms are not always in place to create an environment in which every child has a safety net, and in which no child is forgotten. Although some students can make it through the secondary school years without any personal connections, all students require a supportive environment, some more than others (National Association of Secondary School Principals, 2004).

> On any given day, I think every adolescent is at-risk in some way. How many schools approach such concerns with purposeful, planned, and progressive awareness-building, educational, and intervention strategies in place as opposed to trying to deny these realities or being caught in a reactive, crisis-oriented position?
> — *Marnik, 1997, p. 37*

High schools are often large and impersonal environments. Every teenager needs a significant adult in her or his life to support the challenges presented by school rigor, policies, and socialization pressures. Smaller, more intimate environments ensure that no child goes unnoticed and afford students the ability to make connections with adults. Here's one school's response to creating a personalized, more student-centered experience:

Counselors Making a Difference

Meet Linda Quinn, Michaele Sein-Ryan,
and the Faculty and Staff of Emerald Ridge High School

A Community of Caring

The mission of Emerald Ridge High School is to help all students acquire the skills necessary to be contributing members of a high-quality work force, the critical thinking abilities necessary to be productive citizens, and the social responsibility necessary to be positive community builders. This may sound similar to many other district mission statements, but the faculty at Emerald Ridge has committed to make sure that every student will be

- well known, both personally and academically, by at least one adult staff member;
- challenged to meet rigorous academic standards in an appropriate educational program;

- provided with opportunities to experience the benefits of community membership and to develop and practice leadership skills;
- prepared for whatever he or she chooses to do after graduation, with a strong transcript, a career pathway, a plan, and a portfolio.

How can the faculty and staff possibly accomplish this challenge in a high school of 1,500 students? Linda Quinn, founding principal, and Michaele Sein-Ryan, counselor and career specialist, led a schoolwide initiative to personalize the high-school experience for every student. At the center of each student's day is a commonly shared block of time when she or he meets with an advisory group. Advisory is best described as the "home base" for each student and the key communication vehicle for the school. Advisers are mediators, motivators, and schoolhouse versions of moms and dads. They are college counselors, activities coordinators, and career specialists. They are coaches, and over the course of the three years, they coach their advisees through a variety of activities and lessons related to educational and career planning, leadership development, and community involvement.

The advisory program has recast high-school counselors in new roles, allowing them to serve as staff leaders, curriculum developers, and advisers to the advisers rather than credit counters, clerks, and crisis managers. Advisory helps students feel connected, become part of a peer group, and develop a relationship with at least one caring adult advocate. Students learn to

- understand their learning style and the styles of others;
- collaborate and team on projects;
- experience and apply the "new 3 Rs"—respect, responsibility, and resourcefulness;
- have opportunities to reflect and self-assess their academic, career, and personal-social growth as they transition from grade level to grade level and prepare for life after high school.

The administration and staff of Emerald Ridge have transformed the high-school experience to one of caring connections between and among students and adults. Respect for self and others is part of the undercurrent of the school experience. Violent incidents are practically nonexistent, and discipline incidents have been significantly reduced. No student can get lost at Emerald Ridge—being known and well respected by peers and faculty is part of the culture.

Emerald Ridge High School, located in the Puyallup School District, the twelfth-largest district in the State of Washington, serves a population of approximately 90,000 residents. Approximately 1,500 students attend Emerald Ridge High School in grades 10, 11, and 12. Reprinted with permission by Linda Quinn and Michaele Sein-Ryan.

Advisory programs are an important component of the personalized school experience. Clarke and Frazer (2003) identified six developmental needs of students that can be addressed through personalization (National Association of Secondary School Principals, 2004, p. 70).

- Voice—the need to express their personal perspective
- Belonging—the need to establish individual and group identities
- Choice—the need to examine options and choose a path
- Freedom—the need to take risks and assess effects
- Imagination—the need to create a projected view of self
- Success—the need to demonstrate mastery

Engaging students in the personalization experience allows each student to earn recognition. Advisory models such as the one described at Emerald Ridge High provide opportunities for students to establish an identity and a mechanism for self-expression. School counselors can assume a leadership role in the organization and curricular development of an advisory model that emphasizes affective and life-skills instructional components.

Character Matters

According to the Character Education Partnership (2004), character education is an intentional effort to help students understand, care about, and act upon core ethical values. The absence of the core values of respect, responsibility, trustworthiness, fairness, diligence, self-control, caring, and courage can lead to destructive youth behaviors. Thus schools that do not emphasize these core values are at greater risk of acts of violence or aggressive behaviors.

Connecting Character to Conduct (CCC) (Stein et al., 2001) is a comprehensive methodology that promotes the core values of RICE:

Respect: Showing respect toward ourselves and others

Impulse Control: Doing the right things for the right reasons

Compassion: Showing concern and caring for others

Equity: Treating everyone with fairness

The CCC method includes adult modeling of RICE behaviors and curriculum-specific activities that are initiated anywhere there is an opportunity to learn, including classrooms, hallways, and the cafeteria.

Counselors Making a Difference

Meet Lewis Serra and Susan Sklar, leaders of Grand Avenue Middle School

A Commitment to Core Values

Lewis Serra, principal, and Susan Sklar, chairperson of pupil personnel services, had the data to demonstrate that the students of Grand Avenue Middle School were well behaved, academically successful, and involved in many extracurricular activities. It was a principal's dream. But Mr. Serra agreed with his leadership team, counseling staff, and faculty that the students could do even better. They wanted their students to be kind and respectful, even if no one else was looking. Yet, everyone recognized that they could not force one more thing into the packed academic day. If they were to adopt an approach to character education, it had to be something everyone could do as a seamless, natural part of their role. The faculty chose the process of Connecting Character to Conduct (CCC) to help them develop core values that everyone would abide by.

Through professional development and parent engagement practices, the Grand Avenue middle school team adopted a shared vocabulary to clearly define their purpose, strengthen their sense of membership, and specifically articulate their roles and rules, or guiding principles. Today, everyone at Grand Avenue abides by the guiding principles and core values of RICE. Now every member of the school learning team—faculty, staff, and students alike—are using their shared core values to achieve their individual goals while advancing the purpose of their school, which is to help all students learn well, stay safe, and graduate! Everyone has a specific role to play; roles clearly define areas of responsibility. Every Grand Avenue student has a dual role: to learn well, stay safe, and graduate, and to help other students do the same.

Grand Avenue Middle School is located in the Bellmore-Merrick School District on Long Island, New York.

School Counselors Taking the Next Steps

With virtually almost every youth exposed to a barrage of visual violence in the media—and for some, in their communities and homes—we must recognize that we live in potentially dangerous times (Gabarino, 1999). School violence can manifest itself in many different forms. Once remanded to the playground or streets, the definition of violence is far more than physical assaults in schools and can be displayed as hostility, aggressive language, threats, subtle and overt acts of peer pressure, put-downs, harassment, bullying, intimidation and extortion, and teasing (Leinhardt &

Willert, 2002). The stringent discipline policies and metal detectors may be important security measures, but they do not get at the source of the problem. High morals and strong leadership coupled with organizational and administrative support contribute highly to a school's prevention program (Gottfredson, 2001). Building a level of trust amongst and between all members of our school community can help to identify the shared values that all stakeholders embrace and support.

School counselors, in collaboration with faculty, can help to put more extraordinary measures in place to help students navigate materialism, competitiveness, pressures, insensitivity, failure, and conflicting values. School counselors as responsible and caring adults, and they play a key role in the lives of our youth (Daniels, 2002). "The potential for healing lies not within a system of rules and punishments, but in a system that celebrates curiosity and caring, discovery and joy and in the process, and we will make it (our schools) better and we will make it (our schools) safe" (Bluestein, 2001, p. 381).

To live in a world of hope one must put the fear aside. No longer can caring school personnel always protect children from hate, terrorism, and violence. The fear that some children experience when "bullied" on the playground is similar to the fear used by terrorists for intimidation. Children can learn they cannot act out of hate, anger, and fear.

Alternative ways for children to learn to cope with emotions are possible. School counselors can assume a leadership role to help young children and adolescents build strong character, develop coping and resiliency skills, and set goals for the future. School counselors can help to transform the world of schools and, through intentional efforts in our schools, create a more respectful and peaceful climate than the one in which we live in today.

TechTools

When you become a school counselor, use the power of technology to maximize the efficiency and effectiveness of your contributions to creating a safe and respectful learning environment.

- Use the World Wide Web to explore resources, programs, and research related to character education to promote safe schools.
- What do the data tell us? In addition to sites such as U.S. Department of Education's *Early Warning, Timely Response: A Guide to Safe Schools* (http://www.ed.gov/about/offices/list/osers/osep/gtss.html) and the Centers for Disease Control and Prevention (http://www.cdc.gov/ncipc/factsheets/yvfacts.htm), use the Web to look at statistics for youth abuse of alcohol, or

drugs, or tobacco. You will discover many governmental agencies and organizations collecting data and providing resources.

- The U.S. Department of Educational Research and Improvement (2002) established rigorous criteria to evaluate prevention programs.
- Analyze TV programming for an hour during prime time. Log how many acts of violence children are exposed to, how many explicit sexual comments are made, how many ethical dilemmas are posed. Compare notes with your colleagues.
- Pop culture is represented in many mediums. Watch the Grammys, or spend an hour viewing MTV videos. What can we learn about youth culture from music?
- Looking for resources for your classroom guidance character education program? Check out state education department websites as well as organizations such as Character Counts for ideas and lessons.
- Explore your county or community website for community-based organizations and governmental services that offer prevention programs to reduce or eliminate youth violence.

Internet Resources

Center for Substance Abuse Prevention
http://www.samhsa.gov

The National Institute on Drug Abuse: Preventing Drug Use Among Children and Adolescents: A Research-based Guide. Call 1-800-729-9989.
http://www.nida.nih.gov/Prevention/Prevopen.html

The National Institute of Justice: Preventing Crime: What Works, What Doesn't, What's Promising?
http://www.ncjrs.org/works/index.html

U.S. Department of Education Safe and Drug Free Schools Program
http://www.ed.gov/offices/OESE/SDFS

National Youth Violence Prevention Resource Center
http://www.safeyouth.org/home.htm

D.A.V.E.
http://dave.esc4.net/search/

Indiana Department of Education—Character Education
http://ideanet.doe.state.in.us/charactered/welcome.html

Youth and Violence: Students Speak out for a More Civil Society
http://www.jointogether.org/y/0,2521,553791,00.html?U=83579

Federal Resources

Federal Government:

http://www.ed.gov/about/offices/list/osers/osep/gtss.html

This publication offers research-based practices designed to help school communities identify these early warning signs and develop prevention, intervention, and crisis response plans.

Centers for Disease Control and Prevention: Youth Violence in the United States

http://www.cdc.gov/ncipc/factsheets/yvfacts.htm

This is a fact sheet on youth violence in the United States.

Office of Juvenile Justice and Delinquency Prevention (OJJDP), U.S. Department of Justice

http://ojjdp.ncjrs.org

This page provides links to OJJDP's "Violence and Victimization" summaries.

Office of Juvenile Justice and Delinquency Prevention, U.S. Department of Justice Youth Violence in America

http://www.ojp.usdoj.gov/nij/newsletter/0499chapter.html

The purpose of this National Institute of Justice newsletter is to help the process of comprehending the problem and policy challenges of youth violence by engaging academic researchers in serious efforts to describe and explain the epidemic, and to devise plausibly effective means for combating it.

Office of Juvenile Justice and Delinquency Prevention, U.S. Department of Justice Predictors of Youth Violence

http://www.ncjrs.org/pdffiles1/ojjdp/179065.pdf

This Bulletin describes a number of risk and protective factors of youth violence, including individual, family, school, peer-related, community/neighborhood, and situational factors.

Office of Juvenile Justice and Delinquency Prevention, U.S. Department of Justice: Adolescent Violence: A View from the Street

http://www.ncjrs.org/pdffiles/fs000189.pdf

Researchers at Columbia University's Center for Violence Research and Prevention are conducting a qualitative, multistage study on adolescent violence. This document is a summary of a presentation by Jeffrey Fagen, Ph.D., Center for Violence Research and Prevention.

U.S. Department of Education: Assessing Potentially Violent Students

http://www.ed.gov/databases/ERIC_Digests/ed435894.html

This ERIC digest describes the importance of assessment and diagnosis of potentially violent and violent students.

The National Institute of Health Child and Adolescent Violence Research at the National Institute of Mental Health (NIMH))

http://www.nimh.nih.gov/publicat/violenceresfact.cfm

The fact sheet discusses child and adolescent violence research activities at the NIMH, including studies that focus on gender differences, risk factors, antisocial behavior, and depression.

School Counselor Casebook: Voices From the Field

The Scenario Reviewed

The conversation at today's team meeting focused on a small group of disengaged students. Two of the teachers commented that the students were in different classes and that they were antisocial except with their group. None of the teachers noticed any gang indicia or color display. The social studies teacher spoke up to say that even though she does not have specifics, she is certain she overheard a conversation in the cafeteria in which a few of these disengaged students were "threatening" other students. She turns to you, the school counselor, and asks, "What should we do about this?"

A Practitioner's Approach

Here's how two practicing school counselors responded to the school scenario.

1st Response

A conversation that is "overheard" can often be taken out of context, so it is important to start with some fact-finding. I would meet with the students and ask them about their relationship with the students they may have threatened, and whether threats were made directly. If a teacher heard threats, students probably also heard and will be putting the information into the rumor mill.

Disengaged students have not found a meaningful way to contribute to their school community and need to be connected in some way. As I work to sort out the possible threats, I will also be looking for ways to draw the students constructively into the school community to find a place for themselves.

I am responsible to promote a safe learning environment for all students. If students are threatened or getting word that a threat may have been made, they often feel unsafe at school. My ethical and legal responsibility to each student is to teach skills in conflict resolution, mediation, and peacemaking. I would draw on training already done in the classrooms to guide the students through the steps to a positive outcome. Depending upon the facts of the situation and level of problem intensity, I would use further classroom guidance, group intervention, behavior assessment, peer mediation, parent contact, and referral and/or teacher collaboration. Often, I find that several of these options make the best response. With situations of high intensity I contact an administrator as well, because threats are also a discipline issue.

If indeed a threat has been made, a multifaceted approach is always helpful. The infraction of the rules warrants a discipline response, but the same behavior will continue if it is not explored for precipitating factors and if appropriate interventions are not made.

Linda Eby is a licensed professional counselor who has worked as a child development specialist at the Gordon Russell Middle School in Gresham, Oregon. Active in her professional organizations, Linda is past president of the Oregon School Counselor Association and recently served as the Middle Level vice president for the American School Counselor Association. She is the recipient of several state awards for exemplary service and practice. Reprinted with permission by Linda C. Eby.

2nd response

This scenario calls the counselor to action in several different ways. There is a need to deal with the potential of imminent danger to the safety of students within the school environment. There is a need to explore why a group of students appears disengaged—to find out how to help individuals who may be at risk. Finally, there is a need to step back and look at the "big picture" and to examine how structures that exist within the system can be tapped to help prevent situations like this from occurring in the future.

In response to the overheard threats, as a counselor I would feel compelled to investigate the situation further. This investigation would need to be conducted on several different levels. The first order of business would be fact-finding. Information from other teachers in the building would need to be gathered. In a consulting role, I would make the rounds to all of the teachers who have contact with the identified students and hear what their concerns are regarding these students. Do these teachers share the concerns of the team? Do they see the students as "disengaged" as well? Have they observed any aggressive or threatening behavior? Are these students passing their classes and involved in the learning process? I would take notes on what I heard from the teachers and ask them to be especially vigilant regarding these students in the days and weeks ahead. I would ask them to communicate their concerns back to me.

The next part of the investigation would involve interviewing students. The assistant principal could conduct these interviews. Students who might have overheard the threats should be queried and their statements recorded. I would interview the identified students because I believe a counselor can listen to the facts but also assess the emotions involved. As teachers have expressed concerns that these students appear disengaged, I would want to begin to develop an understanding as to what exactly that means. Are these students socially isolated? Gang involved? Depressed? Academically challenged? Dealing with family issues, which are preoccupying them? The hope would be to use individual counseling to intervene successfully before a threat is acted upon. In a situation like this, individual counseling might need to be complemented by use of our peer mediation program. Peer mediation can be a very powerful tool to assist in conflict resolution. The trained peer mediators bring both parties together with the goal of reaching a level of understanding (sometimes taking the form of a written contract) that prevents friction between students from escalating to violence. Disengaged students might actually be more willing to work with their peers than with adults in the school.

One might think this is an overreaction and question whether using one's valuable time investigating a situation that has not yet erupted is worthwhile. Legally, threats are a form of harassment, which is against not only school rules, but also the law. Ethically, a counselor has a responsibility to respond to hearing about any student who appears disengaged. The research clearly indicates that students who show signs of disconnection from the school community are at greater risk for many problems, ranging from dropping out to suicide.

After responding promptly and thoroughly to the situation at hand, I would then ponder was this an isolated incident or, during the investigation conducted with the assistant principal, did more systemic problems surface? In my school this question would be turned over to the respect committee. This interdisciplinary group was started 4 years ago by the counseling department to find systemic solutions to any problems that interfere with the maintenance of a safe learning environment, which is part of our school mission. The committee has counselors, teachers, administrators, and students as regular members. It provides a forum for counselors to serve as "leaders" on projects designed to promote respect and tolerance among students and for each individual in our school. The personal-social strand of the National Standards for School Counseling lists as its first standard: "Students will acquire the knowledge and skills to help them respect themselves and others." The committee has won the respect of the school community by using data to show the connection between a safe learning environment and increased student achievement. Actions that this committee might initiate in response to an increase in threatening behavior or student disengagement could range from curriculum modifications (to health and/or guidance lessons) to staff in-service to bringing in a speaker for the student body.

This seemingly simple and commonly occurring scenario demonstrates how counselors are challenged daily to use not only their counseling skills but also their collaboration, consultation, and leadership skills to create a safe school environment.

Katie Gray is director of student services at Blackstone Valley Regional Vocational Technical High School in Upton, Massachusetts, and serves as the current president of the Massachusetts School Counselors' Association. Reprinted with permission by Katharine H. Gray.

Chapter Summary

Seeking a Safer Learning Environment

Schools may look the same from the outside of the building as they did in the past; however, violent acts and the impact of trauma, tragedy, and terrorism have moved from the community into the schoolhouse. This constant barrage of violent images reinforces a false message: that violence is an appropriate choice of action. Our public schools must be reclaimed to once again become emotionally and physically safe havens for students.

The Challenge for Educators

Many of our schools are unprepared to address the behaviors or the challenges that arise out of the ever-increasing complexity of societal trends and influences. School personnel struggle to strike a balance between holding all students accountable for their actions yet ensuring that all students receive the necessary resources and supports to achieve and succeed at the highest level. Developing safe and responsive schools is a comprehensive approach that includes acknowledging the risk factors, developing effective strategies, and involving all of the stakeholders.

School Violence Defined

Although the factors and contributors to school violence may present a bleak picture, targeted acts of violence are the exception to the rule (U.S. Department of Education Office of Safe and Drug-Free Schools, 2003; U.S. Department of Education & U.S. Secret Service, 2002a). Yet the public perceives that schools are no longer safe. The research both supports and contradicts this perception. While it is clear that other kinds of problems in American schools are far more common than is targeted violence, high-profile incidents that have occurred in schools over the past decade have resulted in increased fear among students, educators, and parents (U.S. Department of Education & U.S. Secret Service, 2002a).

Violence in schools, including fighting, homicide, suicide, firearm injury, and bullying, is usually the result of a series of factors that build up over a period of time. School violence is the result of an intentional action that leads one to harm oneself or another person. School personnel, including school counselors, work in a focused manner to help keep the school and students safe from harm's way (Dwyer, Osher, & Warger, 1998).

The Etiology of School Violence

Schools can successfully identify students at risk of violent behaviors when effective prevention measures are put in place (U.S. Department of Education & U.S. Department of Justice, 2003). Research has shown that the first steps toward preventing violence are to identify and understand the factors that place youth at risk for violent victimization and perpetration (National Center for Injury Prevention and Control, 2002).

Contributing to a Safe and Respectful School Environment

School counselors can proactively reach out to all students to maximize every student's development; collaborate and team with teachers to develop sensitivities about students who appear alienated or disaffected; consult with teachers on the characteristics of the warning signs of troubled students and lend support to teachers to help them cope with difficult students in their classrooms; and engage all stakeholders in the process to comprehensively address the problem.

Implementing a Respectful Environment

RESPECT is an acronym for a series of steps that can help instill a safe and respectful environment in a school. It stands for **R**eflect on the current climate, **E**ducate the faculty, **S**ecure a commitment, **P**repare for the unexpected, **E**xamine data, **C**ooperate across all the content areas, and **T**ransform the school culture and climate.

Personalizing the School Experience: Advisory Programs

Secondary schools can be large and impersonal environments. Advisory programs can personalize the school experience and provide opportunities for students to establish an identity and a mechanism for self-expression and to participate in school-based experience that emphasizes affective and life-skills instructional components.

Character Matters

Character education is an intentional effort to help students, understand, care about, and act upon core ethical values. These core values of respect, responsibility, trustworthiness, fairness, diligence, self-control, caring, and courage promote school environments that are safe and respectful.

School Counselors Taking the Next Steps

Building trust amongst and between all members of the school community can lead to a climate in which all stakeholders are involved with creating a climate of respect and support. The potential for healing lies not within a system of rules and punishments, but in a system that celebrates student curiosity and caring, discovery and joy. In the process, and school counselors will make it better and make it safe. As school counselors build safe and respectful environments, it is time to make sure that no child will go unattended or unnoticed.

Key Terms

Bullying p. 365
Disruptive student p. 366
Early warning signs p. 369
Imminent warning signs p. 369

Risk factors p. 367
School climate p. 364
School violence p. 363

Learning Extensions

1. Interview a school counselor or school administrator regarding his or her experiences with student violent/aggressive behavior, and discuss effective solutions to these problems.

2. Research your state department of education's policies and procedures regarding safe schools. What is expected of individual schools and systems? What documentation must be kept?

3. Develop one strategy for your school building to identify and intervene with those students who are at risk for aggressive or violent behavior. Consider involving all school personnel. Identify one national standard and one student competency that you will address. Also consider any building policy or procedures that must be considered to successfully implement your strategy.

4. Consider these four student incidents, which you and your colleagues worked with this week:

   a. An angry girl who threatened others.

   b. Bullying in the bathroom.

    c. A student whose boyfriend started a fight in the cafeteria because she ate lunch with another boy.

    d. A student who brought a knife to school.

       For each incident, discuss the feelings associated with the violent/disruptive student. Identify the behaviors manifested by the feelings, and discuss which behaviors are early and/or imminent warning signs. Finally, identify the key issues and implications associated with each scenario.

5. Prepare a 5-minute presentation on fostering connectedness that you could share at a faculty meeting. Give a concrete example of how teachers and staff could utilize these strategies in the classroom:

- Help students get to know each other's (and your) strengths.
- Involve students in planning, problem solving, and identifying issues in the classroom.
- Involve all students in classroom responsibilities.
- Integrate the concepts of self-discipline and respect for each other throughout your lessons.
- Involve students in developing the criteria by which their work will be assessed.

Chapter 14

Transitioning Into the Field of School Counseling

Envisioning Your Future

Planning for Your Success
    Learning About the Home and Community Environment
    Learning About the School Environment

Heading Toward Success
    Organizing Your Physical Environment
    Organizing Your Time
    Organizing Your Resources
    Organizing Your Data Sources
    Organizing Your Support System

Ensuring Your Success
    Professional Development
    Practicing Wellness
    Professional Comportment
    Maintaining Your Professional Commitments

Laying the Foundation for Your School Counseling Program
    Preparing a Mission Statement
    Building a Belief System
    Building Your Team

Making the Shift to a Comprehensive, Transformed
School Counseling Program

One Year Later: Envisioning Your Transformed School
Counseling Program

A Closing Word From the Authors

Chapter Objectives

By the time you have completed this chapter, you should be able to:

- Explain how you will implement the elements of a comprehensive school counseling program.
- Integrate the major themes of the textbook into your own comprehensive school counseling program.
- Identify practical suggestions you will use to strengthen your professional relationships and allies.
- Define how your belief system will be demonstrated in delivering equitable and quality education for all students.
- Explain how you will examine and enhance the physical, academic, and social climates in schools for optimum success.
- Explain how to use a school's power base, your leadership style, and your own power base to enhance student learning.
- Describe specific steps you will take to build your professionalism.

School Counselor Casebook: Getting Started

The Scenario

It is the last day of the school year and you have just finished your first year as a school counselor. You feel very good about what you consider a very successful first year. You believe you have made significant strides in grooming relationships and garnering support from administration and teachers for your program. You wonder if your perceptions of a very successful year match others' evaluations of you and your program. You think about the things that surprised you most about the job. You also think about the things you wish someone had told you before you began your first day in the profession.

Thinking About Solutions

As you read this chapter, imagine yourself as the school counselor in this scenario. When you come to the end of the chapter, you will see how four new counselors (each with 2 to 4 years of experience) and two interns responded to these questions.

Envisioning Your Future

We hope you are excited about the great places this amazing profession is going to take you. Our sincere hope is that this textbook has served not only to inform but also to energize you about your journey ahead. As you move ahead you can be secure in the knowledge that the work you do along the way will improve the lives of hundreds of students. You will make a difference. How many professionals can say this with assurance?

During the past few months you have studied, reflected, and grappled with the traditional and the transformed practices of school counseling. Whether you are preparing for an immediate induction into the profession of school counseling or still have several courses ahead of you, it is our hope that you are developing a strong belief system and formulating in your mind how your beliefs will be demonstrated in your actions. These beliefs are at the core of the authors' belief system:

- Every student can learn and achieve to high standards.
- Every child is entitled to an equitable and quality educational experience in a school environment that is safe and respectful.
- All students can benefit from an effective school counseling program.
- School counseling programs are most successful when delivered in collaboration and in partnership with students, families, community members, educators, and administrators.

We also hope that you are developing strong beliefs about the role and responsibilities of a school counselor. The authors hold these beliefs:

- School counselors, as leaders and advocates, identify and rectify school-based practices that inhibit the success of individuals and groups of students.
- School counselors model behavior that contributes to a climate of caring and academic rigor, and play a significant role in raising aspirations and motivating every student to succeed.
- School counselors help students develop effective interpersonal relationships and establish individual plans to achieve successful futures.
- School counselors, like all educators, are accountable for student success and have a responsibility to contribute significantly to systemic change (Stone, 1996; Stone & Hanson, 2002).

Your entrée into the profession can be facilitated by calculated moves on your part, starting with the first day of school. Following are some suggested guiding principles for maintaining your focus and belief system.

- Act as a *counselor, advocate, leader, collaborator, and consultant* to maximize opportunities for students to succeed academically, emotionally, and socially.
- Strive to develop in all students *ambitious goals* and a *commitment to achievement* and to provide the positive environmental conditions that enable students to realize high aspirations.
- Become a **steward of equity;** be able to use data to recognize *institutional and environmental barriers* that impede students' ability to realize their full academic potential, and be equipped to take the lead in remedying these inequities.
- Provide all students with *academic and career advising* to help them form values and attitudes about the significance of education to their future economic success and their quality of life.
- Become an effective *manager of resources* and partnership builder, enlisting the support of parents, agencies, and community members (Stone, 1996).

Planning for Your Success

Before you begin your new job, spend as much time as you can learning about the physical, structural, academic, and social climate of the school, starting with the community in which it is situated.

Learning About the Home and Community Environment

If possible drive, walk, or ride public transportation around the neighborhoods where your students live. Physically placing yourself in your students' neighborhood can be an eye-opening experience and will help you start to develop a solid understanding of your students' needs. Ask questions of other faculty and community members about the range of socioeconomic levels in the community, about incidents of child abuse, and about the degree of parental involvement. The front-office staff are a good source of valuable information, such as how many students are on free or reduced lunch, which student came in upset, attendance rates, and so on. Letting the front office staff know that you consider them a valuable resource has a dual purpose: you learn a great deal and you start to groom a relationship with a group of people who can considerably smooth your induction into the school. Learn all you can about the stressors and support systems of your school's families so that you can be prepared for the students who walk through your door. First-year counselor Ellen Balent-Golden says, "The front-office staff knows everything. They are my lookout. They know who has been absent or who comes to the clinic sick or hurt a lot. Parents call them and tell them everything, and they alert me when it is something that I need to know" (personal communication, 2004).

Community Standards

Become familiar with the prevailing community standards. Are you in an ultraconservative part of the world, a bastion of liberalism, a solid middle-class suburb, or an urban setting? Remember that ethics are situational. You will need to know the community and institutional standards to discern how to behave ethically in this particular environment. Would your community be respectful of a poster on your door advertising a support group for gay, lesbian, bisexual, and questioning youth? Could you encourage a student to go to a neighborhood health clinic if she tells you she is pregnant? It is important to have a feel for the level of tolerance for school interference in value-laden issues. We have to be highly sensitive to the fact that parents have been given the legal right to be the guiding voice in their children's lives.

Learning About the School Environment

Try to determine the nature of the school environment by asking questions. What is the working climate like at this school? Is there a sense of camaraderie and cohesiveness among faculty, or is the general atmosphere one of strife, tension, and unhealthy competition? Ask questions. Which departments or grade levels are functioning well? Are there problem or model areas?

Leadership and the Power Structure

Leadership and power are important aspects of the school environment and the **school climate**. Where is the power base for decision making on schoolwide issues? How are school counselors involved? Who are the formal leaders, and what is the formal organizational structure of your school? Does the formal organizational structure match the power structure? The informal power base is critically important. Who are the teachers who hold the power, have the principal's ear, or wield the greatest influence among the faculty? You will need these teachers and their influence, even though some of them may have negative attitudes. Think back to the chapter on leadership (Chapter 4). Identify those who have the referent power, connection power, and expert power. These are the people to know and court. Jim MacGregor, a high-school counselor whom you met in Chapter 5, understood the power of buy-in and relationship building. He opened doors for his students to be enrolled in higher level academics because he tenaciously tackled building a relationship with the external and internal community.

Culture and Beliefs of Administration and Faculty

Learn about the culture and belief system of the administration and faculty. What is their belief about student learning? Almost all educators espouse the belief that given the right conditions, all children can achieve to high levels. Do the educators in your school live this belief in programs and actions that support all students to be successful learners? How does the school use data to understand student achievement?

Ask questions about how students are disciplined in your school and look to see if there is a disciplinary plan in place. Read the disciplinary plan and see if you agree with it. Discreetly check to see if the plan is really carried out uniformly. Sejal Parikh, an elementary counselor in Jacksonville, Florida, found that in her school there was a disciplinary plan in need of revisiting. She participated in a committee that formulated a disciplinary plan that had teeth and could be uniformly enforced so that teachers and students both were ultimately winners.

Observe how teachers interact with students. Walk the hallways, listen, and keenly observe. You will be one of the few people in the school who has a finger on the pulse of the school and who understands which teachers have good classroom management, which rule by intimidation, or which employ cooperative discipline. Capitalize on this knowledge by helping other teachers to replicate the practices that result in a safer more respectful school climate for all children.

The Students

Student morale is an aspect of the school environment and the school climate. Are the students engaged, enthusiastic, positive, and motivated? Find out how school spirit is demonstrated. What percentage of the student body feels disenfranchised? To gain a better understanding of the student body, go into the cafeteria and sit down with groups of students to talk to them. By asking students what they think of their school and their school counseling program, you can open a dialogue, learn how the school counseling program is perceived, discover whether the program has any public relations problems, and solicit ideas on areas to include in your program. Students often lament that the adults in the school do not really understand the cliques, gangs, and social order of the school environment (Stone & Isaacs, 2002).

Engage a cross section of the student body—not just the high-achieving, well-behaved students—to answer questions about the real climate of the school (Stone & Isaacs, 2002). Students can tell us who is being bullied, who is in charge, where the bullying is taking place, whether students feel safe, and other important issues that impact the learning and well-being of students (Stone & Isaacs, 2002).

Counselors Making a Difference

Meet Carol McLeod-Orso

Changing the Culture and the Belief System

While a University of North Florida school counseling student, Carol interned at a rural high school that had a history of minimal course offerings in higher level academics. Carol knew that course assignments in high school significantly differentiate students' opportunities beyond high school as well as their economic futures. Carol worked with the administrative team to use the school's database to provide her with information about students' mathematics scores on the state tests. Carol learned that a significant number of students taking the higher level mathematics courses were scoring the highest on the state tests regardless of their grades or success rate in higher level mathematics courses. In other words, she found a direct correlation between taking higher level mathematics and doing better on statewide tests, and no correlation between mathematics course grades and statewide test scores. Carol looked further and found that failures in mathematics were largely due to factors such as not completing homework, excessive absences, and other variables that did not have to do with the students' ability to do higher level mathematics. Armed with this information, Carol started a critical dialogue with her administration about her findings. Using the school's database, she identified ninth graders who made a final grade of D or F in Algebra 1 in eighth grade and therefore were not recommended to take geometry, yet these students had demonstrated solid mathematics scores on their standardized tests! Understanding that knowledge can raise aspirations, she decided to ask the administrative team and chairman of the mathematics department if she could help these students understand the interrelationship between higher level mathematics and their future economic opportunities. Carol will follow this academic advising with student performance contracts and advance them to geometry in 9th grade and Algebra II in 10th grade—the year they take the state test to determine eligibility to graduate. Students at this school who have had poor grades in mathematics in the past—regardless of state test scores—have regularly been scheduled to take low level mathematics courses. Carol is a social justice advocate who used data to give her knowledge and power when advocating for greater opportunities for the students in her school.

Reprinted with permission by Carol McLeod-Orso.

Curriculum/Instruction and Student Support

To the extent possible, learn as much as you can about the school's curriculum offerings, the special education program, and all support systems in place for struggling students. What is the philosophy and belief about what makes effective instruction?

In elementary and middle school, getting advice about resource schedules such as physical education, music, and art can help you develop your classroom guidance schedule and further your understanding of the nature of this particular school.

Heading Toward Success

On or before your first day, begin heading toward success by organizing your space, your time, your resources, your data sources, and your support system.

Organizing Your Physical Environment

You may have little or no control over the physical environment you are assigned. However, try to optimize your environment before the first day of school, because as the year progresses you will have little time to fuss over making changes, moving furniture, and hanging pictures. Set yourself up early in a comfortable arrangement for the year. Vie for an office near equipment and the people you most often need to access. You may have to scavenge if resources and furniture don't meet your needs. Find out what your school district has in the form of a surplus furniture warehouse. Place your furniture with attention to traffic patterns, and have a space that allows you and students to be comfortable and in close proximity to each other without a desk or other barrier between you. A small table with chairs is ideal if you are lucky enough to have an office that will accommodate this.

Organizing Your Time

A weekly, monthly, and yearly calendar can be a support. Establish a weekly calendar and place it on your door. Even if you have no idea as to what your month or year will actually look like, taking the step to have a semblance of organization and voice in your weekly schedule will help establish a feeling of being in control of your time and job assignments. You can make adjustments and changes as you go along, but getting started is an important first step.

Organizing Your Resources

What technology resources are available? The hope is that your school has a wonderful infrastructure for high-speed Internet use, computers on every desk, technology labs, closed-circuit television, and a computer teacher(s). Ideally your equipment will include computers for you and the students, a phone with multiple phone lines, a copy machine, and a fax machine. It is very likely that you will not have the perfect situation. Be resourceful and seek support from business partners and others to help meet the equipment needs of your office. Often you will be hired into an already established program and things will be set up for you. You have to use your judgment about how much change you should ask for right away and which items you will want to table for a more opportune time. You are working to establish an inviting space for yourself and your students.

Organizing Your Data Sources

Chapter 9 covered the rationale and mechanics of identifying and using critical data elements, also known as report card data. As early as possible you will want to study your school's report card data. An easy way to start is to find the person in your school most familiar with the data and capture a few minutes of their time to discuss student performance and other critical data. The principal is usually a great resource for this information and will likely cooperate with vigor and appreciation. Improving student data elements is a "do-or-die" proposition for principals, so when you ask about the school's report card data, you are placing yourself in a positive light as someone who believes that the accountability imperative includes you (Stone & Clark, 2001; Stone & Hanson, 2002).

Organizing Your Support System

Many school systems assign new counselors a buddy or a mentor. This person usually is a talented, seasoned counselor who can assist new professionals in negotiating the first year and avoiding some of the pitfalls. If there is not a formal program in place in your district, reach out to someone and ask whether he or she will mentor you. If your school district does not have a formal mentoring program, find someone to support you in this way.

Find colleagues right in your own building who can support your efforts, such as your fellow counselors, a talented, influential teacher, or a grade-level or department chairperson. Orchestrate success for yourself. For example, present your first classroom guidance lessons in the rooms of teachers who have the best classroom management. Deliver a 5- or 10-minute staff development presentation early in the year on a topic that is sure to be of interest to all and that will place you in a positive, proactive light in the eyes of others. Outside of school, find a sounding board, an ear, someone with whom you can share all the frustrations that you don't want to air at school.

To further prepare for your first day in the profession, attend to some public relations efforts that will help launch your program. Establish a bulletin board and give each teacher a newsletter or flier to distribute to his or her students, highlighting components of your program. Contribute to an invitational environment for students by joining existing efforts or suggesting ways to welcome students. In addition to your bulletin board, flier, or newsletter, greet students with a message over the public address system. The opportunities for public relations are endless.

Ensuring Your Success

As you launch into your first year as a transformed school counselor, attend to your professional skills and knowledge. Develop ways to maintain your energy and resolve to meet your professional commitments. Begin building the relationships that will support you in all of your efforts to develop a successful program.

Professional Development

Professional organizations offer support and can help you increase your **professionalism** in the field. As a new counselor, never miss an opportunity to go to the state conference. Time away with others in your profession reenergizes and excites you about your profession, in addition to bringing back armloads of ideas. Your peers can be your best teachers and motivators. When looking back to the "standard of care" principle in Chapter 11, remember that you increase your commitment to professional growth and raise your standard of care when you are an active member of your professional organization. If you ever find yourself in legal hot water, your attorney is going to ask you about membership in professional organizations and how you demonstrated your commitment to the organization. Your lawyer's intent in this type of situation would be to show that you behaved as the reasonably competent professional in supporting your own professional growth.

Professional organizations such as the American School Counselor Association (ASCA) and the American Counseling Association (ACA) also provide informative publications and listservers as part of your membership. Each and every dollar spent on ASCA and ACA is returned to you in terms of the wonderful benefits you receive in professional development.

District-level in-services, regional workshops, and summer institutes are but a few of the many ways you can continue to grow your professionalism. It is the responsibility of each one of us to seek ways to continue to stay abreast of an ever-changing profession.

Practicing Wellness

What do you do for wellness? School counselors expend considerable energy. How do you sustain your energy? The more you give of yourself to support others, the more you need to take care of your own personal wellness. Every organization has its drawbacks and unfortunately schools are no different and sometimes there can be unhealthy people, toxic environments, bureaucracy, and other drains on a school counselor's emotional well-being. The nature of most school counseling situations is one of satisfaction in knowing that we have made a positive impact on students, but counseling also is a demanding profession because there are too many students with unmet needs. While developing student resiliency, cultivate and guard your own. Find outlets that renew your spirit, and seek opportunities to do them regularly. Do you find renewal in travel, exercise, friends, and family? Does your serenity come from reading, spiritual pursuits, writing, or hobbies? Find allies among your colleagues to help buoy and support your resolve to do all you can for students. Orchestrate opportunities for tangible successes in order to help sustain the enthusiasm necessary for what you are doing.

Professional Comportment

Behave in a professional manner at all times, and be your own best advertisement. Positive self-talk is usually translated into a positive demeanor and hangs a welcome sign on your back that says, "I am approachable." Attitude is everything. Instead of being frustrated with barriers, develop a sense of humor about the absurdities of institutions, people, and bureaucracies. Your work is critically important, but give yourself permission not to be consumed by it. Set boundaries, develop coping skills, and keep whatever comes your way in perspective, because in the end your attitude will affect the beliefs and behaviors from which you operate and assist students.

Build and protect your relationships. A good portion of the coordination, consultation, and theories chapters focused on building relationships; offered here are some cautions about protecting your relationships! Avoid behaving as a divisive element, and be vigilant not to give the appearance of siding with one faction of the administration or faculty over another. Refuse to be a party to tearing down the administration, other faculty members, parents, or students. Build bridges.

Respect the experience of others and share your knowledge. Teachers and staff may look with suspicion on the new person who comes in eager with new ideas, ready to save the world. The undertones of climate and morale may influence their receptivity to your ideas. Respect the traditions and established procedures of the school to the greatest extent possible and astutely make your changes so that you can be as effective as possible in the long run. Find and celebrate the gems in current practices; then, with solid relationship building, you can start to make systemic changes.

Maintaining Your Professional Commitments

Adhering to many of the ideals you learned in graduate school will be tougher than you think. Be prepared to fight the good fight.

Stay Passionate About Advocacy

Advocacy is hard work. Expect support, praise, and ridicule at varying times. How do you stay invigorated when the response from others may be indifference at best, and resistance at worst? One way to stay the course when you feel your resolve wavering is to walk into classrooms and look into the eyes of the students sitting there. Throughout this text you have been presented with the statistics of lost potential. When you feel your advocacy wavering, go into the kindergarten classes, look into the eyes of 100 students, and identify the 47 students that you are willing to sacrifice. By keeping the children's faces in your mind's eye, you will be spurred on to make the system work for all students. When teachers or others say to you, directly or indirectly, that certain students are "a lost cause," find a way to gently, politically, and skillfully remind them that the hopes and dreams they want for their own children are the same as what educators should want for all students. If all of us in our communities and schools would do for each child what we would want done for our own children, then we would have a system committed to finding ways to widen students' opportunities. If as an advocate you can remember that the alternative to making waves is allowing some students to be left out of the success picture, then it will help fuel your passion to stay the course.

Counselors Making a Difference

Jim MacGregor

Changing the Status Quo

Like most school counselors, Jim is outnumbered by a heavy counselor-student ratio. Not content to accept that he would only be able to be a career and academic advisor to a few students, Jim developed a computer-based 4-year plan that interfaced with student-identified career clusters. Using the career cluster as a guide, Jim's program informed students as to which mathematics and sciences they would need to match their career plans. Jim's efforts to help students see that they would have brighter futures if they would stretch and strive academically was made considerably easier when he tied course-taking to a student's career goals, and the 4-year career plan became a living document that changed as the student's career cluster changed. Over the course of six years, Jim's advocacy resulted in a 40% increase in African-American students choosing higher level mathematics and science courses. School counselors who act purposefully to connect students to their future opportunities impact the instructional program and change the status quo regarding which students will reach graduation with a wide range of paths from which to choose.

There have been too many examples of academic success in the face of tremendous adversity to conclude that intelligence and ability are handed out sparingly or based on only genetic endowments, or that they cannot be affected by educational environments. These examples are powerful reminders that great potential exists in all students. What needs changing first are the attitudes, beliefs, and values with which teachers approach their students, and the conditions in schools to support the high-level learning of all students (Nieto, 1999, p. 173).

Support the Instructional Program

Good teaching matters! Throughout the text you have been given many techniques for supporting the instructional program. Constantly think of new ways to implement strategies to support teaching and learning. Send the message at every turn that you respect the tough job teachers have and that you are there to support the instructional program and the teachers' efforts. Be slow to judge. Teaching and school administration are hard jobs, indeed among the hardest jobs in America today, with tough accountability, and oftentimes minimal support. Be a cheerleader, never a thorn, for teachers and administrators.

Counselors Making a Difference

Meet Melissa Hippensteel Howell

Good Teaching Matters

Melissa was assigned to a school in which all previous teachers except the physical education (PE) teacher were removed and replaced by proven master teachers. This school was designated by the state for takeover at the end of the year if test scores did not improve. The PE teacher marveled at the change in the school: "In the past, all the teachers slept or took turns watching each other's class while they left campus. There was no education going on here." Melissa knew how to teach. It was said of Melissa that she could teach anyone to read and could motivate even the most troubled child. She set her jaw with determination, rolled up her sleeves, won her third graders' hearts and, oh, how they worked for her. Test results arrived and the principal called all staff together to inform them that the school had excelled and that they were now off the "F" list. Each teacher received his or her students' scores for sorting into two stacks to indicate which students fell "below basic." Melissa had no sorting to do; none of her students scored "below basic." When Melissa returned her single stack, this reserved, low-key principal let out a whoop, grabbed her, hugged her, and said, "Don't you realize what you have done?" Many students drop out of education in third grade but wait until they are 16 to leave school. In Melissa's class that year, no one dropped out. Good teaching matters!

Reprinted with permission by Melissa H. Howell.

Laying the Foundation for Your School Counseling Program

Every chapter in this text has given you pieces of the puzzle so that you will be able to build a solid school counseling program. Chapter 8 explained the ASCA national models and standards and laid out the components of a comprehensive school counseling program. Chapters on counseling, consultation, leadership, advocacy, theory, and counseling applications gave you the knowledge and skills to implement the components of your school counseling program. This chapter is designed to help you transition into the field and start to build a solid foundation. Let us continue the work by discussing the major components of a successful program.

Preparing a Mission Statement

Study the school's mission statement, then write the mission statement for your counseling program. You will recall from Chapter 9 that the mission of the school counseling program should be closely aligned with the school's mission. For example, "The mission of the school counseling program is to provide professional school counseling expertise to all students, pre-K through 12, to ensure that every student, regardless of race, gender, religion, heritage, ability, or economic status, will be afforded the opportunity to achieve the skills needed to become a lifelong learner and productive member of society." Printing out and displaying your mission statement will serve two purposes: (a) it will provide you with transparency, letting everyone—including students, teachers, and administrators—know what you stand for and what you hope to accomplish, and (b) it will keep you focused by reminding you every day of how your program connects to the mission of the school.

Building a Belief System

As we discussed earlier in this chapter, beliefs shape how we view our world; behaviors reflect our belief system. What we believe, what we hold fast and true about students, families, teachers, and the educational process, drives our ability to support success for every student. Our beliefs are derived from our background and experiences. Earlier in this chapter you had an opportunity to develop a personal belief statement. To develop a core belief system for their programs requires a dialogue among school counselors and their colleagues to explore the complexity of educational issues from all vantage points. A belief statement may read, "We believe that all students can learn and achieve to high levels. We believe that a comprehensive developmental school counseling program will help promote equity and access to educational opportunities. We believe that as leaders in our schools, as advocates for our students, and as collaborators with students, teachers, parents, and administrators, we serve every student and provide equal access to school counseling programs." To launch the building of the school's formal belief system, draft a core belief statement and circulate it among your new colleagues, asking for their comments and contributions.

Building Your Team

The key to the development and implementation of a successful program is readiness! Before charging forward, identify a team that can help to implement your program. The core team members would include administrators, teachers, student service personnel, parents, students, and business and community representatives. Your team can start small and grow as needed. Table 14.1 shows the typical program implementation team and the responsibilities of its members.

Table 14.1 Program Implementation Team

Implementation Team Members	*Responsibilities in a Comprehensive School Counseling Program*
School Counselors	Provide proactive leadership to ensure that every student is served. They manage the comprehensive program and coordinate strategies and activities with others (teachers, support staff, parents, community agencies, business representatives) to meet the stated goals and standards/competencies.
Teachers	Are partners with school counselors. They develop and infuse guidance activities into the instructional program that are integral to good learning, *not* extraneous or disconnected material. They may serve as advisers or mentors to students.
Pupil Personnel Services (school psychologist, social worker, school nurse, etc.)	Collaborate and team with the school's counselors to ensure that school psychologists, school social workers, school nurses, student assistance counselors, and other support personnel are actively involved in supporting each student's academic, career, and personal-social development. They support students and families with information regarding outside agencies and assist students with mental or physical health issues, or with social issues.
Administrators	Provide leadership in developing the program and in the ongoing program improvement. They provide continuous support and emphasize the importance of the program to others. They promote cooperation between and among counselors, faculty, and others. Additionally, they provide facilities and resources and allow time to facilitate the program process.
Parents	Work cooperatively with school personnel in delivering the program. They serve on committees and provide linkages to the community by communicating program goals to others.

Implementation Team Members	Responsibilities in a Comprehensive School Counseling Program
Students	Actively participate and assume responsibility for meeting standards/competencies. They will be able to identify the skills, knowledge, and attitudes they have gained in structured guidance sessions.
Business/Community Representatives	Representatives from business and industry and others in the community serve on committees, talk with classes, act as mentors, provide financial support, and generally serve as partners in the education of youth.

Making the Shift to a Comprehensive, Transformed School Counseling Program

What do you do if you start a new job in a school that does not have a comprehensive, transformed school counseling program as prescribed by ASCA? Ideally you would negotiate the political landscape skillfully and move toward a collaborative effort in which key players will analyze existing practices (Table 14.2). The purpose of the analysis would be to determine to what degree comprehensive

Table 14.2 Analyzing Existing Practices

Current Practice	Analysis
Individual Counseling	How much time have school counselors been spending in individual counseling sessions?
	How many students per year receive individual counseling?
	What program initiatives can be instituted that help more students while lessening the need for individual counseling?
Group Counseling	How many group counseling sessions have counselors been hosting each month? How many students are involved with group counseling?
	How can group counseling be used to meet the needs of all students?
Collaboration	What are the resources available within the district and community to assist students and families, and how do counselors currently collaborate with these services?
	In what ways can collaboration with district and community services be improved?
Consultation	How often do school counselors consult with other members of the school community?
	How could this consultation process be improved?

(continued)

Table 14.2 Continued

Current Practice	Analysis
Leadership	In what manner do the school counselors currently demonstrate leadership?
	How might your leadership skills be better used to help all students reach their potential?
Advocacy	How does the school counseling program advocate for equity and support students who are at risk of failure?
	How can the advocacy component of the program be improved?
Teaming and Collaboration	How often and in what ways do counselors collaborate with members of the school community to assist students?
	How can teamwork and collaboration at this school be improved?
Data-Driven Results	What type of data does the school district collect?
	How can that data be used to drive the comprehensive school counseling program?
Use of Technology	Take an inventory of the technology available at this school.
	Is the available technology sufficient to help you assist students and their families?
	What additional technology do you need, and how will you justify its purchase?

school counseling is in place and to clearly identify aspects of a comprehensive model that need to be implemented.

One Year Later: Envisioning Your Transformed School Counseling Program

In an ideal world, what might your transformed school counseling program look like one year after it is launched? The ASCA school counseling program model forms the foundation of your program, supports the mission of your school, and provides the direction as to how every student will benefit from the school counseling program. The implementation team has determined a mission statement, philosophy, and guiding beliefs in line with the school, district, and ASCA mission. The team has identified an appropriate delivery system, to include classroom teachers and support personnel. Parents, students, teachers, and support staff are aware of their roles within the delivery system. Newsletters, parents' nights, and presentations to faculty and community members promote the delivery system, and career and business partners are included in the delivery model.

The implementation team meets regularly to discuss implementation at each level, acting as a support team, sharing the burden of change, and celebrating the victories achieved. Additionally, the members monitor whether one or more aspects of the pre-K through 12 comprehensive counseling program have *not* been addressed. If components of the program are lacking, discussions take place to ensure that implementation progresses holistically and remains focused upon improving student academic success.

Your comprehensive school counseling program is in a constant state of growth and change so that it will continue to address the specific needs of all students each year. A concerted effort is made to meet students in small and large groups. School counselors are now more visible to a greater number of students and faculty and are viewed as leaders, advocates, and team players working toward school improvement and systemic change.

Your newly developed program supports the school's academic mission by promoting and enhancing the learning process for all students through an integration of academic, career, and personal-social development. The comprehensive school counseling program is an integral component of the total educational experience of all students. The program fosters student achievement and school improvement and is developmental and systematic in nature, sequential, clearly defined, and accountable. By addressing student needs in academic, career, and personal-social development throughout their pre-K through 12 schooling, the comprehensive school counseling program promotes and enhances the learning process for all students.

Your school counseling program is now organized as an integral and essential part of the broader school mission (Gysbers & Henderson, 2000; Schmidt, 2000; Wittmer, 2000). The program promotes educational excellence through individual excellence, provides preventive and intervention programs and experiences, creates a collaborative model that integrates the expertise of school counselors and other pupil services personnel as well as business and community into the total program, and is current with the needs and expectations of the education agenda and societal issues (Dahir, 2001; Gysbers & Henderson, 2000; Myrick, 2003b).

A Closing Word From the Authors

Traditionally, professional school counselors have been ancillary to the mission of schools. The ASCA model and standards and the Transforming School Counseling Initiative place professional school counselors at the forefront of school reform. With current data indicating achievement and opportunity gaps between low socioeconomic students and their more advantaged peers, there is an ethical and moral imperative for professional school counselors to utilize all resources available to acquire the knowledge, skills, and attitudes to close the gaps and to support all students.

You are preparing to be a professional school counselor, an educator who, like your colleagues, will be at the heart and soul of the educational process; not a visitor whose job it is to be a clinician, but an educator who will bring unique counseling skills and specialized knowledge to the school setting. You will have a major impact upon your students through a repertoire of powerful roles: counselor, leader, advocate, collaborator, team builder, consultant, data analyzer/consumer, systemic change agent, steward of equity and access, manager of resources, career and academic advisor, and didactic counselor. This text has introduced you to school counselors who understand that they are uniquely positioned to touch all the students in their schools through their skills.

Emulate these role models and embrace your future as a counselor, consultant, collaborator, leader, advocate, and systemic change agent, wielding influence and contributing to student success. Find your focus and implement your belief system. Being a counselor and an educator is an amazing privilege that allows us to use our skills to give our young people the gift of access and success in learning—a gift that will carry them beyond the school walls. How exciting to be part of this crucial profession and touch the future through the lives of our students!

As a newly minted school counselor, build a support base so that you can attack barriers to student success and tackle the daunting task of changing attitudes and beliefs about students and their ability to learn. Make that mythical level playing field your sparring ground, where you tackle institutional and environmental barriers that continue to adversely stratify students' opportunities. Embrace a social justice agenda and kick dirt in the proverbial eye of inequity.

TechTools

This TechTools section offers suggestions to help you maximize the goals of your program when you become a practicing school counselor. However, when appropriate and possible, learn and implement these "tech tools" before you enter the field.

- Contact Educational Testing Services of the College Board and the ACT organization to learn what they have available in disaggregated student data and survey information that will help you better understand your students' test scores and their survey responses.
- Use a search engine to look for grants to purchase equipment for your school counseling office and for other needs.
- Find the data wizard in your school—the person who can help you better understand which groups of students successfully mastered the annual achievement exams and provide other critical data.

- Read how school counselors could benefit from "E-government Solutions: The Case of Paperwork," which is posted on the Indiana School Counselor Association website, to gain further insights into streamlining and automating cumbersome "paper-pushing processes."
- Join a listserver so that you have colleagues to consult with readily.
- Earmark websites that will prove especially helpful to you by putting them in the "My Favorites" category on your computer's desktop. Some examples of such websites are www.Schoolcounselor.com, electronic versions of Education Week, and www.cyberguidance.net.
- Develop an electronic newsletter for your students and parents.
- Learn to use the closed-circuit television equipment or find someone who can help you, so that you can deliver daily messages to students.
- Attend to your professional development by taking advantage of the American Counselor Association courses that are available on video. Many are excellent and can contribute mightily to increasing your knowledge on everything from brief therapy to legal and ethical issues.

School Counselor Casebook: Voices From the Field

The Scenario Reviewed

It is the last day of the school year and you have just finished your first year as a school counselor. You feel very good about what you consider a very successful first year. You believe you have made significant strides in grooming relationships and garnering support from administration and teachers for your program. You wonder if your perceptions of a very successful year match others' evaluations of you and your program. You think about the things that surprised you most about the job. You also think about the things you wish someone had told you before you began your first day in the profession.

A Practitioner's Approach

Four new counselors (each with 2 to 4 years of experience) and two interns responded to this question.

I never could have imagined the amount of serious family issues that elementary children must deal with (i.e., divorce, domestic violence, single parents, death, drugs and alcohol, sexual/physical abuse, neglect in varying degrees, lack of parenting skills, and patterns of blame. Before becoming a school counselor I wish I had known the time spent (and very much needed) as a sounding board (listener and problem solver) for parents, teachers, and administrators. I have found it so important to work with the parents and teachers to provide interventions and accommodations for children. It is because of the special needs of my students that classroom guidance, systemic changes, and grant writing are a big part of my life as a school counselor.

Laura Lee Kinard is an elementary counselor at a rural school in Bryceville, Florida. Laura graduated from the University of North Florida School Counseling Program in 2003.

Before becoming a counselor I never could have imagined how much I would worry about my students' future, especially my high-school and continuing education students. I work with students who are all deaf or blind with additional special needs. As I work on their final Transition Individual Education Plans it is like a huge scavenger hunt to try to research resources for these students, who are from all over the state of Florida. I want my students to experience the best opportunities out there, because they deserve the best. I am constantly amazed at how much trust the parents put in the school counselor. Parents have a huge responsibility and they need all the support that school counselors can offer them. In the preparation program we talked about the importance of working as part of the team and collaborating with others. I never would have imagined how huge this part of the job is. Learning how to relate with students, school staff, parents, community agencies, and local businesses in positive ways is so important. I've also been amazed at how valuable my relationships with the other students in my counselor preparation program have become. We are always there for each other and can offer support and feedback.

I never imagined how important it was going to be to be creative and to be able to take initiative. I've learned in this job that if you can dream it, you can make it happen. If you have supportive administration, teachers, support staff, and parents, the sky is the limit. Sometimes it may be a balancing act, but always working on building positive relationships allows me to attain these dreams.

I wish I had known just how important time management really is! Each year that I perform my job, my skills and techniques for time management grow and improve. I am able to do so much more this third year as compared to my first year. At the end of a year, I now sit down with my planner and pencil in the entire next year, making sure I have time for classroom guidance sessions, transition planning/counseling sessions, career fair, red ribbon activities, testing/assessment training/consultation, special projects, and team meetings. I get so much more done if I plan out my year in advance rather than just taking each day as it comes. I have learned that it is so important to take care of myself and to nurture a wonderful support group (friendships) beyond school and get plenty of rest so that I can meet the demands of a job I truly love.

Karen Kolkedy is a counselor at The School for the Deaf and Blind in St. Augustine, Florida. Karen graduated from the University of North Florida School Counseling Program in 2002. Reprinted with permission by Karen E. Kolkedy.

I would never have imagined the extent to which there are inequities in our public schools. The problem is compounded because so many educators are not trained to teach low socioeconomic, urban students. The resiliency of elementary students to survive and thrive under adverse conditions always surprises me and gives me hope. I wish I would have known before becoming a school counselor how better to work with fellow educators who are not invested in their school and their students. This daily struggle has been very taxing.

Sejal Parikh has worked as both an urban elementary school counselor and a suburban high-school counselor in the Jacksonville, Florida, area. Sejal graduated from the University of North Florida School Counseling Program in 2001. Sejal is now a doctoral candidate at the University of North Carolina, Charlotte.

I never could have imagined how rewarding it is to work with students. Each day I learn something new from them. I'm always on my toes! As a counselor, we have more freedom to work with students without having the curriculum constraints that teachers have and can impact a student as a whole. I have been very surprised about how entrenched school counseling departments can be. Entering into an already established school counseling office makes it difficult to implement schoolwide comprehensive guidance programs; buy-in is difficult to obtain as a new counselor.

Shirin Mitsis is an urban high-school counselor in Jacksonville, Florida, and is in her first year as a school counselor. Shirin graduated from the University of North Florida School Counseling Program in 2004. Reprinted with permission by Shirin Mitsis.

Making the transition from the graduate school classroom to the counseling department may leave you feeling a bit unprepared, but there is no time to hesitate. There is simply no substitute for being in the school environment and watching events unfold. I know I have a lot to learn, even though I feel well prepared. There never seems to be enough time. I learned fairly early that counseling, especially at the elementary level, is not a linear process. The truth is that as I grow as a school counselor, I will be more able to define where the book knowledge ends and the real-life knowledge begins. Every experience is a learning experience, even though it might not feel that way at the time. Internship has taught me the value of small steps. I can think of no better preparation for new counselors than spending time "on-the-job" as interns.

Julie Van Nostrand interned at Southampton High School and Southampton Elementary School and graduated from the New York Institute of Technology School Counseling Program in 2004. Reprinted with permission by Julie Van Nostrand, School Counselor Intern.

Some counselors initially question the intern's abilities, and the intern needs to prove himself or herself. I feel that my abilities were at the level necessary to be a contributing and valued member of the counseling staff. We were well prepared by the books. We know our alphabet soup of policies, interventions, and committees. Gysbers, Gladding, Turba, and Stone are like old friends, and we can plan out a way to implement the ASCA national model with the best of them. The foundation was strong. Theory and planning took a back seat when a child's family was evicted, a father passed away, college applications were due and New York State changed the graduation requirements, and we were in the midst of it all trying to be a rock of stability and a source for answers. This is not a case study, and practicum hours don't allow an individual to truly wrestle with these issues.

The theoretical foundation is useful, but learning on the job is going to be an on-going process for years and years to come. Being a seasoned counselor will be worth more than all the printed knowledge in the end. Theoretically, a feather and a brick fall at the same rate, but we know that isn't what actually occurs in real life. We need to understand a little Newtonian physics to have the big picture make sense and know where to go from there. The books and the internship experience have the same sort of relationship. Theoretically, we know where we need to go and how we may get there, but is takes a bit of pizzazz and chutzpah to get there in an actual school.

It is scary to think that students will be looking to me solely next year, but I am con-fident that I can handle it. "When in doubt, consult, consult, consult!" That is a les-son from first semester, but probably one of the most valuable in over two years. That needs to be a way of life as a counselor.

Philip Petrone interned at Westbury High School and Westbury Middle School and graduated from the New York Institute of Technology School Counseling Program in 2004. Reprinted with permission by Philip Petrone, School Counselor Intern.

Chapter Summary

Envisioning Your Future

For the past few months you have studied, reflected on, and grappled with the tra-ditional and the transformed practices of school counseling. You probably have de-veloped a strong belief system founded on the worth and dignity of each student, and have formulated in your mind how your beliefs will be demonstrated in your actions. The school counselor who believes that every student can learn and succeed will make this the compass and direction for his or her behavior in day-to-day work. Establish your focus by defining your guiding principles and belief system.

Preparing for Success as a School Counselor

Learn about your new school, beginning with your students' home and community environments. Try to determine the climate at your school to determine if there is a sense of camaraderie and cohesiveness among the faculty. Determine whether stu-dents are engaged, enthusiastic, positive, and motivated. Try to understand the cliques, gangs, and social order of the school environment. Determine the power base for decision making as well as the formal and informal organizational structure of your school. Try to understand what the administration and faculty's core belief systems are regarding student learning. Determine whether the school uses data to understand student achievement. Observe how teachers interact with students. Walk the hallways, listen, and keenly observe.

Build your support system and your professionalism. You increase your commitment to professional growth when you are an active member of your professional organization. Practice personal wellness, because the school counseling job demands both physical and emotional stamina. Try to optimize your physical environment before the first day of school. Set yourself up early in a comfortable arrangement for the year. Get psyched for advocacy by visiting classrooms and reminding yourself of why you are there.

Developing Your School Counseling Program

Write the mission statement for your school counseling program in coordination with the mission statement of the school. Identify an implementation team, whose purpose is to institutionalize the pre-K through 12 comprehensive counseling program. Design the program and, with the help of the implementation team, put the program into operation. Respect the traditions and the established procedures of the school to the greatest extent possible, and astutely make your changes so that you can be as effective as possible in the long run. Your comprehensive school counseling program should be in a constant state of growth and change so that it will continue to address the specific needs of all students each year. Make your school counseling program an integral component of the total educational experience of all students.

Key Terms

Professionalism p. 405   Steward of equity p. 399
School climate p. 400

Learning Extensions

1. Design a student and parent newsletter to distribute for a school's opening using word processing, graphics, and photos.

2. Create a resource list of websites to distribute to students, and a list of websites to use for your own professional development.

3. Visit a school and start to ask questions about how they use relational databases to inform their decision making around school improvement issues. Write up your findings in a 2-page summary.

4. Make a list of school report card critical data elements and write up a 2-page report explaining how and why you will discuss these data elements with your principal.

5. Design and deliver a presentation on an issue related to school counseling using presentation software.

6. Put together a mock purchase order describing the equipment you will want for your school counseling office, and present a rationale for the purchase of each piece of equipment. Give details, such as the components you will want on your computer. Visit equipment retailers via the Internet to learn all you can about the equipment you are ordering.

7. Put together a mock weekly, monthly, and yearly calendar. Do as Karen Kolkedy described, and pencil in your activities for the coming year.

References

Adelman, H. S. (2002). School counselors and school reform: New directions. *Professional School Counseling, 5*, 235–248.

Adelman, H., & Taylor, L. (2003). Commentary: Advancing mental health science and practice through authentic collaboration. *School Psychology Review, 32*(1), 53–56.

AEL, Inc. (2000, November). *School counselors: Emerging vanguards of student safety and success.* Policy Briefs. Charleston, WV: AEL Regional Educational Laboratory.

Aiken, L. R., Jr. (2000). *Psychological testing and assessment* (10th ed.). Boston: Allyn & Bacon.

Alexander, F. (1993, February). National standards: A new conventional wisdom. *Educational Leadership,* 9–10.

Allen-Meares, P., Washington, R. O., & Welsh, B. L. (2004). *Social work services in schools* (4th ed.). Englewood Cliffs, NJ: Prentice Hall.

American Association of University Women. (1993). *Hostile hallways.* Washington, DC: Author.

American Association of University Women. (2001). *Hostile hallways: Bullying, teasing and sexual harassment in school.* Washington, DC: Author.

American Counseling Association. (1987). *School counseling: A profession at risk.* Alexandria, VA: American Association for Counseling and Development.

American Counseling Association. (1993a). *Counseling minor students.* Alexandria, VA: Author.

American Counseling Association. (1993b). *The crisis in school counseling.* Alexandria, VA: Author.

American Counseling Association. (1994). Avoiding lawsuits and legal problems. *Legal Aspects of Counseling.* Washington, DC: Author.

American Counseling Association. (1995). *Code of ethics and standards of practice.* Retrieved December 12, 2001, from www.counseling.org

American Counseling Association. (1997b). *Sexual harassment in the schools: Background on Title IX of the education amendments of 1972 and guidance issued by the office of civil rights.* Alexandria, VA: Author.

American Counseling Association. (2004). *Draft position statement on high stakes testing.* Task Force on High Stakes Testing. Alexandria: VA.

American Psychiatric Association. (2000). *Diagnostic and statistical manual of mental disorders* (4th ed.). Text revision. Washington, DC: Author.

American School Counselor Association. (1979). *Standards for guidance and counseling programs.* Falls Church, VA: American Personnel and Guidance Association.

American School Counselor Association. (1990). *Role of the school counselor.* Alexandria, VA: Author.

American School Counselor Association. (1994). *The school counselor's role in educational reform*. Alexandria, VA: ASCA Press.

American School Counselor Association. (1996). *The school counselor's role in school to work*. Professional Development Series. Alexandria, VA: Author.

American School Counselor Association. (1997a). *Definition of school counseling*. Alexandria, VA: Author.

American School Counselor Association. (1997b). *Executive summary: The national standards for school counseling programs*. Alexandria, VA: Author.

American School Counselor Association. (1998). *Ethical standards for school counselors*. Retrieved May 30, 2004, from www.schoolcounselor.org

American School Counselor Association. (1999a). *Position statement: The professional school counselor and comprehensive school counseling*. Alexandria, VA: Author.

American School Counselor Association. (1999b). *Position statement: The role of the professional school counselor*. Alexandria, VA: Author.

American School Counselor Association. (2002). *The professional school counselor and high stakes testing*. Alexandria, VA: Author.

American School Counselor Association. (2003). *American school counselor association national model: A framework for school counseling programs*. Alexandria, VA: Author.

American School Counselor Association. (2004). *Ethical standards for school counselors*. Retrieved September 28, 2004, from www.schoolcounselor.org

American Youth Policy Forum. (2000). *High schools of the millennium*. Washington, DC: American Youth Policy Forum.

Anastasi, A. (1992). What counselors should know about the use of psychological tests. *Journal of Counseling and Development, 70*, 610–615.

Anastasi, A. & Urbina, S. (1997). *Psychological testing* (7th ed.). New York: Macmillan.

Anderson-Butcher, D., & Ashton, D. (2004a). Innovative models of collaboration to serve children, youths, families, and communities. *Children and Schools, 26*(1), 39.

Anderson-Butcher, D., & Ashton, D. (2004b). Reinventing a school. *Principal Leadership 26*, 1.

Annie Casey Foundation. (1996). *Kids count data book*. Baltimore, MD: Author.

Archibald, R. (2000, September 3). On the stump: The hot topic is education. *New York Times*, p. A31.

Arman, J. F. (2000). In the wake of the tragedy of Columbine High School. *Professional School Counseling, 2*, 218–220.

Arnold v. Board of Education, 880 U.S. F.2d 305 (1989).

Arredondo, P., & Arciniega, G. M. (2001). Strategies and techniques for counselor training based on the multicultural counseling competencies. *Journal of Multicultural Counseling and Development, 29*, 263–273.

Arredondo, P., Toporek, R., Brown, S. P., Jones, J., Locke, D., Sanchez, J., & Stadler, H. (1996). Operationalization of the multicultural counseling competencies. *Journal of Multicultural Counseling and Development, 24*, 42–78.

Arriaza, G. (2004). Making changes that stay made: School reform and community involvement 1. *The High School Journal, 87*(4), 10.

Atkins, M., Graczyk, P., Frazier, S., & Abdul-Adil, J. (2003). Toward a new model for promoting urban children's mental health: Accessible, effective, and sustainable school-based mental health. *School Psychology Review, 32*(4), 503.

Atkins, M., McKay, M., Arvanitis, P., London, L., Madison, S., Costigan, C., et al. (1998). An ecological model for school-based mental health services for urban low-income aggressive children. *The Journal of Behavioral Health Services & Research, 5*, 64–75.

Axelson, J. (1999). *Counseling and development in a multicultural society.* (3rd ed.). Pacific Grove, CA: Brooks/Cole.

Bailey, S. M. (1993). The current status of gender equity research in American schools. *Educational Psychologist, 28,* 321–339.

Baker, S. B. (2000). *School counseling for the 21st century* (3rd ed.). Upper Saddle River, NJ: Merrill Prentice Hall.

Ballard, M. B., & Murgatroyd, W. (1999). Defending a vital program: School counselors define their roles. *NASSP Bulletin, 83*(603), 19–26.

Banach, W. (2004). *What students, parents, and staff are saying about schools.* Ray Township, MI: Banach, Banach & Cassidy, Inc.

Bandura, A. (1986). *Social foundations of thought and action.* A social cognitive theory. Upper Saddle River, NJ: Prentice Hall.

Bandura, A. (1993). Perceived self efficacy in cognitive development and functioning. *Educational Psychologist, 28,* 117–148.

Bandura, A., & Jeffrey, R. W. (1977). Roles of symbolic coding and rehearsal processes in observational learning. *Journal of Personality and Social Psychology, 26,* 122–130.

Banks, J. A. (2001). *Multicultural education: Issues and perspectives.* (4th ed.). Boston: Allyn & Bacon.

Bart, M. (1998, September). Creating a safer school for gay students. *Counseling Today, 26,* 36–39.

Barth, K., Heinzmann, G. S., Casey-Doecke, J., Kahan, D. (2003). Is parental involvement a liability in youth sports? *Journal of Physical Education, Recreation & Dance, 74,* 41–42.

Bass, B. (2000). The future of leadership in learning organizations. *Journal of Leadership Studies, 7*(3), 18–38.

Beale, A., & Scott, P. (2001). "Bullybusters": Using drama to empower students to take a stand against bullying behavior. *Professional School Counseling, 4,* 300–305.

Bellotti v. Baird, 443 U.S. 622, S. Ct. 3035 (1979).

Bemak, F. (2000). Transforming the role of the counselor to provide leadership in educational reform through collaboration. *Professional School Counseling, 3,* 323–331.

Bennet, C. J. (1995). *Comprehensive multi-cultural education: Theory in practice.* (4th ed.) Boston: Allyn & Bacon.

Benson, P. L., Scales, P. C., Effort, N., & Roehikeepartain, E. C. (1999). *A fragile foundation: The state of developmental assets among American youth.* Minneapolis, MN: The Search Institute.

Bergin, J. W., & Bergin, J. J. (2000). Consultation and counseling strategies to facilitate inclusion. *Counseling and Human Development, 33*(2), 1.

Bettis, R. A. (1998). Commentary on "redefining industry structure for the information age" by J. L. Sampler. *Strategic Management Journal, 19,* 357–361

Bilzing, D. (1996). *Wisconsin Developmental Guidance Model.* Madison, WI: Wisconsin Department of Education.

Black, S. (2004). Stroking stressed-out teachers. *The Education Digest, 69*(5), 28.

Blackorby, J., & Wagner, M. M. (1997). The employment outcomes of youth with learning disabilities. In P. J. Gerber & D. S. Brown (Eds.), *Learning Disabilities and Employment* (pp. 57–74). Austin, TX: PRO-ED, Inc.

Blackwell, T. L. (2001). Woodcock-Johnson III test. *Rehabilitation Counseling Bulletin, 44*(4), 232–235.

Bloom, B. (1992). *Planned short-term therapy.* Boston: Allyn & Bacon.

Bluestein, J. (2001). *Creating emotionally safe schools.* Deerfield Beach, FL: Health Communications.

Borders, D. L., & Drury, R. D. (1992). Comprehensive school counseling programs: A review for policy makers and practitioners. *Journal of Counseling and Development, 70*(4), 487–498.

Bowers, J., Hatch, T., & Schwallie-Giddis, P. (2001, September/October). The brain storm. *ASCA School Counselor, 42,* 17–18.

Boyer, E. L. (1988). Exploring the future: Seeking new challenges. *Journal of College Admissions, 118,* 2–8.

Brammer, L. M. (1993). *The helping relationship: Process and skills* (5th ed.). Boston: Allyn & Bacon.

Brewer, J. M. (1932). *Education as guidance: An examination of the possibilities of curriculum in terms of life activities in elementary and secondary schools and colleges.* New York: Macmillan.

Brigman, G., & Campbell, C. (2003). Helping students improve academic achievement and school success behavior. *Professional School Counseling, 7,* 91–99.

Brown v. Board of Education, 347 U.S. 483, 74 S. Ct. 686 (1954). (Supreme Court, May, 17) nexis.com/universe

Bruce, M. A. (1995). Brief counseling: An effective model for change. *The School Counselor, 42,* 353–363.

Bryan, J., & Holcomb-McCoy. (2004). School counselors' perceptions of their involvement in school-family-community partnerships. *Professional School Counseling, 7*(3), 162–171.

Bureau of Labor Statistics. (2000). Occupational employment projections to 2008. *NAB Workforce Economics, 6.* Washington, DC: U.S. Department of Labor (October). The outlook for college graduates, 1998–2008. In *Getting Ready Pays Off!* Washington, DC: U.S. Department of Labor, Bureau of Labor Statistics.

Bureau of Labor Statistics (U.S. Dept. of Labor). (May 14, 2002). *College enrollment and work activities of the year 2001 high school graduates.* Retrieved December 4, 2002, from http://www.bls.gov/news/release/gsgec.nr0.htm

Bureau of Labor Statistics (U.S. Dept. of Labor). (September 3, 2004). *Employment status of the civilian population.* Retrieved September 11, 2004, from http://www.bls.gov/news/release/empsit.t04.htm

Burnham, J. J., & Jackson, C. M. (2000). School counselor roles: Discrepancies between actual practice and existing models. *Professional School Counseling, 4,* 41–49.

Burns, M. (1999). Effectiveness of special education personnel in the intervention assistance team model. *The Journal of Educational Research, 92*(6), 354.

Burtnett, F. (1993, April 28). Move counseling off the back burner of reform. *Education Week, 32,* 22.

Bush, G. W. (2001). *No child left behind.* Washington, DC: U.S. Department of Education.

Butcher, J. N., Dahlstrom, W. G., Graham, J. R., Tellegen, A., & Kraemmer, B. (1989). Minnesota multiphasic personality inventory-2 (MMPI-2): Manual for administration and scoring. Minneapolis, MN: University of Minnesota.

Campbell, C., & Dahir, C. (1997). *Sharing the vision: The national standards for school counseling programs.* Alexandria, VA: American School Counselor Association.

Capuzzi, D., & Gross, D. R. (2000). I don't want to live: The adolescent at risk for suicidal behavior. In D. Capuzzi & D. R. Gross (Eds.), *Youth at risk: A prevention resource for counselors, teachers, and parents* (3rd ed., pp. 319–352). Alexandria, VA: American Counseling Association.

Capuzzi, D., & Gross, D. R. (2003). *Counseling and psychotherapy: Theories and interventions.* (3rd ed.). Upper Saddle River, NJ: Merrill Prentice Hall.

Career Institute for Education and Workforce Development. (2002). *Decisions without direction: Career guidance and decision making among American youth.* Lansing: MI: EPIC-MRA.

Carey, K. (2004). *A matter of degrees: Improving graduation rates in 4 year colleges and universities. A report for the education trust.* Washington DC: Education Trust.

Carkhuff, R. (1985). *The art of helping.* (6th ed.). Amherst, MA: Human Resource Development Press.

Carnegie Forum on Education and the Economy. (1986). *A nation prepared: Teachers for the 21st century.* Author.

Carnevale, A., & Desrochers, D. M. (2003a). *Standards for what: The economic roots of k-16 reform.* Princeton, NJ: Educational Testing Service.

Carnevale, A., & Desrochers, D. M. (2003b). Preparing students for the knowledge economy: What school counselors need to know. *Professional School Counseling, 6*(4), 228–236.

Casey, J. A. (1995). Elementary school guidance & counseling. *Development Issues for School Counselors Using Technology, 30,* 26–34. *Counselor, 41* (2), 6–7.

Center on Education Policy. (1998). *Public schools: A place where children can learn to get along with others in a diverse society.* Washington, DC: Author.

Centers for Disease Control and Prevention. (2002). *HIV+ Children and schooling.* Retrieved January 20, 2002, from http://www.cdc.gov

Character Education Partnership. (2004). *Eleven principles of character education.* Retrieved September 12, 2004, from www.goodcharacter.com

Cheek, J., Bradley, L., Reynolds, J., & Coy, D. (2002). An intervention for helping elementary students reduce text anxiety. *Professional School Counseling, 73,* 311–316.

Chen-Hayes, S. (2001). Counseling and advocacy with transgendered and gender-variant persons in schools and families. *Journal of Humanistic Counseling, Education and Development, 40*(1), 34.

Children's Defense Fund. (2004). *The state of America's children: Yearbook 2004.* Washington, DC: Author.

Chisholm, I., & Trumbull, E. (2001, March). The diverse challenges of multiculturalism. *Education Update, 43,* 1–3.

Chung, Y. B., & Katayama, M. (1998). Ethnic and sexual identity development of Asian-American lesbian and gay adolescents. *Professional School Counseling, 1* (3), 21–25.

Clark, M., & Stone, C. (2000). The developmental school counselor as educational leader. In J. Wittmer (Ed.), *Managing your school counseling program: K-12 developmental strategies* (2nd ed., pp. 75–81). Minneapolis, MN: Educational Media.

Clarke, J. H., & Frazer, E. (2003). Making learning personal: Educational practices that work. In J. DiMartino, J. Clarke, & D. Wolk (Eds.), *Personalized learning: Preparing high school students to create their futures* (pp. 174–193). Latham, MD: Scarecrow Press.

Clinchy, E. (1991, November). America 2000: Reform, revolution, or just more smoke and mirrors. *Phi Delta Kappan,* 210–218.

Cobia, C., & Henderson, D. (2003). *The handbook of school counseling.* Columbus, OH: Merrill Prentice Hall.

Coker, K., & Schrader, S. (2004). Conducting a school-based practicum: A collaborative model. *Professional School Counseling, 7*(4), 263–267.

Commission on Precollege Guidance and Counseling. (1986). *Keeping the options open: Recommendations.* New York: College Entrance Examination Board. (ERIC Document Reproduction Service No. ED275948)

Conger, R. D., Conger, K. J., & Elder, G. (1997). Family economic hardship and adolescent academic performance: Mediating and moderating processes. In G. Duncan & J. Brooks-Gunnan (Eds.), *Consequences of growing up poor* (pp. 288–310). New York: Russell Sage Foundation.

Conley, S., & Muncey, D. (1999). Teachers talk about teaming and leadership in their work. *Theory into Practice, 38*(1), 46.

Conoley, C. K., & Impara, J. C. (Eds.). (1998). *Mental measurement yearbook* (Vol. 13). Lincoln, NE: University of Nebraska Press.

Constantine, M. G., & Gainor, K. A. (2001). Emotional intelligence and empathy: Their relation to multicultural counseling knowledge and awareness. *Professional School Counseling, 5,* 131–137.

Cooper, C. R. (1998). *The weaving of maturity: Cultural perspectives on adolescent development.* New York: Oxford University Press.

Cooper, C. R., & Denner, J. (1998). Theories linking culture and psychology: Universal and community specific processes. *Annual Review of Psychology, 49,* 559–584.

Corey, G. (2001). *The theory and practice of counseling and psychotherapy* (6th ed.). Pacific Grove, CA: Brooks/Cole.

Corey, G., Corey, M. S., Callanan, P., & O'Phelan, M. L. (1998). *Issues and ethics: In the helping professions.* Pacific Grove, CA: Brooks/Cole.

Corsini, R., & Wedding, D. (1995). *Current psychotherapies* (5th ed). Itasca, IL: F. E. Peacock.

Council for Accreditation of Counseling and Related Educational Programs. (2001). *The 2001 standards.* Alexandria, VA: Author.

Covey, Stephen. (1990). *The 7 habits of highly effective people.* New York: Simon & Schuster.

Coy, D. R. (1999). The role and training of the school counselor: Background and purpose. *NASSP Bulletin, 83*(603), 2–8.

Cunanan, E., & Maddy-Bernstein, C. (1994, August). *The role of the school counselor.* BRIEF v. 1, 1, NCRVE: Berkeley.

Cunanan, E., & Maddy-Bernstein, C. (2000). Individualized career plans: Opening doors for all students. BRIEF, v. 7, 1, NCRVE: Berkeley.

D'Andrea, M., & Daniels, J. (1999). *Youth Advocacy.* Alexandria, VA: American Counseling Association.

Daggett, W. (2003). School counselors and information literacy from the perspective of Willard Daggett. *Professional School Counseling, 6*(4), 238–242.

Dahir, C. (2000, May). The national standards for school counseling programs: A partnership in preparing students for the new millennium. *NASSP Bulletin, 616*(84), 68–76.

Dahir, C. (2001). The national standards for school counseling programs: Development and implementation. *Professional School Counseling, 4*(5), 320–327.

Dahir, C. (Ed.). (2001). *Planning for life: A resource guide for counselors.* Fort Knox, KY: American School Counselor Association & the U.S. Army Recruiting Command.

Dahir, C. (2002, Winter). *We have all become important in one day.* NYSSCA Gram-Fall, 2002. Albany, NY: New York State School Counselor Association.

Dahir, C. (2004). Supporting a nation of learners: The development of the national standards for school counseling programs. *Journal of Counseling and Development, 82*(3), 344–353.

Dahir, C., Campbell, C., Johnson, L., Scholes, R., & Valiga, M. (1997, March). *Supporting a nation of learners: The development of national standards for school counseling programs.* Paper presented at the annual meeting of the American Educational Research Association, Chicago, IL.

Dahir, C., & Stone, C. (2003). Accountability: A m.e.a.s.u.r.e. of the impact school counselors have on student achievement. *Professional School Counseling, 6,* 214–221.

Dahir, C., & Stone, C. (2004). No school counselor left behind. *VISTAS: Perspectives on counseling 2004.* Greensboro, NC: CAPS Press.

Dahir, C. A., Sheldon, C. B., & Valiga, M. J. (1998). *Vision into action: Implementing the national standards for school counseling programs.* Alexandria, VA: American School Counselor Association.

Daniels, J. (2002). Assessing threats of school violence: Implications for counselors. *Journal of Counseling and Development, 80,* 215–218.

Darling-Hammond, L. (1992). *Standards of practice in learner-centered schools.* Albany, NY: New York State Education Department.

Davis v. Monroe County Board of Education et al. 120 F.3d 1390. (Supreme Court, May 24, 1999). Retrieved July 1, 1999 from http://web.lexis-nexis.com/universe

Davis, T. E., & Osborn, C. J. (2000). *The solution-focused school counselor: Shaping professional practice.* Philadelphia, PA: Accelerated Development.

DeBoer, A. (1995). *Working Together: The art of consulting and communicating.* Longmont, CO: Sopris West.

Delaney, E. M., & Kaiser, A. P. (2001). The effects of teaching parents blended communication and behavior support strategies. *Behavioral Disorders, 26*(2), 93–116.

de Shazer, S. (1985). *Keys to solution in brief therapy.* New York: W. W. Norton.

Dettmer, P., Thurston, L. P., & Dyck, N. (2002). *Consultation, collaboration, and teamwork for students with special needs.* Boston: Allyn & Bacon.

Dettmer, P., Thurston, L. P., & Dyck, N. (2005). *Consultation, collaboration, and teamwork for students with special needs* (5th ed.). Boston: Allyn & Bacon.

Dimmitt, C. (2003). Transforming school counseling practice through collaboration and the use of data: A study of academic failure in high school. *Professional School Counseling, 6*(5), 340–349.

Dinkmeyer, D., & Caldwell, E. (1970). *Developmental counseling and guidance: A comprehensive school approach.* New York: McGraw-Hill.

Dinkmeyer, D., Sr., McKay, G., & Dinkmeyer, D., Jr. (1997). *Systematic Training for Effective Parenting.* Circle Pines, MN: American Guidance Services Publishing.

Dorn, M. (2002, February). Ten common mistakes districts make when developing emergency response plans. *School Superintendent's Insider,* 14.

Dorsey, J. (2000). *Ending school violence: Solutions from America's youth.* Nashville, TN: Archstone Press/Golden Ladder Productions.

Doyle, L. (2004). Leadership for community building: Changing how we think and act. *The Clearing House, 77*(5), 196.

Dreikurs, R., & Soltz, V. (1990). *Children: The challenge.* New York: Plume.

Drury, S. S. (1984). Counselor survival in the 1980s. *School Counselor, 31,* 234–240.

Dryfoos, J. (1994). *Full service schools: A revolution in health and human services for children, youth and families.* San Francisco: Jossey-Bass.

Duffey, T. (1998). Applying resiliency philosophy. *Student Assistance Journal.* September/October, 1998, 20–23.

Dunn, K., & Dunn, R. (1987). Dispelling outmoded beliefs about student learning. *Educational Leadership, 45,* 55–63.

Dwyer, K., Osher, D., & Warger, C. (1998). *Early warning, timely response: A guide to safe schools.* Washington, DC: U.S. Department of Education.

Education of All Handicapped Children Act. (1973). Title 20 United States Code Section 1400 *et seq.* (20 USC 1400). U.S. Department of Education Public Law 94-142.

Education Trust. (1997). *Working definition of school counseling.* Washington, DC: Author.

Education Trust. (1999). *Transforming school counseling.* Retrieved December 29, 2004, from http://www.edtrust.org/main/school_counseling.asp

Education Trust. (2001a). *Achievement in America*. Retrieved January 11, 2005 from http://www2.edtrust.org/edtrust/

Education Trust. (2001b). *National commission on the high school senior year youth at crossroads: Facing high school and beyond*. Washington, DC: Author.

Education Week. (2003). *Quality counts*. Washington D.C.: Author.

Edwards, J., Green, K., & Lyons, C. (2002). Personal empowerment, efficacy, and environmental characteristics. *Journal of Educational Administration, 40*(1), 67.

Edwards, M. A. (1994). Foreword. In D. G. Burgess & R. M. Dedmond (Eds.), *Quality leadership and the professional school counselor*. Alexandria, VA: ASCA.

Egan, G. (1994). *The skilled helper* (5th ed.). Monterey, CA: Brooks/Cole.

Eisel v. Board of Education of Montgomery County, 324 Md. 376, 597 A. 2d 447 (Md. Ct. App. 1991).

Eisner, E. W. (1993). Why standards may not improve schools. *Educational Leadership, 51*, 22–24.

Epstein, J., & Sheldon, S. (2002). Present and accounted for: Improving student attendance through family and community involvement. *The Journal of Educational Research, 95*(5), 308.

Epstein, J. L. (1988). How do we improve programs for parent involvement? *Educational Horizons, 66*, 58–62.

Epstein, J. L. (2001). *School, family, and community partnerships: Preparing educators and improving schools*. Boulder, CO: Westview Press.

Equal Employment Opportunity Commission. (1986). *Guidelines on discrimination because of sex*, 29 C.F.R. 1604.11, 25 C.F.R 700.561.

Ericksen, K. (1997). *Making an impact: A handbook on counselor advocacy*. Philadelphia, PA: Taylor & Francis Group.

Erickson, E. H. (1963). *Childhood and society*. New York: W. W. Norton

Erickson, E. H. (1968). *Identity, youth and crisis*. New York: W. W. Norton.

Ettinger, J., Lambert, R., & Rudolph, A. (1994). *Career counseling for change: Helping students transition from school to work*. Madison, WI: Career Development and Training Institute, Center on Education and Work, University of Wisconsin, Madison.

Everett, D., Tichenor, M., & Heins, E. (2003). A profile of elementary teachers involved in a professional development school. *Journal of Research in Childhood Education, 18*(1), 37.

Feller, R. W. (2003). Aligning school counseling: The changing workplace, and career development assumptions. *Professional School Counseling*, [Internet] Retrieved January 4, 2005 from http://www.findarticles.com/cftrvgnt/

Feller, R. W., & Davies, T. G. (2002). Changing the career planning context. In T. Harrington (Ed.), *Handbook for career planning for students with special needs* (3rd ed.). Austin, TX: PRO-ED, Inc.

Fink, E., & Resnick, L. B. (2001). Developing principals as instructional leaders. *Phi Delta Kappan, 82*, 598–606.

Fischer, G. P., & Sorenson, L. (1996). *School law for counselors, psychologists and social workers* (3rd ed.). White Plains, NY: Longman.

Fischer, K., & Kettl, P. (2001). Trends in school violence: Are our schools safe? In M. Shafii & S. L. Shafii (Eds.), *School violence: Assessment, management, prevention*. Washington, DC: American Psychiatric Publishing, Inc.

Fitch, T., & Marshall, J. (2004). What counselors do in high-achieving schools: A study on the role of the school counselor. *Professional School Counseling, 7*(3), 172–178.

Fitch, T., Newby, E., Ballestero, V., & Marshall, J. L. (2001). Counselor preparation: Future school administrators' perceptions of the school counselor's role. *Counselor Education and Supervision, 41*(2), 89.

Forsyth, S. (1999). The data game: Collecting dependable information for school safety planning. *The Challenge, 8* (3). New York: American Council for Drug Education.

Frankl, V. L. (1963). *Man's search for meaning.* Boston: Beacon.

Franklin, J. (2001). The diverse challenges of multicultural education. *Education Update, 43,* 2.

Fredrickson, B. L. (2001). The role of positive emotions in positive psychology. *American Psychologist, 56,* 218–226.

French, J. R. P., & Raven, B. H. (1959). The basis of social power. In D. Cartwright (Ed.), *Studies in social power* (pp. 150–167). Ann Arbor, MI: University of Michigan, Institute of Social Research.

Friend, M., & Cook, L. (2003). *Interactions: Collaboration skills for school professionals.* Boston: Allyn & Bacon.

Fullan, M. (1993). Innovation, reform and restructuring strategies. Challenges and Achievements of American Education, the 1993 ASCD Yearbook. *Association of Supervision in Curriculum and Development, 4,* 14.

Fullan, M. (2004). *Leadership and Sustainability.* Thousand Oaks, CA: Corwin Press.

Gable, R., Mostert, M., & Tonelson, S. (2004). Assessing professional collaboration in schools: Knowing what works. *Preventing School Failure, 48*(3), 4–8.

Galassi, J., & Akos, P. (2004a). Déjà vu and moving the conversation: Reactions to an underutilized partnership. *The Counseling Psychologist, 32,* 215–244.

Galassi, J., & Akos, P. (2004b). Developmental advocacy: twenty-first century school counseling. *Journal of Counseling and Development, 82,* 146–157.

Garbarino, J. (1999). *Lost boys: Why our sons turn violent and how we can save them.* Chicago: Simon & Schuster.

Garbarino, J., & Stott, F. M. (1989). *What children can tell us.* San Francisco: Jossey-Bass.

Garcia, J., Adams, J., Friedman, L., & East, P. (2002). Links between past abuse, suicide ideation, and sexual orientation among San Diego students. *Journal of American College Health, 51*(1), 9.

Gardiner, H. (1999). *Intelligence reframed: Multiple intelligences for the 21st century.* New York: Simon & Schuster.

Garrett, P., Ng'andu, N., & Ferron, J. (1994). Poverty experiences of young children and quality of their home environment. *Child Development, 65,* 331–345.

Gati, I. (1996). Computer assisted counseling: Dilemmas, problems, and possible solutions. *Journal of Counseling and Development, 73,* 51–56.

George, R. L., & Cristiani, T. S. (1990). *Counseling: Theory and practice* (3rd ed.). Englewood Cliffs, NJ: Prentice Hall

Gerler, E. R. (1992). What we know about school counseling: A reaction to Borders and Drury. *Journal of Counseling and Development, 70,* 499–500.

Gerler, E. R., Jr., Kinney, J., & Anderson, R. (1985). The effects of counseling on classroom performance. *Journal of Humanistic Education and Development,* 155–162.

Geroski, A. M., & Knauss, L. (2000). Addressing the needs of foster children in a school counseling program. *Professional School Counseling, 3,* 152–161.

Gilligan, C. (1993). *In a different voice: Psychological theory and women's development.* Cambridge, MA: Harvard University Press.

Gladding, S. T. (2004). *Counseling: A comprehensive profession* (5th ed.). Upper Saddle River, NJ: Pearson Education, Inc.

Glasser, W. (2000a). *Reality therapy in action.* New York: HarperCollins.

Glasser, W. (2000b). School violence from the perspective of William Glasser. *Professional School Counseling, 4,* 77–80.

GLSENTalk. (1998, October). *GLSEN Hudson Valley co-sponsors youth conference.* Available by e-mail from Glsentalk@glsen.org

Goldstein, A., & Kodluboy, D. (1998). *Gangs in schools: Signs, symbols and solutions.* Champaign, IL: Research Press.

Goleman, D. (1995). *Emotional intelligence.* New York: Bantam.

Gordon, T. (2000). Parent effectiveness training: The proven program for raising responsible children. Three Rivers, MI: Three Rivers Press.

Gore, P. A., & Leuwerke, W. C. (2000). Information technology for career assessment on the Internet. *Journal of Career Assessment, 8*(1), 3–19.

Grotberg, E. (1998). I am, I have, I can: What families worldwide taught us about resilience. *Reaching Today's Youth: The Community Circle of Caring, 1*(3), 36–39.

Gottfredson, D. (2001). *School-based crime prevention of problem behavior: what works . . . under what conditions?* Paper presented at the 2001 Office of Safe and Drug Free Schools Technical Assistance Meeting. Washington, DC.

Graham, S., & Taylor, A. Z. (2002). Ethnicity, gender and the development of achievement values. In A. Wigfield & J. S. Eccles (Eds.), *Development of achievement motivation: A volume in the educational psychology series* (pp. 121–146). San Diego, CA: Academic Press.

Greene, J. P. (2002). *Graduation rates.* New York: Manhattan Institute for Policy Research.

Guerra, P. (1998, April). Reaction to DeWitt Wallace grant overwhelming: Readers sound off on February Counseling Today article. *Counseling Today 40,* 13–20.

Guindon, M. H. (2003). Assessment. In B. T. Erford, *Transforming the school counseling profession.* Upper Saddle River, NJ: Merrill Prentice Hall.

Gysbers, N. C., & Henderson, P. (1994). *Developing and managing your school guidance program* (2nd ed.). Alexandria, VA: American Counseling Association.

Gysbers, N. C., & Henderson, P. (Eds.). (1997). *Comprehensive guidance programs that work—II.* Greensboro, NC: ERIC/CASS.

Gysbers, N. C., & Henderson, P. (2000). *Developing and managing your school guidance program* (3rd ed.). Alexandria, VA: American Counseling Association.

Gysbers, N. C., & Henderson, P. (2001). Comprehensive guidance and counseling programs: A rich history and a bright future. *Professional School Counseling, 4,* 246–256.

Gysbers, N. C., & Henderson, P. (2002). *Leading and managing comprehensive school guidance programs.* Greensboro, NC: ERIC/CASS Digest. (ERIC Document Reproduction Service No. ED462670)

Gysbers, N. C., & Moore, E. J. (1981). *Improving guidance programs.* Englewood Cliffs, NJ: Prentice-Hall.

Hackman, R. (2002). *Leading teams: Setting the stage for great performances.* Boston, MA: Harvard Business School Press.

Halford, J. M. (1999). A different mirror: A conversation with Richard Takaki. *Educational Leadership, 56*(7), 8–13.

Handy, C. (2002). *The elephant and the flea.* London: Hutchinson.

Harris, M. B., & Bliss, K. G. (1997). Coming out in a school setting: Former students' experiences and opinions about disclosure. In M. B. Harris (Ed.), *School experiences of gay and lesbian youth* (pp. 85–100). New York: Harrington Park Press.

Harris/Scholastic Research. (1993). *Hostile hallways: The AAUW survey on sexual harassment in America's schools*. Washington, DC: American Association of University Women Educational Foundation.

Hart, P., & Jacobi, M. (1992). *Gatekeeper to advocate*. New York: College Board Press.

Hawkins, J. D., Catalano, R. E., Kosterman, R., Abbott, R., & Hill, K. G. (1999). Preventing adolescent health risk behaviors by strengthening protection during childhood. *Archives of Pediatric and Adolescent Medicine, 153*, 226–234.

Hawkins, J. D., Farrington, D. P., & Catalano, R. F. (1998). Reducing violence through the schools. In D. S. Elliott, B. A. Hamburg, & K. R. Williams (Eds.), *Violence in American schools: A new perspective* (pp. 188–216). Cambridge, England: Cambridge University Press.

Hawkins, J. D., Herrenkohl, T., Farrington, D. B., Catalano, R., Harachl, T., & Cothern, L. (2000, April). Predictors of youth violence. *Juvenile Justice Bulletin*. Retrieved May 14, 2005 from http://ncjrs.org/html/jojdp/jjbul2000_04_5/contents.html

Hay Management Consultants. (2000). *The lessons of leadership*. London: Author.

Haycock, K. (2001). Closing the achievement gap. *Educational Leadership, 58*(6), 6–11.

Haycock, H. (2002, June). *Improving achievement and closing gaps between groups*. Paper presented at the annual Education Trust's Summer Institute on Transforming School Counseling, Chicago, Illinois.

Heinzmann, G. S. (2002). Parental violence in youth sports: Facts, myths and videotape. *Parks & Recreation, 37*, 66–73.

Henderson, N., & Milstein, M. (1996). *Resiliency in schools: Making it happen for students and educators*. Thousand Oaks, CA: Corwin Press.

Herr, E. L. (1979). *Guidance and counseling in the schools. Perspectives on the past, present, and future*. Falls Church, VA: American Personnel and Guidance Association.

Herr, E. L. (1997). *Career development and work-bound youth*. University of North Carolina at Greensboro, NC: ERIC/CASS. (ERIC Document Reproduction Service Document No. ED051199)

Herr, E. L. (2001). The impact of national policies, economics, and school reform on comprehensive guidance programs. *Professional School Counseling, 4*(4), 236.

Hitchings, W., & Retish, P. (2000). Career development needs of students with learning disabilities. In D. Luzzo (Ed.),*Career Counseling of College Students* (pp. 217–231). Washington, DC: American Psychological Association.

Holcomb-McCoy, C. (2003). Multicultural competence. In B. T. Erford (Ed.), *Transforming the school counseling profession* (pp. 317–330). Upper Saddle River, New Jersey: Merrill Prentice Hall.

Holcomb-McCoy, C. (2004). Assessing the multicultural competence of school counselors: A checklist. *Professional School Counseling, 7*, 178–186

Holland, J. L. (1994). *Self-Directed Search*. Odessa, FL: Psychological Assessment Resources.

Holland, J. L. (1997). *Making vocational choices. A theory of vocational personalities and work environments* (3rd ed). Odessa, FL: Psychological Assessment Resources.

Holland, J. L., Daiger, D., & Power, P. (1980). *My vocational situation: Description of an experimental diagnostic form for the selection of vocational assistance*. Palo Alto, CA: Consulting Psychologists Press.

Holland, J. L., Fritzsche, B. A., & Powell, A. B. (1994a). *The self-directed search technical manual*. Odesssa, FL: Psychological Assessment Resources.

Holt-Otten, E. (2002). *Character education*. Retrieved January 25, 2005 from http://www.Indiana.edu/%7Essdc/chardig.htm

House, R., & Martin, P. (1998a). Advocating for better futures for all students: A new vision for school counselors. *Education, 119*, 284–286.

House, R. M., & Hayes, R. L. (2002). School counselors: Becoming key players in school reform. *Professional School Counseling, 5*, 249–256.

House, R. M., Martin, P. J., & Ward, C. C. (2002). Changing school counselor preparation: A critical need. In C. D. Johnson & S. K. Johnson (Eds.), *Building stronger school counseling programs: Bringing futuristic approaches into the present* (pp. 185–208). Greensboro, NC: ERIC Clearinghouse on Counseling and Student Services.

Howe, H. (1991, November). America 2000: A bumpy ride on four trains. *Phi Delta Kappan*, 192–203.

Howe, N., & Strauss, W. (2000). *Millenials rising: The next great generation*. New York: Vintage Books.

Hoye, J. D. (1998, October). Moving from School to Work Keynote address presented at the meeting of the Long Island School to Careers Conference. Huntington, NY.

Hoyt, K. B. (2001). Helping high school students broaden their knowledge of postsecondary options. *Professional School Counseling, 5*, 6–12.

Hoyt, K. B. (2002). The right tools. *ASCA School Counselor, 39*, 19–23.

Hoyt, K. B., & Wickwire, P. N. (2001). Knowledge-information-service era changes in work and education and the changing role of the school counselor in career education. *Career Development Quarterly, 49*, 238–249.

Hoyt, M. F. (1995). Brief psychotherapies. In A. S. Gurman & S. B. Messer (Eds.), *Essential psychotherapies: Theories and practice* (pp. 441–487). New York: Guilford.

Huey, W. C., & Remley, T. P., Jr. (1988). Confidentiality and the school counselor: A challenge for the 1990s. *The School Counselor, 41*, 23–30.

Hughes, D., & James, S. H. (2001). Using accountability data to protect a school counseling program: One counselor's experience. *Professional School Counseling, 4*, 306–310.

HyperDictionary's Dictionary Results. (n.d.). Retrieved February 24, 2003, from http://www.hyperdictionary.com/dictionar?

Idol, L., & Baran, S. (1992). Elementary school counselors and special educators consulting together: Perilous pitfalls or opportunities to collaborate. *Elementary School Guidance and Counseling, 3*(26), 202–213.

Isaacs, M. L. (2003). Data-driven decision making: The engine of accountability. *Professional School Counseling, 6*(4), 288–295.

Isaacs, M. L., & Stone, C. (1999). School counselors and confidentiality: Factors affecting professional choices. *The Professional School Counselor, 2*, 258–266.

Isaacs, M. L., & Stone, C. (2001). Confidentiality with minors: How mental health counselors manage dangerous behaviors. *The Journal of Mental Health Counseling, 23*(3), 342–356.

Ivey, A. E. (2003). *Intentional interviewing and counseling: Facilitating client development in a multicultural society* (5th ed.). Pacific Grove, CA: Brooks/Cole.

Ivey, A. E., Ivey, M. B., & Simek-Downing, L. (1993). *Counseling and psychotherapy: A multicultural perspective*. Boston: Allyn & Bacon.

Jackson, A., & Davis, G. (2000). *Turning points 2000: Educating adolescents in the 21st century.* A Report of Carnegie Corporation of New York. New York: Teachers College Press.

Johnson, C. D., & Johnson, S. K. (1991). The new guidance: A system approach to pupil personnel programs. *CACD Journal, 11,* 5–14.

Johnson, C. D., & Johnson, S. K. (2001). *Results-based student support programs: Leadership academy workbook.* San Juan Capistrano, CA: Professional Update.

Johnson, C. D., & Johnson, S. K. (2002). *Building stronger school counseling programs: Bringing futuristic approaches into the present.* Greensboro, NC: Caps Publications.

Johnson, L. S. (1995). Enhancing multicultural reactions: Intervention strategies for the school counselor. *The School Counselor, 43*(2), 103–113.

Johnson, L. S. (2000). Promoting professional identity in an era of educational reform. *Professional School Counseling, 4,* 31–40.

Jurich, S., & Estes, S. (2000). *Raising academic achievement.* Washington, DC: American Youth Policy Forum.

Kachgal, M., Romano, J. L., & Peterson, J. (2001). *Changes in counseling preparation programs: Early findings.* Minneapolis, MN: University of Minnesota, Center for Applied Research and Educational Improvement.

Kahn, B. B. (2000). A model of solution-focused consultation for school counselors. *Professional School Counseling, 3,* 248–254.

Kaiser, A., & Hancock, T. (2003). Teaching parents new skills to support their young children's development. *Infants and Young Children, 16*(1), 9–21

Kampwirth, T. (2003). *Collaborative consultation in the schools: Effective practices for students with learning and behavior problems.* Upper Saddle River, NJ: Prentice-Hall.

Kaplan, L. S. (1996). Outrageous or legitimate concerns: What some parents are saying about school counseling. *The School Counselor, 43,* 165–170.

Keeling, R. (2001). Is college dangerous? *Journal of American College Health, 50*(2), 53.

Keeling, R. (2002). Asking the right question. *Journal of American College Health, 51*(1), 5.

Kenny, P. (2003). Unalterable Factors for Children: Let Us not Bless their Hearts to Death. Training video.

Keogh, B. K., & MacMillan, D. L. (1996). Exceptionality. In D. Berliner & R. Calfee (Eds.), *Handbook of educational psychology* (pp. 311–330). New York: Macmillan.

Keys, S. G., & Lockhart, E. J. (1999). The school counselor's role in facilitating multisystemic change. *Professional School Counseling, 3,* 101–107.

Keys, S. G. (2000). Living the collaborative role: Voices from the field. *Professional School Counseling, (3)*5, 332.

Kimmel, M. (2003). I am not insane; I am angry. In M. Sadowski (Ed.), *Adolescents at school: Perspectives on youth, identity, and education.* Cambridge, MA: Harvard University Press.

Kiselica, M., & Robinson, M. (2001). Bringing advocacy counseling to life: The history, issues, and human dramas of social justice work in counseling. *Journal of Counseling and Development, 79,* 387–397.

Kitchener, K. S. (1986). Teaching applied ethics in counselor education: An integration of psychological processes and philosophical analysis. *Journal of Counseling and Development, 64,* 306–310.

Kohlberg, L. (1984). *The psychology of moral development: The nature and validity of moral stages.* San Francisco: Harper & Row.

Kortering, L., & Braziel, P. (2000). A look at the expressed career ambitions of youth with disabilities. *Journal for Vocational Special Needs Education, 23*(1), 24–33.

Koss, M. P., & Butcher, J. N. (1986). Research on brief psychotherapy. In S. L. Garfield & A. E. Bergin (Eds.), *Handbook of psychotherapy and behavior change* (3rd ed.). New York: John Wiley and Sons.

Koss, M. P., & Shiang, J. (1994). Research on brief psychotherapy. In S. L. Garfield & A. E. Bergin (Eds.), *Handbook of Psychotherapy and Behavior Change* (4th ed., pp. 664–700). New York: John Wiley and Sons.

Kottler, J. A. (2000). *Doing good: Passion and commitment for helping others.* Philadelphia, PA: Taylor & Francis Group.

Kratochwill, T. R., & Bergan, J. R. (1990). *Behavioral consultation in applied settings: An individual guide.* New York: Plenum Press.

Krumboltz, J. D. (1998). Counselor actions needed for the new career perspective. *British Journal of Guidance and Counseling, 26,* 559–564

Krumboltz, J. D., & Levin, A. S. (2004). *Luck is no accident.* Atascaddero, CA: Impact Publishers.

Krumboltz, J. D., Mitchell, A. M., & Jones, G. B. (1976). A social learning theory of career selection. *Counseling Psychologist, 6,* 71–81.

Lane, K. L., Mahdavi, J. N., & Borthwick-Duffy, S. (2003). Teacher perceptions of the pre-referral intervention process: A call for assistance with school-based interventions. *Preventing School Failure, (47)*4, 148.

Langhout, R. D., Rappaport, J., & Simmons, D. (2002). Integrating community into the classroom: Community gardening, community involvement, and project-based learning. *Urban Education, 37*(3), 323.

Lapan, R. T. (2001). Results-based comprehensive guidance and counseling program: A framework for planning and evaluation. *Professional School Counseling, 4,* 289–299.

Lapan, R. T., Gysbers, N. C., & Petroski, G. (2001). Helping seventh graders be safe and successful: A statewide study of the impact of comprehensive guidance programs. *Journal of Counseling and Development, 79,* 320–330.

Lawhorn, W. (2004, Spring). The 2002–12 job outlook in brief. *Occupational Outlook Quarterly.* Spring 2004, Vol. 48, Number 1. Washington, DC: U.S. Department of Labor.

Lawson, H. A., & Barkdull, C. (2000). Gaining the collaborative advantage and promoting systems and cross-systems change. In A. Sallee, K. Briar-Lawson, & H. A. Lawson (Eds.), *New century practice with child welfare families* (pp. 245–270). Las Cruces, NM: Eddie Bowers Education.

Lee, C. (1998). *Counseling for diversity: A guide for school counselors and related professionals.* Alexandria, VA: American Counseling Association.

Lee, C. (2001). Culturally responsive school counselors and programs: Addressing the needs of all students. *Professional School Counseling, 4,* 163–171.

Lee, C. (2002). *Multicultural issues in counseling* (3rd ed.). Alexandria, VA: American Counseling Association.

Lee, C. C., & Walz, G. R. (Eds.). (1998). *Social action: A mandate for counselors.* Alexandria, VA: American Counseling Association.

Leffert, N., & Scales, P. (1999). *Developmental assets.* Minneapolis, MN: Search Institute.

Lehmanowsky, M. (1991). Using counseling skills to effectively serve students. *School Counselor, 38*(5), 385–392.

Leinhardt, A. M., & Willert, H. J. (2002). Involving stakeholders in resolving school violence. *NASSP Bulletin, 86,* 32–43.

Leithwood, K., Begley, P., & Cousins, J. B. (1992). *Developing expert leadership for future schools.* Washington, DC: The Falmer Press.

Leithwood, K., Jantzi, D., & Steinbach, R. (in press). Leadership practices for accountable schools. In K. Leithwood & P. Hallinger (Eds.), *Second international handbook of educational leadership and administration.* Dordecht, Netherlands: Kluwer Press.

Lent, R. W., Brown, S. D., & Hackett, G. (1996). Career development from a sociocognitive perspective. In D. Brown & L. Brooks (Eds.), *Career choice and development* (3rd ed., pp. 373–421). San Francisco, CA: Jossey-Bass.

Lesko, N. (2001). *Act your age! A cultural construction of adolescence.* New York: Routledge Falmer.

Lewis, A., & Forman, T. (2002). Contestation or collaboration? A comparative study of home-school relations. *Anthropology and Education Quarterly, 33*(1), 60.

Lewis, J., & Bradley, L. (Eds.). (2000). *Advocacy in counseling: Counselors, clients, & community.* Greensboro, NC: CAPS Publications and ERIC/CASS.

Lewis, J. A., Lewis, M. D., Daniels, J. A., & D'Andrea, M. J. (1998). *Community counseling: Empowerment strategies for a diverse society* (2nd ed.). Pacific Grove, CA: Brooks/Cole.

Lieberman, A. (2004). Confusion regarding school counselor functions: School leadership impacts role clarity. *Education, 124*(3), 552.

Likona, T. (2004). *Character matters.* Carmichael, CA: Touchstone Press.

Likona, T., Schaps, E., & Lewis, C. (2000). *Eleven principles of effective character education.* Retrieved October 19, 2003 from www.character.org

Lilly Endowment. (1994). *High hopes, long odds.* Chicago: Public Policy Research Consortium and The Indiana Youth Institute.

Lipkin, A. (2004). *Beyond diversity day: A Q & A on gay and lesbian issues in schools.* Lanham, NY: Rowman & Littlefield.

Lipsyte, R. (2000, April 30). An icon recast: Support for gay athlete. *New York Times,* pp. A1, A18.

Littrell, J. M. (1998). *Brief counseling in action.* New York: W. W. Norton.

Lockhart, E. J., & Keys, S. G. (1998). The mental health counseling role of school counselors. *Professional School Counseling, 1,* 3–6.

Louis, K. S., Jones, L. M., & Barajas, H. (2001). *Evaluation of the transforming school counselor initiative: Districts and schools as a context for transformed counseling roles.* Minneapolis, MN: University of Minnesota, Center for the Applied Research and Educational Improvement.

Loveless, T. (1999). *The tracking and ability group debate.* Washington, DC: Thomas B. Fordham Foundation.

Lowry, R., Powell, K. E., Kann, L., Collins, J. L., Kolbe, L. J. (1998). Weapon carrying, physical fighting and fight related injuries among U.S. adolescents. *American Journal of Preventive Medicine, 14,* 122–129.

Luongo, P. F. (2000). Partnering child welfare, juvenile justice and behavioral health with children. *Professional School Counseling, 3,* 308–314.

Lynch, R. L. (2000). *New directions or high school career and technical education in the 21st century.* Columbus, OH: ERIC Clearinghouse on Adult, Career and Technical Education.

MacGregor, J. (2004). Unpublished video. September 15, 2003.

Maddy-Bernstein, C. (2000). Career development issues affecting secondary schools. *The Highlight Zone Research @ Work.* Retrieved from http://www.nccte.org/publications/infosynthesis/highlightzone/highlight01/highlight01-careerdevelopment.pdf

Maital, S. L. (1996). Integration of behavioral and mental health consultation as a means of overcoming resistance. *Journal of Educational and Psychological Consultation, 7*(4), 291–303.

Marnik, G. (1997). *A glimpse at today's high schools.* Presented at Successful Transitions conference by the College of Education and Human Development, University of Maine, Orono.

Martin, P. (1998). *Transforming School Counseling.* Unpublished manuscript. Washington, DC: The Education Trust.

Martin, P. J. (2004). *The school counselor's role in closing the achievement gap.* Presentation delivered at the Teaching and Learning Academy. March 16, 2004. Memphis, TN.

Martinez v. School Board, 711 F. Supp. 1066 (1989).

Marzano, R. J. (2000). Implementing standards in schools. *National Association of Secondary School Principals Bulletin, 82,* 2–4

Mathewson, R. H. (1962). *Guidance policy and practice.* New York: Harper & Bros.

May, R. (1950). *Love and will.* New York: W. W. Norton.

May, R., & Yalom, I. (1995). Existential psychotherapy. In R. Corsini & D. Wedding (Eds.), *Current Psychotherapies* (5th ed., pp. 262–292). Itasca, IL: Peacock.

McCullough, L. (1994). Legislation enhances school-to-work initiatives. *ACA Guidepost, 36,* 1.

McDevitt, T., & Ormond, J. (2002). *Child development and education.* Upper Saddle River, NJ: Merrill Prentice Hall.

McDonald, G., & Sink, C. (1999). A qualitative developmental analysis of comprehensive guidance programmes in schools in the United States. *British Journal of Guidance and Counseling, 27,* 415–430.

McEachern, A. (2003). School counselor preparation to meet the guidance needs of exceptional students : A national study. *Counselor Education and Supervision, 42*(4), 314.

McFarland, W. P., & Dupuis, M. (2001). The legal duty to protect gay and lesbian students from violence in schools. *Professional School Counseling, 4,* 171–179.

McLeod, J. (1995). *Ain't no making it.* Boulder, CO: Westview Press.

McLoyd, V. C. (1998). Socio-economic disadvantage and child development. *American Psychologist, 53*(2), 185–204.

McNeely, C. A., & Blum, R. W. (2002). Promoting student connectedness to school: Evidence from the national longitudinal study of adolescent health. *Journal of School Health, 72,* 4.

McWhirter, E. H. (1997). Empowerment, social activism, and counseling. *Counseling and Human Development, 29,* 1–14.

Menning, C. (2002). Absent parents are more than money: The joint effect of activities and financial support on youths' educational attainment. *Journal of Family Issues, 23*(5), 648.

Metcalf, L. (1995). *Counseling towards solutions: A practical solution-focused program for working with students, teachers and parents.* West Nyack, NY: Center for Applied Research.

Michaels, C. A. (1997). Preparation for employment. In P. J. Gerber & D. S. Brown (Eds.), *Learning Disabilities and Employment* (pp. 187–212.) Austin, TX: PRO-ED, Inc.

Mitchell, K. E., Levin, A. S., & Krumboltz, J. D. (1999). Planned happenstance: Constructing unexpected career opportunities. *Journal of Counseling and Development, 77,* 115–124.

Mitchell, L. K., & Krumboltz, J. D. (1996). Krumboltz's learning theory of career choice and counseling. In D. Brown, L. Brooks, & Associates (Eds.), *Career choice and development* (3rd ed., pp. 233–276). San Francisco: Jossey-Bass.

Moe, J. (2001, June). *Helping students build their strength.* Paper presented at the American School Counselor Association Annual Conference, Portland, OR.

Moore, D. (2003). Community Partners. *Leadership for Student Activities, 32*(3), 27.

Morgan, A. (2003). No school is an island. *Leadership for Student Activities, 32*(3), 9.

Mortenson, T. G. (2001, June). High school graduation trends and patterns 1981–2000. *Postsecondary Education Opportunity, 108,* 2.

Moss-Greenberg, J., & Shaffer, S. (1991). *Elements of equity: Criteria for equitable schools.*

Murphy, J. J. (1997). *Solution-focused counseling in middle and high schools.* Alexandria, VA: American Counseling Association.

Murrow-Taylor, C., Foltz, B. M., McDonald, A. B., Ellis, M. R., & Culbertson, K. (1999). A multicultural career fair for elementary school students. *Professional School Counseling, 2,* 241–243.

Myrick, R. D. (1997). *Developmental guidance and counseling: A practical approach* (3rd ed.). Minneapolis, MN: Educational Media Corporation.

Myrick, R. D. (2000). *Developmental guidance and counseling: A practical approach* (4th ed). Minneapolis, MN: Educational Media Corporation.

Myrick, R. D. (2003a). Accountability: Counselors count. *Professional School Counseling, 6*(3), 174–179.

Myrick, R. D. (2003b). *Developmental guidance and counseling: A practical handbook.* Minneapolis, MN: Educational Media Corporation.

National Association of Secondary School Principals. (1996). *Breaking ranks: Changing an American institution.* Reston, VA: Author.

National Association of Secondary School Principals. (2004). *Breaking ranks II: Strategies for leading high school reform.* Reston, VA: Author.

National Career Development Guidelines. (2004). Retrieved September 11, 2004, from www.acrnetwork.org

National Center for Education Statistics. (1997). *Condition of Education.* Washington, DC: U.S. Department of Education.

National Center for Education Statistics. (2001). *Executive summary: Dropout rates in the United States: 2000.* NCES 2002–114. Washington, DC: Author.

National Center for Education Statistics. (2002). *Student completion rates.* Washington, DC: Author.

National Center for Education Statistics. (2000, August). *NAEP 1999 trends in academic progress.* 108. Washington, DC: U.S. Department of Education.

National Center for Education Statistics. (2003). *Condition of Education.* Washington, DC: Author.

National Center for Education Statistics. (2004). Projections of education statistics to 2013. *The Education Statistics Quarterly, 5,* 5.

National Center for Injury Prevention and Control. (2002). *National youth violence resource center.* Atlanta, GA: Author.

National Center for Missing and Exploited Children. (2001). Retrieved October 19, 2003 from www.missingkids.com

National Commission on Excellence in Education. (1983). *A nation at risk: The imperative for educational reform.* Washington, D.C.: Author.

National Consortium for State Guidance Leadership. (2000). *A national framework for state programs in guidance and counseling.* Columbus, OH: Author.

National Governor's Association. (1995). *Strategies for linking school finance and students' opportunity to learn.* Washington, DC: Author.

National Institute on Drug Abuse. (1997). *The individual will be more resilient, prevent problems and promote a healthy life-style.* Washington, DC: Author

National Occupational Information Coordinating Committee. (1989a). U.S. Department of Labor. *The national career development guidelines project.* Washington, DC: Author.

National Occupational Information Coordinating Committee. (1989b). *National career development guidelines: Local handbook.* Washington, DC: Author. (ERIC Document Reproduction Service No.: Elementary School Level—ED317879; Middle School/Junior High School Level—ED317878; High School Level—ED317877; Postsecondary Level—ED317876; Community and Business Organizations—ED317875)

National Occupational Information Coordinating Committee. (1989c). *National career development guidelines: Trainer's guide.* Washington, DC: Author. (ERIC Document Reproduction Service No. ED317874)

Neukrug, E. (1999). The *world of the counselor: An introduction to the counseling profession.* Pacific Grove, CA: Brooks/Cole.

New York State Education Department. (2004). *Special education in New York State for children ages 3–21: A parent's guide.* Albany, NY: The University of the State of New York; The State Education Department; Vocational and Educational Services for Individuals with Disabilities.

New York State Office of Mental Health. (2000). *Violence prevention: Violence prevention strategies.* Retrieved April 4, 2005, from http://www.omh.state.ny.us/omhweb/sv/strategies.htm

Nieto, S. (1999). *The light in their eyes: Creating multicultural learning communities.* New York: Teachers College Press.

Niles, S. G., & Goodnough, G. (1996). Life long salience and values: A review of recent research. *Career Development Quarterly, 45,* 65–86.

Niles, S. G., & Harris-Bowlsbey, J. (2002). *Career development intervention in the 21st century.* New Jersey: Prentice-Hall.

Nugent, F. A. (1994). *An introduction to professional counseling.* New York: Merrill.

O'Connor, C. (1997). Dispositions towards struggle and educational resilience in the inner city: A case analysis of six African-American high school students. *American Educational Research Journal, 34,* 593–629.

O'Day, J. (2002). Complexity, accountability, and school improvement. *Harvard Educational Review, 72*(3), 293.

Office for Civil Rights. (1973). *Section 504 of the Rehabilitation Act of 1973.* Washington, DC: Author.

Office for Civil Rights. (1997). *Sexual harassment policy guidance: Harassment of students by school employees, other students or third parties.* Washington, DC: U.S. Department of Education.

Office for Civil Rights. (2001). *Revised sexual harassment policy guidance: Harassment of students by school employees, other students or third parties.* Retrieved June 13, 2004, from www.ed.gov/offices/OCR/shguide/index.html

Office of Special Education Programs. (2000). *Twenty-second annual report to Congress on the implementation of the Individuals with Disabilities Education Act.* Washington, DC: Author.

Olson, L. (2001, January 10). *Quality Counts* explores standards in the classroom. *Education Week,* 3.

Orfield, G., Losen, D., Wald, J., Swanson, C. (2004). *Losing our future: How minority youth are being left behind by the graduation rate crisis.* Cambridge, MA: The Civil Rights Project at Harvard University.

Ormsbee, C. (2001). Effective pre-assessment team procedures: Making the process work for teachers and students. *Intervention in School and Clinic, (36)*3, 146.

Osborne, J. L., Collison, B. B., House, R. M., Gray, L. A., Firth, J., & Lou, M. (1998). Developing a social advocacy model for counselor education. *Counselor Education and Supervision, 37*, 190–202.

Owings, W., & Kaplan, L. (2000). Learning of standards. *Virginia ASCD, 3*, 1–6.

Page v. Rotterdam-Mohonasen Central School District, et. al., 109 Misc. 2d 1049, 441 N.Y.S.2d 323 (1981).

Paisley, P. O. (1999). The next evolution in school counselor practice and preparation: A national initiative, local example, and personal reflection. *The Journal of the Pennsylvania Counseling Association, 1*(1), 7–15.

Paisley, P. O., & McMahon, G. (2001). School counseling for the 21st century: Challenges and opportunities. *Professional School Counseling, 5*, 106–115.

Parrott, J. (2002). Are advisors risking lawsuits for misadvising students? *The mentor: an academic advising journal.* (2001, July 9). Retrieved January 20, 2002, from www.psu.edu/dus/mentor

Payne, K. J., & Biddle, B. J. (1999). Poor school funding, child poverty, and mathematic achievement. *Educational Researcher, 28*(6), 4–12.

Pedersen, P. B. (1991). Multiculturalism as a generic approach to counseling. *Journal of Counseling & Development, 70*, 6–12.

Peebles-Wilkins, W. (2003). Collaborative interventions. *Children and Schools, 25*(4), 195.

Perls, F. (1969). *Gestalt therapy verbatim.* Lafayette, CA: Real Person.

Perry, N. (1991). The school counselor's role in education reform. *NASSP Bulletin, 79*, 24–29.

Perry, N., & Schwallie-Giddis, P. (1993). The counselor and reform in tomorrow's schools. *The Journal of Counseling and Human Development, 25*, 1–8.

Pérusse, R., Goodnough, G. E., & Noel, C. J. (2001a). A national survey of school counselor preparation programs: Screening methods, faculty experiences, curricular content, and fieldwork requirements. *Counselor Education and Supervision, 40*, 252–262.

Pérusse, R., Goodnough, G. E., & Noel, C. J. (2001b). Use of the national standards for school counseling programs in preparing school counselors. *Professional School Counseling, 5*, 49–55.

PFLAG. Retreived June 24, 2004 from Parents and Youth's website: www.pflag.org/education/schools.html

Phillips, P. P. (2002). Retaining your best employees. Alexandria, VA: Society for Human Resource Management.

Piaget, J. (1952). *The origins of intelligence in children.* New York: International Universities Press.

Pollack, W. (1998). *Real boys: Rescuing our sons from the myths of boyhood.* New York: Henry Holt.

Ponec, D. L., & Brock, B. L. (2000). Relationships among elementary school counselors and principals: A unique bond. *Professional School Counseling, 3*, 208–217.

Pope, M. (2004). Sexual minority youth in the schools: Issues and desirable counselor responses. In G. Walz & R. Yep (Eds.), *Vistas: Perspectives on counseling 2004.* Alexandria, VA: American Counseling Association.

Porter, G., Epp, L., & Bryant, S. (2000). Collaborating among school mental health professions: A necessity, not a luxury. *Professional School Counseling, (3)*5, 315.

Postsecondary Education Opportunity. (2000, February). *Academic preparation for college by gender, race and family income, 1983 to 1999. 02*, Retrieved September 25, 2004 from www. Postsecondary.org

Postsecondary Education Opportunity. (2000, December). *Family income by educational attainment of householder. 02*, Retrieved September 25, 2004 from www. Postsecondary.org

Psychological Corporation. (1991; 2003). The Differential Aptitude Test. San Antonio, TX: Harcourt Assessment.

Quigney, T. A., & Studer, J. R. (1998). Touching strands of the educational web: The professional school counselor's role in inclusion. *Professional School Counseling, 2*(1), 77–81.

Raelin, J. (2004). Preparing for Leaderful Practice. *T + D, 58*(3), 64–70.

Raven, B. (1965). Social influence and power. In I. D. Steiner & M. Fishbein (Eds.), *Current studies in social psychology* (pp. 371–382). New York: Holt Rinehart & Winston.

Reid, K. (2001, May 2). Iowa's high court holds counselors liable. *Education Week*. Retrieved January 20, 2002, from http://www.edweek.org/ew/ewstory.cfm?slug=33guide.h20

Remley, T., Jr., & Herlihy, B. (2001). *Ethical, legal, and professional issues in counseling*. Upper Saddle River, NJ: Merrill Prentice Hall.

Remley, T. P., & Sparkman, L. B. (1993). Student suicides: The counselor's limited legal liability. *School Counselor, 40*(3), 164–169.

Rhode Island Department of Education. (1997). *School accountability for learning and teaching* (SALT). Providence, RI: Author

Ripley, V., Erford, B., & Dahir, C. (2002). Planning and implementing a 21st century comprehensive, developmental professional school counseling program. In B. Erford, *Transforming School Counseling*. Columbus, OH: Merrill Prentice Hall.

Roberts, M. E. P. (1997, October 31). Who's looking out for Tiffany? *Washington City Paper*, p. 23.

Rogers, C. (1961). *On becoming a person*. Boston: Houghton Mifflin.

Rogers, C. (1980). *A way of being*. Boston: Houghton Mifflin.

Rose, L., & Gallup, A. (September, 2004). Phi Delta Kappan/Gallup poll of the public's attitudes toward the public schools. *Phi Delta Kappan*, September, 2004.

Rosenbaum, J. E. (1976). *Making inequality: The hidden current of high school tracking*. New York: Wiley.

Rubin, H. (2002). *Collaborative Leadership: Developing Effective Partnerships in Communities and Schools*. National Association of Secondary School Principals, September 2002.

Ruble, D., & Martin, C. (1998). Gender development. In W. Damon (Editor-in-Chief) & N. Eisenberg (Vol. Ed.), *Handbook of child psychology* (Vol. 3): *Social, emotional, and personality development* (5th ed., pp. 993–1016). New York: Wiley.

Ryan, T., & Zeran, F. (1972). *Organization and administration of guidance services*. Danville, IL: Interstate.

Sadker, M., & Sadker, D. (1994). *Failing at fairness: How America's schools cheat girls*. New York: Scribner.

Sadker, M., & Sadker, D. (2005). *Teachers, schools, and society* (7th ed.). New York: McGraw-Hill.

Safeyouth.org (2004). National Youth Violence Prevention Resource Center. Retrieved January 8, 2005 from http://www.safeyouth.org/home.htm

Sain v. Cedar Rapids Community School District, 626 N.W.2d 115 (Iowa 2001).

Salo, M. M., & Shumate, S. G. (1993). Counseling minor clients. *The ACA Legal Series, 4,* 9–10.

Sampson, J. P. (1997). *Helping clients get the most from computer assisted career guidance systems.* Retrieved December 27, 2002, from http://www.career.fsu.edu/techcenter

Sanders, M. G. (2000). *Schools, families, and communities: Partnerships for school success.* Reston, VA: National Association of Secondary School Principals. Retrieved September 30, 2004 from http://www.principals.org/pdf/schls_fmles_Cmntes.pdf

Sandhu, D. S. (2000). Alienated students: Counseling strategies to curb school violence. *Professional School Counseling, 4,* 81–85.

Sanford, S. (2001, January). General Colin Powell: Keeping America's promise. Retrieved May 14, 2005 from http://www.centerdigitaled.com/converge/?pg=magstory&id=3284

Santa Rosa County School District. (2000). *Know your rights.* Santa Rosa County, Florida: Santa Rosa School District.

Sapon-Shevin, M. (2001). Schools fit for all. *Educational Leadership, 58,* 34–39.

Scales, P., & Taccogna, J. (2000). Caring to try: How building students' developmental assets can promote school engagement and success. *NASSP Bulletin, 84,* 69–78.

Schmidt, J. J. (1999). *Counseling in schools: Essential services and comprehensive programs* (3rd ed.). Needham Heights, MA: Allyn & Bacon.

Schmidt, J. J. (2003). *Counseling in schools: Essential services and comprehensive programs.* 4th edition. Boston: Allyn & Bacon.

Schneider, B., & Stevenson, D. (1999). *The ambitious generation—America's teenagers: Motivated but directionless.* New Haven: Yale University Press.

Schwallie-Giddis, P., & Kobylarz, L. (2000). Career development: The counselor's role in preparing K–12 students for the 21st century. In J. Wittmer (Ed.), *Managing your school counseling program: K–12 developmental strategies* (2nd ed., pp. 211–218). Minneapolis, MN: Educational Media Corporation.

Schwallie-Giddis, P., ter Maat, M., & Park, M. (2003). Initiating leadership by introducing and implementing the ASCA national model. *Professional School Counseling, 6*(3), 170.

Sciarra, D. T. (2004). *School counseling: Foundations and contemporary issues.* Belmont, CA: Brooks/Cole.

Scott, T. M., DeSimone, C., Fowler, W., & Webb, E. (2000). Using functional analysis to develop interventions for challenging behaviors in the classroom: Three case studies. *Preventing School Failure, 44,* 51–56.

Search Institute. (1997). *The forty developmental assets.* Minneapolis, MN: Author. Retrieved February 25, 2004 from http://www.search-institute.org/assets/40Assets.pdf

Search Institute. (1998). *Developmental assets: An overview.* Retrieved February 25, 2004 from http://www.search-institute.org/assets

Search Institute. (2004). *Making a difference for young people: The power of one.* Minneapolis, MN: Author.

Sears, S. (1999). Transforming school counseling: Making a difference for students. *NASSP Bulletin, 83*(603), 47–53.

Secretary's Commission on Achieving Necessary Skills. (1991). *What work requires of schools: A SCANS report for America 2000.* Washington, DC: U.S. Department of Labor.

Seligman, L. (2001). *Systems, strategies, and skills of counseling and psychotherapy.* Columbus, OH: Merrill Prentice Hall.

Sewall, G. (1991, November). America 2000: An appraisal. *Phi Delta Kappan, 72,* 204–209.

Shafii, M., & Shafii, S. L. (1992). Clinical manifestations and developmental psychopathology of depression. In Shafii, M., & Shafii, S. L. (Eds.), *Clinical guide to depression in children and adolescents* (pp. 3–42). Washington DC: American Psychiatric Press.

Shafii, M., & Shafii, S. L. (2001). *School violence: Assessment, management, prevention.* Washington, DC: American Psychiatric Press.

Sheldon, C., & Morgan, C. D. (1984). The child development specialist: A prevention program. *Personnel and Guidance Journal, 62,* 470–474.

Sheldon, S. B., & Epstein, J. L. (2002). Improving student behavior and school discipline with family and community involvement. *Education and Urban Society, 35*(1), 4–26

Shore, K. (2001). Success for ESL students. *Instructor, 110,* 30–32.

Silins, H., & Mulford, B. (2002). Leadership and school results. In K. Leithwood & P. Hallinger (Eds.), *International handbook of educational leadership and administration* (pp. 561–612). Norwell, MA: Kluwer.

Simpson, M. (1999). Student suicide: Who's liable? *National Education Association, 5*(17), 1–25.

Sink, C. A., & Stroh, H. R. (2003). Raising achievement test scores of early elementary school students through comprehensive school counseling programs. *Professional School Counseling, 6,* 352–364.

Sink, C. A., & McDonald, G. (1998). The status of comprehensive guidance and counseling in the United States. *Professional School Counseling, 2,* 88–94.

Sistek-Chandler, C. (2001, May). The incredible expanding classroom of Marco Torres. *Converge, 4,* 44.

Skiba, R. J., & Peterson, R. L. (1999). The dark side of zero tolerance: Can punishment lead to safe schools?. *Phi Delta Kappan, 80,* 372–382.

Sklare, G. B. (1997). *Brief counseling that works: A solution focused approach for school counselors.* Thousand Oaks, CA: Corwin Press.

Snyder, T., & Hoffman, C. (2001). Digest of education statistics 2001. *Education Statistics Quarterly, 4,* 1. Washington DC: National Center for Education Statistics.

Spinetta, A. (2002, October). Where's the conversation? *Converge, 5,* 24. Folsum, CA: e.Republic, Inc.

Sprinthall, N. A. (1981). A new model for research in the science of guidance and counseling. *Personnel and Guidance Journal, 59,* 487–493.

Staley, W. L., & Carey, A. L. (1997, May). The role of school counselors in facilitating a quality twenty-first century workforce. *The School Counselor, 44,* 377–381.

Stanciak, L. (1995). Reforming the high school counselor's role: A look at developmental guidance. *NASSP Bulletin, 79,* 60–68.

Staton, A. R., & Gilligan, T. D. (2003). Teaching school counselors and school psychologists to work collaboratively. *Counselor Education and Supervision, (42)*3, 1962.

Steenbarger, B. N. (1992). Toward science-practice integration in brief counseling and therapy. *Counseling Psychologist, 20,* 403–450.

Stein, R., Richin, R., Banyon, R., Banyon, F., & Stein, M. (2001). *Connecting character to conduct: Helping students do the right things.* Alexandria, VA: Association of Supervision and Curriculum Development.

Sternberg, R. J. (1985). *Beyond IQ: A triarchic theory of human intelligence.* New York: Cambridge University Press.

Stevens-Smith, P., & Remley, T. (1994). Drugs, AIDS and teens: Interventions and the school counselor. *School Counselor, 41*(3), 180–185.

Stickel, S. A. (1996). *Developing teambuilding skills for collaborative schools: Using school counselors as a resource.* Greensboro, NC: Eastern Michigan University, Department of Leadership and Counseling. (ERIC Document Reproduction Service No. ED396202).

Stone, C. (1996). Unpublished successful grant application for the Transforming School Counseling DeWitt-Wallace Grant.

Stone, C. (1998). Leveling the playing field: An urban school system examines access to mathematics curriculum. *Urban Review, 30*(4), 295–307.

Stone, C. (2000). Confidentiality: Counselors caught up in other responsibilities. In L. Tyson & P. Pedersen (Eds.), *Critical incidents in school counseling* (2nd ed., pp. 51–60). Boston, MA: Allyn & Bacon.

Stone, C. (2001, 2002, 2003). Unpublished interviews with the students of the Expo Program, Yale University.

Stone, C. (Speaker). (2001b). *Legal and ethical issues in working with minors in schools* [Film]. Alexandria, VA: American Counseling Association.

Stone, C. (2002). Negligence in academic advising and abortion counseling: Courts rulings and implications. *Professional School Counselor: Special Issue on Legal and Ethical Issues, School Counselor, 6* (1).

Stone, C. (2003, April). The new school counselor: Agent of change. *The College Board Review,* #199, 45–48.

Stone, C. (2003, September). School counselors: Educators first with mental health expertise. *Counseling Today, 46*(3), 14–15.

Stone, C. (2003a). Leadership and advocacy in personal/social development: Sexual harassment (pp. 353–377). In R. Pérusse & G. Goodnough (Eds.), *Leadership and Advocacy in School Counseling.* Belmont, CA: Brooks/Cole.

Stone, C. (2003b). Ethical and legal considerations for students, parents, and professional school counselors. In B. T. Erford (Ed.), *Professional school counseling: A handbook of theories, programs, and practices* (pp. 57–64). Austin, TX: PRO-ED, Inc.

Stone, C. (2003c). Philosophical counselor as social justice advocate. *Journal of Canadian Philosophical Practice.* Retrieved January 6, 2005 from http://web.ustpaul.uottawa.ca/fr/fac_philosophie/revue/articles/stone_0310.html

Stone, C. (2003d). Point-counterpoint. *Counseling Today, 46*(3), 15.

Stone, C. (2003e). School counselors as advocates for gay, lesbian, and bisexual students: A call for action from the U.S. Supreme Court. *Journal of Multicultural Counseling and Development, 31*(2), 143–155.

Stone, C. (2003f). Advocacy in academic advising: Behaving legally and ethically. *ASCA School Counselor, 44*(1), 8–9.

Stone, C. (2003g). Case notes, educational records and subpoenas. *ASCA School Counselor, 41*(2), 6–7.

Stone, C. (2003h). Group work: What's appropriate, what's not? *ASCA School Counselor, 41*(6), 6–7.

Stone, C. (2003i). Sexual harassment: The legal muscle to support victims. *ASCA School Counselor, 41*(5), 6–7.

Stone, C. (2003j). Suicide: A duty owed. *ASCA School Counselor, 40*(4), 12–13.

Stone, C. & Clark, M. A. (2001). School counselors and principals: Partners in support of academic achievement. *National Association of Secondary School Principals Bulletin, 85*(624), 46–53.

Stone, C., & Dahir, C. (2004). *School counselor accountability: A measure of student success.* Upper Saddle River, NJ: Pearson Education.

Stone, C., & Hanson, C. (2002). Selection of school counselor candidates: Future directions at two Universities. *Counselor Education and Supervision, 41*(3), 175–192.

Stone, C., & Isaacs, M. (2002a). Involving students in violence prevention: Anonymous reporting and the need to promote and protect confidences. *National Association of Secondary School Principals Bulletin, 86*(633), 54–65.

Stone, C., & Isaacs, M. (2002b). Confidentiality with minors: The effects of Columbine on counselor attitudes regarding breaching confidentiality. *The Journal of Educational Research, 96*(2), 140–150.

Stone, C., & Turba, R. (1999). School counselors using technology for advocacy. *The Journal of Technology in Counseling, 1*(1). Available from http://jtc.colstate.edu/vol1_1/advocacy.htm

Stone, C. B., & Clark, M. (2001). School counselors and principals: Partners in support of academic achievement. *National Association of Secondary School Principals Bulletin, 85*(624), 46–53.

Sue, D. W., Arredondo, P., & McDavis, R. J. (1992). Multicultural counseling competencies and standards: A call to the profession. *Journal of Counseling and Development, 70,* 447–483.

Super, D. E. (1980). A life-span approach to career development. *Journal of Vocational Behavior, 16,* 282–298.

Super, D. E., Savickas, M. L., & Super, C. M. (1996). The life span, life-space approach to careers. In D. Brown & L. Brooks (Eds.), *Career choice and development: Applying contemporary theories to practice* (3rd ed., pp. 121–178). San Francisco: Jossey-Bass.

Taylor, L. (2000). Connecting schools, families, and communities. *Professional School Counseling, (3)*5, 298.

Teaching Tolerance. (2003). *Responding to hate at school.* Southern Poverty Law Center. Montgomery, AL: Author.

Thompson, C. L., & Rudolph, L. B. (2000). *Counseling children* (5th ed). Pacific Grove, CA: Brooks/Cole.

Thorn, A. R., & Mulvenon, S. W. (2002). High-stakes testing: An examination of elementary counselors' views and their academic preparation to meet this challenge. *Measurement and Evaluation in Counseling and Development, 35*(3), 195

Thornburg, H. D. (1986). The counselor's impact on middle grade students. *School Counselor, 33,* 170–177.

Title IX, Education Amendments of 1972. Washington, DC: U.S. Department of Labor.

Toporek, R. (2000). Developing a common language and framework for understanding advocacy in counseling. In J. Lewis & L. Bradley (Eds.), *Advocacy in counseling: Counselors, clients, & community* (pp. 5–14). Greensboro, NC: ERIC/CASS (ERIC Document Reproduction Service No. ED435905).

Turba, R. (1998). From supporters of academic rigor. In C. B. Stone, *School counselors: supporters of academic rigor.* Unpublished article, University of North Florida.

Turner S., & Lapan, R. T. (2002). Career self-efficacy and perceptions of parent support in adolescent career. *Career Development Quarterly, 51,* 44–55.

Tyler, J. M., & Sabella, R. A. (2004). *Using technology to improve counseling practice: A primer for the 21st century.* Alexandria, VA: American Counseling Association.

U.S. Census Bureau. (2002). *Statistical Abstract of the United States* (Section 4: Education, pp. 198–282). Retrieved December 10, 2003, from http://www.census.gov/prod/2003pubs/02statab/educ.pdf

U.S. Census Bureau. (2003). *Population Projections.* Washington, DC: U.S. Department of Education.

U.S. Department of Education. (1973). *Family education and privacy rights.* Washington, DC: Author.

U.S. Department of Education. (1975). *The education for all handicapped children act* Washington, DC: Author.

U.S. Department of Education. (1987). *What works: Research about teaching and learning.* Washington, DC: Author

U.S. Department of Education. (1990). *America 2000: An education strategy.* Washington, DC: Author.

U.S. Department of Education. (1994a). *Safe and drug free schools and community act* Washington, DC: Author

U.S. Department of Education. (1994b). *Goals 2000: The educate America act.* Washington, DC: Author.

U.S. Department of Education. (1994c). *School to work opportunities act.* Washington, DC: Author.

U.S. Department of Education. (1998a). *Gaining early awareness and readiness for undergraduate programs.* Washington, DC: Author.

U.S. Department of Education. (1998b). *Early warning, timely response: A guide to safe schools.* Washington, DC: Author.

U.S. Department of Education. (2001). *The no child left behind act.* Washington, DC: Author.

U.S. Department of Education. (2002a). *Exemplary and promising safe, disciplined, and drug free schools.* Washington, DC: Author.

U.S. Department of Education. (2002b). *No child left behind: A desktop reference.* Washington, DC: Author.

U.S. Department of Education. (2002c). *Preventing bullying: A manual for schools and communities.* Washington, DC: Author.

U.S. Department of Education, Office of Civil Rights. Sexual harassment policy guidance: Harassment of students by school employees, other students, or third parties, March 13, 1997 (volume 62, number 49, pages 12034–12051).

U.S. Department of Education, Office of Safe and Drug Free Schools. (2002). *Safe disciplined and drug free schools expert panel findings.* Retrieved September 18, 2004 from www.ed.gov/offices/OESE/SDFS

U.S. Department of Education, Office of Safe and Drug-Free Schools. (2003). School connectedness means less risky behavior. *The Challenge, 11,* 6–7.

U.S. Department of Education, Office of Special Education and Rehabilitative Services, Office of the Assistant Secretary. (2004). *National symposium on learning disabilities in English language learners: Symposium summary.* Symposium conducted October 14–15, 2003. Washington, DC: Author.

U.S. Department of Education & U.S. Department of Justice. (2003). *Annual report on school safety.* Washington, DC: Author.

U.S. Department of Education, U.S. Department of Justice, & American Institute of Research. (2002). *Safeguarding our children: An action plan.* Washington, DC: Author.

U.S. Department of Education & U.S. Secret Service. (2002a). *The final report and findings of the safe school initiative: Implications for the prevention of school attacks in the United States.* Washington, DC: Author.

U.S. Department of Education & U.S. Secret Service. (2002b). *Threat assessment in schools: A guide to managing threatening situations and creating safe school climates.* Washington, DC: Author.

U.S. Department of Educational Research and Improvement. (2002). *Safe and drug free schools.* Washington, DC: Author. Program descriptions available from www.ed.gov/offices/OESE/SDFS

U.S. Department of Health and Human Services. (2002). *Safe, supportive and successful schools: Step by step.* Washington, DC: Author.

U.S. Department of Labor. (2002). *Occupational Outlook Quarterly.* Spring 2002. Washington, DC: Author.

U.S. Department of Labor. (2003a). *Occupational Outlook Handbook, 2003–2004.* Bureau of Labor Statistics. Washington, DC: Author.

U.S. Department of Labor. (2003b). *Occupational Outlook Quarterly.* Spring 2003. Washington, DC: Author.

U.S. Department of Labor. (2004). *Occupational Outlook Quarterly.* Spring 2004. Washington, DC: Author.

Vigoda, E. (2002). From responsiveness to collaboration: Governance, citizens, and the next generation of public administration. *Public Administration Review, 62*(5), 527.

Welfel, E. R., & Lipsitz, N. E. (1983). Wanted: A comprehensive approach to ethics research and education. *Counselor Education and Supervision,* (22), 320–332.

Wellman, M. M. (1984). The school counselor's role in the communication of school ideation by adolescents. *The School Counselor, 2*(32), 104–109.

Werner, E, & Smith, R. (1992). *Overcoming the odds: High risk children from birth to adulthood.* Cornell Press: New York.

Wesley, D. C. (2001, February). The administrator-counselor team: The relationship between counselor and administrator can enhance or exhaust a school's ability to meet the needs of its students. *Principal Leadership,* 60–63.

West, J. F., & Idol, L. (1987). School consultation: An interdisciplinary perspective on theory, models, and research. *Journal of Learning Disabilities, 20*(7), 385–408.

Whiston, S. C. (2000). *Principles and applications of assessment in counseling.* Belmont, CA: Wadsworth.

Whiston, S. C. (2002). Response to the past, present, and future of school counseling: Raising some issues. *Professional School Counseling, 5,* 148–155.

Whiston, S. C., & Sexton, T. L. (1998). A review of school counseling outcome research: Implications for practice. *Journal of Counseling and Development, 4*(76), 412–426.

Wiggins, G. (1991). Standards, not standardization: Evoking quality student work. *Educational Leadership,* 18–25.

Wilkinson, L. (2003). Using behavioral consultation to reduce challenging behavior in the classroom. *Preventing School Failure, 47*(3), 100.

William T. Grant Commission on Work, Family and Citizenship. (1988). *The forgotten half: Pathways to success for America's youth and young families.* Washington, DC: Author.

Wittmer, J. (Ed.). (2000). *Managing your school counseling program: K–12 developmental strategies* (2nd ed.). Minneapolis, MN: Educational Media.

Woodcock, R., McGrew, K., & Mather, N. (2001). Woodcock-Johnson III Tests of Achievement. Riverside Publishing: Itasca, Ill.

Woods, A., & Weasmer, J. (2004). Maintaining job satisfaction: Engaging professionals as active participants. *The Clearing House, 77*(3), 118.

Woolfolk, A. (2001). *Educational psychology* (8th edition). Boston: Allyn & Bacon.

Woolfolk, A. (2004). *Educational psychology* (9th edition). Boston: Allyn & Bacon.

Worthington, R. L., & Juntunen, C. L. (1997). The vocational development of non–college bound youth: Counseling psychology and the school to work transition movement. *Counseling Psychologist, 25*, 323–363.

Wubbolding, R. E. (2000). *Reality therapy for the 21st century.* Bristol, PA: Accelerated Development.

Wyke v. The Polk County School Board, 129 F.3d 560 (11th cir. 1997).

Yalom, I. (1980). *Existential psychotherapy.* New York: Basic Books.

Zehr, M. (2004, January 14). Report updates portrait of LEP students 2004. *Education Week, 23*(18), 3.

Zide, M. R., & Gray, S. W. (2001). *Psychopathology: A competency-based assessment model for social workers.* Belmont, CA: Wadsworth.

Zins, J. (2004). *Building academic success on social and emotional learning: What does the research say?* New York: Teachers College Press.

Zins, J., Kratochwill, T., & Elliott, S. (1993). *Handbook of consultation services for children: Applications in educational and clinical settings.* San Francisco: Jossey-Bass.

Zirkel, P. (1991, April). End of story. *Phi Delta Kappan, 72*(8), 640–642.

Zirkel, P. (1999, June). Fatal suspension. *Phi Delta Kappan, 10*(80), 791–792.

Zirkel, P. (2001a, March). A pregnant pause? *Phi Delta Kappan, 82*(7), 557–558.

Zirkel, P. (2001b, September). Ill advised. *Phi Delta Kappan, 83*(1), 98–99.

Name Index

Subject Index